Child and Adolescent Mental Health: Theory and Practice

Child and Adolescent Mental Health: Theory and Practice

Editor: Lauren Davies

MURPHY & MOORE
www.murphy-moorepublishing.com

www.murphy-moorepublishing.com

MURPHY & MOORE

Cataloging-in-Publication Data

Child and adolescent mental health : theory and practice / edited by Lauren Davies.
p. cm.
Includes bibliographical references and index.
ISBN 978-1-63987-104-9
1. Child mental health. 2. Teenagers--Mental health. 3. Mental health. 4. Child psychology.
5. Developmental disabilities. I. Davies, Lauren.
RJ499 .C45 2022
618.928 9--dc23

Murphy & Moore Publishing,
1 Rockefeller Plaza,
New York City, NY 10020, USA

ISBN 978-1-63987-104-9 (Hardback)

Contents

Preface

Childhood and adolescence are sensitive periods in a person's life since it is during this time that they gain social-emotional and cognitive skills which have a profound impact on their mental health as adults. Some of the prominent reasons behind mental health conditions in children and adolescents are childhood epilepsy, behavioral disorders, depression, developmental disabilities and anxiety. There are several factors which can affect the mental health such as mental illness of parent, poverty, bullying or exposure to violence. A few of the different types of mental health disorders which are studied in relation to child and adolescent mental health are eating disorders, psychosis, suicide and self-harm, and risk-taking behaviors. This book unfolds the researches on child and adolescent mental health which will be crucial for the progress of this field in the future. It presents researches and studies performed by experts across the globe. This book aims to equip students and experts with the advanced topics and upcoming concepts in this area.

The information contained in this book is the result of intensive hard work done by researchers in this field. All due efforts have been made to make this book serve as a complete guiding source for students and researchers. The topics in this book have been comprehensively explained to help readers understand the growing trends in the field.

I would like to thank the entire group of writers who made sincere efforts in this book and my family who supported me in my efforts of working on this book. I take this opportunity to thank all those who have been a guiding force throughout my life.

Editor

1

Marijuana, Experience of Temporality, and School Performance from a Qualitative and Quantitative Approach

Anneliese Dörr, Sandra Viani and
María Elena Gorostegui

Abstract

The study aims at knowing how low marijuana doses affect cognitive ability in postprimary students. The objective of the quantitative research was to analyze the results of neuropsychological and Neuro-SPECT tests comparing schoolchildren who smoke marijuana with those who do not, with emphasis on the effects on cognitive functions involved in learning. We wanted to assess the effects on the cerebral function of marijuana-only users. It was a comparative study based on the total sample of 565 school adolescents coming from four schools in the metropolitan area of Santiago, Chile. All were interviewed in order to select a sample that was stratified by sex, class and consumption of marijuana. The following two groups were made: 40 marijuana-only users and 40 nonusers. We took as a reference a study performed by the authors in 2007, in which the correlation between the consumption of marijuana and effects on cognitive functions involved in scholastic learning were established. The findings show statistically significant differences in the following areas: subgenual bilateral hypoperfusion, more marked on the left side (Brodmann area 25), frontal bilateral hypoperfusion (Brodmann's areas 10 and 32), front cingulate gyrushypoperfusion (Brodmann area 24) and hypoperfusion of Brodmann area 36 that projects to the hippocampus. The results are highly matched with the neuropsychological tests given in the sense that, like with the 2007 study, significant differences are found between the two groups as far as the tests measuring cognitive functions are concerned. A qualitative research: we wanted to investigate the experience of time in high school students who regularly smoke marijuana, given that this substance has effects on the prefrontal lobe and on the hippocampus, brain areas related to the ability to plan tasks (executive function) and to memory. Moreover, adolescence is a delicate stage in regard to planning of the future. At the same time, the idea was to understand and make use of the concepts of temporariness and anticipation, which as a general rule will be handled only by philosophical theories. Our guiding principle is the ability to "anticipate oneself," proposed by Sutter, a phenomenological psychiatrist. Data were analyzed from the autobiographies of the students through the hermeneutical phenomenological method developed by Lindseth, based on Ricoeur. Results allow answering the question of the study about the temporary experiencing of the young abusive marijuana consumer. The results showed poverty in the temporary dimensions referring to the past and the future, while in the report, it is more developed in the present moment. They appear detained in a more childish stage, in which the present predominates, and the future seemed not to be united with the past, which impresses as if it were "avoided." What has been (past) does not link with what is wanted to be, so, elements of the past have no relation with future project.

Keywords: cannabis, marijuana, adolescents, Neuro-SPECT, HMPAO, neuropsychological tests, temporality, time, hermeneutical phenomenological method, anticipation, projection capacity

1. Introduction

From a historical point of view, cannabis or marijuana consumption has been related to cultural and worldview aspects that confer different meanings. Marijuana is a recreational drug that comes from the marijuana plant: the hemp plant Cannabis sativa. Marijuana has 489 known constituents, only 70 of which are cannabinoids with the remainder including potentially neuroactive substances. Tetrahydrocannabinol (THC) is the most common phytocannabinoid and is psychoactive. CBD is the best studied of the nonpsychoactive cannabinoids [1, 2]. Consumption has been common since ancient times, but it never seemed to be a social problem. Nowadays, without discussing its characteristics and biochemical structure, its consumption seems to be tied to both positive and negative connotations that arise from social, historical and cultural circumstances. These circumstances determine and define what a society or era regards as a social problem [3]. Regarding this topic, scientific research reports the negative effects and potential benefits of marijuana consumption. These findings do not have an impact on the discussion, which has turned into a political matter, instead of a public health matter.

In order to discuss the benefits or negative effects of marijuana consumption, and especially its medicinal use, first we need to clarify that marijuana cannot be regarded as medicine. This confusion comes from various studies on the medicinal properties of marijuana, but this study considers the cannabinoids only, which are some of the components of this plant. This means that we must make a difference between the plant and some of its components, which are used in studies on pain management, for instance. Assigning medicinal properties to marijuana is the same as assigning the analgesic properties of morphine to poppy plants: morphine is used to manage the pain, not the hallucinogen effects of opium. This conceptual error is the base argument in the defense of the medicinal use of marijuana plants [4] and, by extension, for its consumption at a population level.

Regarding its use as medication in the palliative treatment of pain in terminal cases, chronic pain reduction is described without a determined cause. The same happens with the increase in mobility in multiple sclerosis patients with spasticity reduction, as well as in arthritis and musculoskeletal ailments. In low doses, it could stimulate the appetite of AIDS patients [5–7].

It is used to relief oncological pain as a palliative strategy (compassionate), even though specialists do not consider it to be better than morphine derivatives. It has been used to treat vomit and secondary effects of chemotherapy, without evidence to defend its use in this cases, nor comparative studies to confirm it to be better than the recommended medication to treat vomit and nausea associated with chemotherapy. It has never been proven to be better than conventional antiemetics, yet only in placebo studies.

It is worth mentioning that, without denying some possible benefits of its medicinal use, none of these studies addresses its use in adolescents directly. Additionally, to this day, the food and drug administration (FDA) has not approved cannabis to treat any disease; therefore, the investigation for its medicinal use, focused on cannabinoids, and the evidence on its medical usefulness are still limited [4], while the discussion regarding the medical benefits of marijuana is still present. The risks associated with the medicinal use of the plant have not been determined accurately [8], and there is a lack of comparative studies to validate its use as a replacement for scientifically approved drugs [9].

Regarding the negative effects related to the early consumption of marijuana, evidence suggests that consumption before the age of 17 may cause neurobiological changes, more serious than in cases of later consumption [10–13]. A deterioration of the neuronal connectivity in specific brain zones has been described in this line of studies, such as the precuneus and hippocampus, zones involved in learning and memory, as well as in the prefrontal networks [14, 15], which can lead to a poor school performance and school desertion [4, 16]. In turn, alterations in the neuronal organization of the nucleus accumbens and the amygdala, as well as in their volume and shape, have been reported in young marijuana smokers [17]. Cognitive deficiencies and reduced IQs have been observed in adults that smoked marijuana regularly during their adolescence [18]. Some other consequences of the consumption of cannabis during adolescence (before the age of 17) that can be observed in adults are pointed out, such as underperformance in academic activities, an increase in the dependence of marijuana and other illegal drugs, as well as a greater number of suicide attempts [19]. On the other hand, in the case of genetic vulnerability, cannabis facilitates the triggering of psychosis [20, 21] and, in addition, it aggravates the course of the disease in patients with schizophrenia and fosters the first psychotic episode [22, 23].

According to the DSM-5 [24], the amotivational syndrome, pathognomonic symptom of marijuana consumption, is characterized by the loss of energy and abulia, which affects the normal performance of everyday activities. This decrease in energy, abulia and demotivation of the young consumer affects their capacity to efficiently plan and organize their time for a determined objective or life goal. This is valid, even though occidental societies have extended the period for youngsters to begin their adult lives and meet the responsibilities entailed in this new stage. This postponement is known as social moratorium.

The studies of Quiroga [25] conclude that consuming cannabis permanently may lead to a state of passivity and indifference, with a subsequent generalized dysfunction of social capabilities;

in addition, the consumption of marijuana can cause addiction: it has been claimed that one in six people that started to consume marijuana in their adolescence develops an addiction, as well as 25–50% of the daily consumers [26]. The cannabis abstinence syndrome is widely known, characterized by irritability, trouble sleeping, dysphoria, need of consuming and anxiety [4, 26].

In order to reveal the social and cultural meaning of cannabis, it is worth mentioning that in the last four decades, there has been a notable change regarding the ways and situations in which it is consumed. During 1960, consumption was relatively normal among university students that defined themselves as rebels or avant-garde, while school pupils practically did not consume. Commonly, they only experimented with alcohol and tobacco in order to look indifferent and defy the status quo. This shows that the environment and the scope of consumption have changed, from a restricted consumption culturally circumscribed to some groups for artistic, ritual or religious purposes, to massive consumption, becoming a part of the everyday lives of many youngsters [27, 28], to the point that we can claim that nowadays marijuana is the most produced, trafficked and consumed illegal drug.

Cannabis is consumed and grown in almost every country, and the produced quantities are higher than the total of other drugs [29]. Additionally, the type of marijuana that is available today for consumption is stronger, since clandestine laboratories have achieved changes at the genetic level through sophisticated biotechnology methods, achieving a higher concentration of THC. This concentration has been increasing from 3% in the 80s to 12% in 2012 [4]. This leads to the hypotheses that the negative consequences of its consumption may be greater.

Regarding risk perception, studies carried out in Spain and Chile [27, 29, 30] show that in the last 10 years the perception of risk associated with consumption has decreased considerably, especially among secondary students, this is adolescents. A report by SENDA in 2015 claims that the risk perception regarding consumption shows significant changes, decreasing from 46.8% to an even lower 34.4%. These data coincide with the findings of recent investigations, such as data in the study on marijuana and learning disorders carried out in 2007 [31], in which the risk perception associated with marijuana consumption was very low. This decrease in the risk perception among youngsters contributes to the fact that in Latin America there is a significant number of free magazines that advertise the benefits of marijuana consumption, ways to consume and acquire the product and different ways of cultivating it, in order to grow better plants at home, or even for commercial production. These magazines are distributed in places with high concentration of youngsters and adolescents, such as concerts, cinemas, art events or simply on the streets or outside schools [29].

The results of the investigation carried out by the Inter-American Drug Abuse Control Commission [32] show that marijuana consumption among youngsters increased in all countries in the continent, except Peru, with Chile as the country with the highest consumption in the region. In Uruguay, marijuana consumption doubled during the 2003–2014 period. An increase of roughly 20% in marijuana consumption among adolescents, 12 years and older, has been observed in Colorado and Washington [33]. Likewise, between 2008 and 2014, the Children's Hospital Colorado reported a significant increase in the number of consultations for high marijuana intake [59]. The 2015 World Drug Report published by United Nations [60] points out that in Chile the consumption level in 13-year-old kids reaches 15.7%, compared to 3% in 1995 and reaches 38.9% for 17-year-old youngsters, while in 1995, it reached 21.4%. It is worth mentioning that this 38.9% of consumption in 17-year-old youngsters represents the highest figure in the world related to age. According to figures reported by SENDA [27], the consumption of marijuana in the 12–18 age group increased from 6.7% in 2012 to 13.5% in 2014. With respect to the group of youngsters aged between 19 and 25, the consumption also increases significantly from 17.5 to 24%.

In Chile, the socially shared belief, especially among youngsters, is that consumption has no negative effects on behavior, mental health or school performance. However, two lines of research carried out recently in the country have empirically proven the existence of negative effects that deny the belief of harmless consumption, especially in school adolescents, who represent the most vulnerable segment of the population.

2. Two studies

Two parallel studies are carried out, one aimed at studying the subjective experience of the young consumer, through the analysis of the temporality variable [34], and a second study that analyses the effects on basic cognitive functions for the school learning process [28, 30]. These studies are carried out in a scenario where Chile is the country with the highest consumption levels in school pupils in Latin America, with a tendency to decrease the age of first consumption.

First, we have a line of research aimed at studying the subjective experience of the temporality variable in young consumers. This approach to the problem represents pioneering work in Chile in terms of addressing the problem in parallel from the individual experience of the adolescent, derived from the analysis of the information that they provide (qualitative approach), and a quantitative study with a representative sample of the consumer adolescent population.

The future experience (qualitative approach) represents a decisive variable in terms of the current behavior of the young adolescent student, their motivation to work and study, and, in general, to plan and achieve their life projects in a society that expects certain competences for them to be prepared to develop in a quintessentially competitive and individualistic world [35]. Very important future aspects are defined in this stage of life, with youngsters freely and consciously deciding the path that will give meaning to their lives.

This planning takes us to the temporal dimension as an existential category of human beings, and therefore decisive in their life history. When we talk about the temporal dimension, we refer to the experience of temporality, this is, their capacity of moving through time, shaping the past through memory and shaping the future through the present [36], in such a way that the subjective experience of time would be equal to the internal temporal happenings [37] in a synthesis of past, present and future. From this perspective, it is not the past, but the future, that determines the actions of the young adolescent. Ortega even claims that we live from the future, which comes to life in our project, and that the future forces us to select everything in our past that is related to our future [38–40].

The study of the experience of temporality in the young consumers should have privileged the qualitative methodology, based on psychological discipline and philosophy, especially in the phenomenological trends, due to its contribution to the understanding of the time experience in human beings. The key concept was the "anticipation," developed by Sutter [41], who presents the centrality of the future and the capacity to anticipate, and how it can be altered in the different psychopathological conditions.

The second parallel investigation presented uses the classic quantitative methodology procedures to study the behavior of a group of nearly 600 high school students, belonging to three schools in Santiago, Chile. These students were evaluated by psychologists through psychometric tests and by medical professionals, qualified specialists, through hi-tech neuroimaging procedures.

These two lines of research address the problem from two different disciplinary and methodological perspectives, which allows us to widen our range of view and add certainty to the conclusions related to the effects of marijuana consumption in young students in Chile.

2.1. Qualitative study about marijuana and temporality experience in adolescents

Psychology has developed the idea that the acquisition of formal thought in the adolescent generates the dimension of future, which is expressed through the life project [42–47]. However, the philosophical phenomenological current offers an analysis of temporality experience allowing a better approach to the study of the experience of the young consumer, generally socially disadvantaged or left at the margin of the work market. This group shows a tendency to remain trapped in an "extended present," with scarce capacity to think in the future and even less to plan it [48–53].

For answering the question about the temporality experience in a group of young Chilean consumers [34], their biographic narratives are analyzed, using for it qualitative methodology validated by the scientific community [54, 58]. This methodology consists in gathering information, starting from autobiographies, about perceptions, feelings and actions and about their capacity to anticipate themselves in the realization of their projects and of their way of experiencing temporality.

The narratives of 15 young consumers [55] who meet the specifications of being school adolescents, men and women, coming from different social contexts are gathered. Among other requirements, they had to be usual marijuana consumers (and not of other drug) with ages fluctuating between 16 and 19 years old. This stage corresponds to the period of late middle adolescence, characterized by the search of reaffirmation of the project and need of social insertion for accomplishments of goals [45, 46, 56, 57].

2.2. Quantitative study with respect to marijuana consumption in pupils and its effects in cognitive functions through neuropsychological tests and Neuro-SPECT

This second study answers the question about the effects over the brain function of exclusive marijuana consumption in adolescents not labeled as addicts, by means of neuropsychological tests, such as Benton Visual Retention Test, Rey Words Memory, Rey Complex Figure Test and

Wisconsin Test. Added to the previous, Neuro-SPECT was used and the information obtained was analyzed with the purpose of identifying regions and sub-regions of altered perfusion as consequence of the consumption.

For purposes of this study, it was considered consumer the student who declares a minimum of four episodes of exclusive cannabis consumption during the last month and minimum usual consumption of 18 months. The ages of the groups forming the sample fluctuated between 15 and 18 years old, with an average of 16 years old.

In accordance with quantitative investigation norms accepted by the scientific community, two groups were conformed: 40 exclusive marijuana consumers and 40 not consumers, and the results obtained were compared in both groups in neuropsychological tests and Neuro-SPECT technology.

3. Results

3.1. Qualitative study of the temporal variable

The so-called naive reading of the biographic narratives delivered by the adolescents show that almost all of them were a production of brief texts, in which it stands out the poverty of the descriptions of past situations, with abundance of experiences associated to losses (death of a close relative), solitude and, specially, feeling of not being recognized by significant figures (father). The temporal dimension of the present appears as richer in details, especially related with present friendships, felt as refuge. In what refers to interests, they showed lack of clarity, frequent changes of goals and objectives and a dimension of future that impresses for absences and losses in almost all the analyzed ambits: family, image of themselves, interests, relationship with pairs and goals or projects. It seemed as if the future was not related with what they did in the present, that is, as if the future was not bound to the present or to the past and as if what was done today was not related with what one wanted to accomplish in the future.

In the following stages of the process of narrative analysis, the same results are confirmed, especially lack of capacity to visualize the future in the areas related with family, pairs, image of oneself and interests. In general, the tendency corresponded to postpone the future, not to assume it, leaving it for later. It is verified that the temporality experience is characterized by centering in the immediate here and now, and an impaired experience of the future. The anticipation capacity, determinant of the acting in favor of the accomplishment of the proposed goals, is absent, is so that although in fact they have some projects, there is no way of visualizing how they anticipated their conduct to reach them.

3.2. Quantitative study of the effect of the consumption in learning

The results obtained in neuropsychological tests individually applied to the selected consumers and nonconsumers show significant differences in yield in favor of the nonconsumer group in comparison with the consumer group.

(a) Rey words memory evaluates immediate verbal memory. The consumer group yields in average 15% less than the nonconsumer group.

(b) Benton Visual Retention Test. The nonconsumer group reaches scores significantly superior in comparison to the consumers in tasks involving capacity of attention, concentration, immediate retention, perception, visual memory and visoconstructive aptitudes, confirming an alteration in the consumers with respect to integration and organization of the spatial stimuli. The adolescent consumers make in average 3.8 mistakes per test in contrast with 1.7 mistakes of the nonconsumers, which means that the quantity of mistakes made by the consuming group is 21% higher. This difference is statistically significant, which reveals an impoverishment of the capacities of attention, concentration and of work spatial memory.

(c) Rey Complex Figure Test. The scores obtained by both groups show significant differences in favor of the nonconsumers in tasks involving ability and strategies of execution in the visoperceptive level, visual memory, capacity of hierarchical structuring and organization of visual information. A difference close to 7 points was verified in the average obtained by both groups revealing clear evocation difficulties and limitations in the fidelity of the visual memory of the consumers. The scores of the test show that the consumers use execution strategies of inferior quality to that expected for age, for copy and visual memory.

(d) Wisconsin Test. It evaluates executive functions, that is, mental flexibility, planning strategies, organized inquiries and utilization of the environmental feedback to change schemes, in addition to capacity of inhibition of the answer in course. It showed that in the category total mistakes 30% of the consumer group is located in the level of moderate to intermediate impairment. In persevering mistakes, 26% scored in the level of medium or inferior impairment. With respect to the percentage of persevering answers, 17.2% of the school consumers obtain scores of impairment superior to the media.

3.3. Results of the evaluation with Neuro-SPECT

The individual results obtained were compared with normal population of the same age. The results were expressed in standard deviations (SD) over and under normal average. It is verified that there are focuses within some Brodmann areas that are hyperperfused to 5 SD over the normal average: areas 9, 10, 46 (frontal lobe) of the right hemisphere, areas 23, 30 and 31 (posterior cingulated, cognitive circuit) bilaterally, and area 17 of the left hemisphere, corresponding to the visual area of association. Hypoperfusion focuses are observed, at less than 5 SD under normal average, bilaterally in Brodmann area 24, in the left hemisphere in area 25, bilaterally in the projection of the hippocampus and Brodmann area 36 and in the frontal lobes in Brodmann areas 10 and 11. Deep hypoperfusion is also observed in bilateral temporal inferior gyrus and 23 right.

Although the understanding of these results is not within reach of everybody, it is clear that marijuana consumers showed brain alterations and dysfunctions that result consistent with the behavior showed in neuropsychological tests and that move them away from the results obtained by adolescents in accordance to demographic norms.

4. Discussion and conclusions

The results of the two presented studies add evidence to the negative effects of marijuana consumption both in the adolescent life project—in a moment in which that project is a key in his psychological development—and in their present school performance, base of their future social, professional, work, family development. Both studies coincide in the fact that marijuana consumption in pupils has harmful effects in the capacities for school learning and in temporality, lived without an explicit connection between the past, the present praxis and the yearning of future.

The lack of capacity for anticipating interferes with the possibility of transcending the present and confines them in themselves. This state of being in captivity in their own intimacy is translated in the evasion of obligations and responsibilities, in not assumed tasks, in largely postponed decisions, for example, with respect to what to study or to what actions to initiate for preparing themselves for adult life.

The fulfillment of the young consumers in neuropsychological tests shows an increased capacity of mistakes in the execution of the proposed tasks. These results can be transferred to situations of their school life and explain their deficient fulfillment in cognitive tests and demands in the classroom. Their diminished capacity of attention and concentration explains their omissions, mistakes and confusion in the moment of answering to the task. Their work strategies, inferior in quality to those expected in relation to their age and cognitive development, bring them to work by trial and error, to improvise answers, not to evaluate nor self-correct their work, in any way, to deliver infantile, improvised solutions, only for answering without demanding themselves farther. Without doubt, the executive functions affected by the consumption compromise learning and in general, school performance.

The results of the application of neuropsychological tests and evaluations by images (Neuro-SPECT) confirm the association between marijuana consumption in adolescents and harmful effects over brain functioning, especially in executive and cognitive functions. It is added to the previous the compromise of the immediate verbal memory or of work, indispensable in the classroom if one considers that most part of the content is orally delivered.

This compromise has its correlate in neuroimaging tests (Neuro-SPECT) by means of which it concluded that marijuana produces, in brain cortex, multifocal functional alterations. It is especially compromised the cognition, the mood control and the executive function for frontal abnormality in area 10 and 11 of bilateral Brodmann. It is necessary to outline that the frontal cortex participates in the range of human conducts related with the ethical dimension, function that would also influence on the work and the social conduct of the pupils consuming marijuana. Functional alterations are also observed in the form of multifocal hypofunction of disorganized distribution in marijuana smokers, although of lower statistical significance (less severity) than the observed in cocaine consumers. These findings allow us to pose the presence of neurotoxicity in marijuana consumers since, when comparing their results with a normative data base for persons of the same age group, none of the Neuro-SPECT studies of the young consumers was normal.

The results of neuroimaging tests showing effects in brain areas related with learning are highly coincidental with the scores obtained by the same subjects in neuropsychological tests, which adds evidence to the negative effects of marijuana consumption in learning, central theme of this study. Especially important is the fact that these results correspond to adolescents who have not been diagnosed nor labeled as addicts and who, therefore, do not yet constitute a public health problem, nor are perceived as adolescents in social risk. If one considers that these youngsters come from socially vulnerable populations associated to poverty, there are aggravated consequences or effects that can have for them the school failure bound to usual marijuana consumption, thinking that education should be the medium that allows them a greater social mobility, and it is in fact a protector factor against social risk.

The nonperception of risk in consumption, the easy access to cannabis, the unquestionable harmful effect over the cognitive functions involved in learning and school performance, the increase of the number of adolescent women consumers, the evidence gathered about cannabis as inductor or facilitator of the use of other substances and the diminution of the age of beginning of consumption constitute a problem for public health policies, compromising school, adolescents and their families. In relation to this challenge, it is again confirmed the debt of the institutions, especially of the family and of the school, in the sense that adolescent consumers do not perceive risk awareness by their parents or by their teachers, nor social control over the consumption.

With respect to qualitative investigations about the altered temporality experience, the results become relevant when coinciding with the also altered functioning of the hippocampus associated to memory and to the prefrontal lobe responsible for planning. The findings about the alterations in temporality experience explain how it is that in these youngsters there is a verifiable connection between the past and the future projections or possibilities. The past, which brings the subjects toward their future and which determines the course of his actions, appears impoverished. Instead of a possible future, it is a matter of a future full of unrealizable projects, of empty possibilities, that do not consider feasibility arguments and that change with facility to replace them by others equally unrealizable. They live, then, an inauthentic future, with an irresponsible treatment of the future, without interest for reaching goals. They verbalize unrealizable and fantastic plans, such as being famous, or that the world recognizes their value, but without planning actions for reaching those unrealizable goals, imprisoned in a present without hope or yearnings.

Finally, it is not difficult to think that this attitude in front of life, this demotivation, has its correlate in school performance, that is, in the most proper task of the adolescent life stage. The circle is then closed and is fed back with negative signs: marijuana consumption, real difficulties in cognitive capacities, closing of the future experience, absence of plans, school failure, verification of the inutility of the effort, withdrawal to the present facilitated by the consumption and more consumption. The cycle is reinitiated.

Although the presented results impact the common sense of the parents and the social sensibility of the teachers who work with adolescents, it is necessary to outline that there is no real discussion on the part of the scientific community with respect to the damages and benefits carried by its use, but rather a debate at the level of public policies, which leads to confusion and to a contradictory discourse between the socially internalized and the message transmitted on one side by the authorities and on the other, by the academic and scientific world.

Cannabis consumption in adolescents is a complex and multidetermined theme, but what the population does with respect to this is simplified and dichotomic without considering the context, the age of onset, who, how much, when good or bad, legal or illegal, beneficial for health or innocuous marijuana. This lack of agreement among the responsible adults leads the young adolescent to adopt the belief and the discourse of the majority who consider themselves avant-garde in relation to the values: "it is not harmful, it is cool, it is a natural herb and the power elites are trying to prescribe it or to restrict its consumption for very determined cases and persons." This contradiction is very real and is clearly reflected in the arguments used by the youngsters: why is the cigar permitted in circumstances that it kills? Why is marijuana illegal? Finally, this situation leads to the fact that its prohibition is seen as empty, without support and believable norms.

Author details

Anneliese Dörr*, Sandra Viani and María Elena Gorostegui

*Address all correspondence to: anneliesed@gmail.com

Psychiatry and Mental Health Department, University of Chile, Santiago, Chile

References

[1] Elsohly MA, Slade D. Chemical constituents of marijuana: the complex mixture of natural cannabinoids. Life Sciences. 2005;78:539–548.

[2] Izzo AA, Borrelli F, Capasso R, Di Marzo V, Mechoulam R. Non-psychotropic plant cannabinoids: new therapeutic opportunities from an ancient herb. Trends Pharmacol Sci 2009; 30: 515–527.

[3] Slapak, S; Grigoravicius, M. (2006). "Consumo De Drogas: La Construcción de un Problema Social". Anuario de Investigaciones. Facultad de Psicología – UBA. Volumen XIV. http://www.scielo.org.ar/pdf/anuinv/v14/v14a23.pdf

[4] Volkow ND, Baler RD, et al. Adverse health effects of marijuana use. The New England Journal of Medicine. 2014;370:2219–2227.

[5] Grant I, Cahn BR. Cannabis and endocannabinoid modulators: therapeutic promises and challenges. Clinical Neuroscience Research. 2005;5:185–199.

[6] Ben Amar M. Cannabinoids in medicine: a review of their therapeutic potential, Journal of Ethnopharmacology. 2006;105(1–2):1–25.

[7] Lakhan SE, Rowland M. Whole plant cannabis extracts in the treatment of spasticity in multiple sclerosis: a systematic review. British Medical Journal Neurology. 2009;9(59): 9–59.

[8] Hill, K. Medical marijuana for treatment of chronic pain and other medical and psychiatric problems: a clinical review. Clinical Review and Education. 2015;313(24): 2474–2483.

[9] Health Canada (2013) Information for Health Care Professionals, Cannabis (marihuana, marijuana) and the cannabinoids, prepared by Health Canada.

[10] Pope Jr. HG, Gruber AJ, Hudson JI, Cohane G, Huestis MA, Yurgelun-Todd D. Early-onset cannabis use and cognitive deficits: what is the nature of the association? Drug and Alcohol Dependence. 2003;69:303–310.

[11] Pattij T, Wiskerke J, Schoffelmeer AN. Cannabinoid modulation of executive functios. European Journal of Pharmacology. 2008;585(2–3):458–463.

[12] Large M, Sharma S, Compton MT, Slade T, Nielssen O. Cannabisuse and earlier onset of psychosis: a systematic meta-analysis. Archives of General Psychiatry. 2011;68:555–561.

[13] Arias F, et al. (2012). Cocaine abuse or dependency and other pyschiatric disorders. Madrid study on dual pathology. Rev Psiquiatr Salud Ment (Barc.). http://dx.doi.org/10.1016/j.rpsm.2012.09.0002

[14] Zalesky A, Solowij N, Yucel M, et al. Effect of long-term cannabis use on axonal fibre connectivity. Brain. 2012;135:2245–2255.

[15] Batalla A, Bhattacharyya S, Yucel M, et al. Structural and functional imaging studies in chronic cannabis users: a systematic review of adolescent and adult findings. PLoS One. 2013;8(2):e55821.

[16] Pistis M, Perra S, Pillolla G, Melis M, Muntoni A, Gessa G. Adolescent exposure to cannabinoids induces long lasting changes in the response to drugs of abuse of rat midbrain dopamine neurons. Biological Psychiatry. 2004;56(2):86–94.

[17] Gilman J, Kuster J, Lee S, Lee MJ, Woo K, Makris N, Kouwe, Blood A, Breiter H. Cannabis use is quantitatively associated with nucleus accumbens and amygdala abnormalities in young adult recreational users. The Journal of Neuroscience. 2014;34(16):5529–5538.

[18] Meier MH., Caspi A, Ambler A.et al. (2012) Persistent cannabis users show neuropsychological decline from childhood to midlife, PNAS,109 (40)

[19] Silins E, Horwood J, Patton G, et al. Young adult sequelae of adolescent cannabis use: an integrative analysis. Lancet Psychiatry. 2014;1:286–293.

[20] Dragt S, et al. Cannabis use and age at onset of symptoms in subjects at clinical high risk for psychosis. Acta Psychiatrica Scandinavia. 2012;125: 45–53.

[21] Degenhardt L, Hall W. Extent of illicit drug use and dependence, and their contribution to the global burden of disease. Lancet. 2012;379:55–70.

[22] Caspi A, Moffitt TE, Cannon M, et al. Moderation of the effect of adolescent-onset cannabis use on adult psychosis by a functional polymorphism in the catechol-O-methyltransferase gene: longitudinal evidence of a gene X environment interaction. Biological Psychiatry. 2005;57:1117–1127.

[23] Di Forti M, Sallis H, Allegri F, et al. Daily use, especially of high-potency cannabis, drives the earlier onset of psychosis in cannabis users. Schizophrenia Bulletin. 2014;40(6):1509–1517.

[24] American Psychiatric Association (APA). Diagnostic and statistical manual of mental disorders, 5th edition. Arlington (VA): American Psychiatric Association. 2013.

[25] Quiroga, M. (2002). Cannabis y psicopatología comórbida [Cannabis and comorbic psychopathology]. Adicciones, 14(2), 191-200.

[26] Hall W, Degenhardt L. Adverse health effects of non-medical cannabis use. Lancet. 2009;374(9698):1383–1391.

[27] SENDA.2014. Décimo Estudio de Drogas en Población Escolar. Observatorio Chileno de Drogas. (National Study of Drugs in Chilean School Population) http://www.senda.gob.cl/observatorio/estadisticas/

[28] UNODC, World Drug Report 2012. United Nations publication, Sales No. E.12.XI.1. Available from: http://www.unodc.org/unodc/en/data-and-analysis/WDR.html

[29] Dörr A, Gorostegui M.E, Viani S & Dörr M.P. (2009). Teenage consumers of marijuana: implications for the family and the school. Revista Salud Mental México, 32 (4), 275-277 http://www.revistasaludmental.mx/index.php/salud_mental/article/view/1293

[30] Ministerio de Sanidad (2014) Servicios Sociales e Igualdad, Informe anual del Sistema Nacional de Salud. Disponible en www. msssi.gob.es,España

[31] Mena I; Dörr A; Viani S; Neubauer S; Gorostegui ME; Dörr P. (2013). Effects of marijuana consumption in students on brain functions demonstrated by means of neuropsychological tests and neuro-SPECT imaging. Salud Mental Mexico, Vol. 36, No. 5. http://www.revistasaludmental.mx/index.php/salud_mental/article/view/SM.0185-3325.2013.045/2201

[32] OID . Inter-American Drug Abuse Control Commission. Informe del Uso de Drogas en las Américas 2015 : http://www.cicad.oas.org/apps/Document.aspx?Id=3209

[33] National Survey on Drug Use and Health, NSDUH. (2014). Substance use and mental health estimates from the 2013 National Survey on Drug Use and Health: overview of findings. Recuperated from Internet on July 29, 2015: http://www.samhsa.gov/data/sites/default/files/NSDUH-SR200-RecoveryMonth-2014/NSDUH-SR200-RecoveryMonth-2014.htm.

[34] Dörr A, Espinoza A, Acevedo J. Adolescentes consumidores habituales de marihuana y su vivencia de la temporalidad, (The experience of time in habitual teenage marijuana smokers). Revista Actas Españolas de Psiquiatría. 2014;42(2):49–56.

[35] Côté, J. (1996). Sociological perspectives on identity formation: the culture-identity link and identity capital, Journal of adolescence, 19 (5), 417-428.

[36] Pifarré L. El itinerario del ser. Revista Filosófica Arvo.net, Barcelona, España. 2012. Recuperated from Internet on December 12, 2012 from the web page: http://arvo.net/seccion-martin-heidegger/heidegger-y-la-pregunta-por-el/gmx-niv550-con11973.htm

[37] Binswanger, L. (1957). Schizophrenie, Ed. Pfullingen: Neske.

[38] Heidegger, Martin (2005). Being and Time. Santiago, Published by Editorial Universitaria Press, Santiago, Chile.

[39] Acevedo, J. (1994). La sociedad como proyecto, Ed. Universitaria, Santiago de Chile.

[40] Ricoeur P. (1995). Time and Narrative, Volume 1, 2, 3. Published by Siglo XXI Editores, Mexico

[41] Sutter, J (1983). L'anticipation, Psychologie et psychopatologie Published by Press Universitaires de France

[42] Spranger E. (1955). Psychologie des Jugendalters.(Psychology of Youth) Published by Quelle & Meyer

[43] Piaget, J. (1973). Seis estudios de Psicología. (Six psychological studies). Published by Barcelona: Seix Barral

[44] Arciero, G. (2002). Estudios y diálogos sobre la identidad personal: Reflexiones sobre la experiencia humana. Published by Bollati Boringhieri, Italy.

[45] Irribarne, M. (2003). Desarrollo psicológico del adolescente. En Almonte, C., Montt, M.E., Correa, A. Psicopatología infantil y de la adolescencia , pg. 37- 47. Ed. Mediterraneo, Santiago, Chile

[46] Sepúlveda G. (2006), Desarrollo psicológico en la edad juvenil: construcción de la identidad personal hacia la autonomía. En Valdivia M., Condeza, M. (eds). Psiquiatría del Adolescente, pp.19-35 Editorial Mediterráneo, Santiago, Chile

[47] Sepúlveda G. (2011). Psicoterapia evolutiva con niños y adolescentes: Enfoque cognitivo. En Almonte, Montt, C., Correa, Psicopatología infantil y de laadolescencia, Editorial Mediterráneo, Santiago, Chile

[48] Anderson M, Bechhofer F. Timespans and plans among young adults, Sociology. 2005; 39(1):139–155. Recuperated from Internet on November 24, 2011 from the web page: http://www.uk.sagepub.com/home.nav.

[49] Brannen J, Nielsen A. Young people's time perspectives: from youth to adulthood. Review of Sociology. 2002;36:513. Recuperated from Internet on September 24, 2011 from the web page: http://www.uk.sagepub.com/home.nav.

[50] Brannen J, Nielsen A. Young people, time horizons and planning: a response to Anderson et al. British Sociological Association. 2007;41:153. Recuperated from Internet on November 24, 2011 from the web page: http://www.uk.sagepub.com/home.nav

[51] Cole J, Durham D. Figuring the future: globalization and the temporalities of children and youth. Santa Fe, NM: School for Advanced Research Press. 2008.

[52] Devadason, R. To plan or not to plan? Young adult future orientations in two European cities. British Sociological Association. 2008;42(6):1127–1145. Recuperated from Internet on April 23, 2013 from the web page: http://www.sagepublications

[53] Reiter H. Past, present, future biographical time structuring of disadvantaged young people. Nordic Journal of Youth Research (Young); 2003;11(3): 253–279.

[54] Lindseth A, Norberg A. A phenomenological hermeneutical method for researching lived experience. Nordic College of Caring Sciences. Scandinavian Journal of Caring Science. 2004;18:145–153.

[55] Scharager, J y Armijo, I. (2001). Metodología de la Investigación para las Ciencias Sociales, Programa computacional. Published by Pontificia Universidad Católica de Chile.

[56] OMS,. (2000). Informe sobre la Salud en el Mundo. World Health Report, Switzerland. http://www.who.int/whr/2000/en/whr00_es.pdf?ua=1.

[57] Krauskopf, D. (2000). El desarrollo psicológico del adolescente. En: Montenegro, H. y Guajardo, H. Psiquiatría del Niño y del Adolescente. Published by Editorial Mediterráneo, Santiago de Chile

[58] Bertaux, D. (1993). La perspectiva biográfica: validez metodológica y potencialidades. En La historia oral: métodos y experiencias. Published by Editorial Debate, Madrd, España.

[59] Children's Hospital of Colorado Emergency Department. (2015). Research About Medical Marijuana. Recuperated on July 29, 2015: http://www.childrenscolorado.org/research/medical-marijuana-research

[60] Observatorio Chileno de drogas. Decimo Primer Estudio Nacional de Drogas en población General de Chile 2014. 2015 http://www.senda.gob.cl/wp-content/uploads/2015/07/Informe-Ejecutivo-ENPG-2014.pdf

2

Prevention of Internalized Problems of Children and Youth in Academic Setting

Miranda Novak and Josipa Mihić

Abstract

Research of internalized problems during school years shows their stability and tendency of enhancement during the period of growing up. There are many challenges children and adolescents have to face: greater academic expectations, changes in relationships with parents and peers, physical changes, and transitions. Given the context and their background, students' feelings such as shy or withdrawn behavior, frequent worrying, sadness, loneliness, and low sense of self-worth are unavoidable part of every classroom. Childhood and adolescence seem to be a critical age for prevention of internalized problems, and schools seem as a natural setting to support the accumulation of positive experiences that outweigh risks. When thinking about general evidence-based approach to internalized problems, findings show that is crucial to educate youth how to develop active coping strategies and to cope with negative thoughts. Schools can be good environments to do that. The aim of this chapter is to offer an overview of critical epidemiological data on internalized disorders of children and youth as well as a summary of evidence-based practices focused on their prevention in schools, going from universal to targeted programs and highlighting mindfulness-based interventions. Finally, Croatian example of investments in socio-emotional learning is presented, examining its effects on students' internalizing symptoms.

Keywords: internalized problems, prevention, school prevention programs, mental health

1. Introduction

1.1. Internalized problems of children and youth

Internalized problems are defined as group of emotional symptoms turned toward individual that reveals more prevalent effortful control of behavior, feelings of sadness, low self-esteem, behavioral inhibition, and fears. A substantive body of research indicates that although children and youth are a healthy subpopulation group, 20% of them could experience mental health issue until early twenties, anxiety and depression being the most prevalent [1–3]. That statement is not so surprising if we are aware of the fact that puberty and adolescence bring more sensitivity to social clues, seeking approval from important others, immaturity of neurobiological system connected with emotions, progressive reduction of parental control, and greater importance of peers. Half of all lifetime mental disorders begin before the age of 14, anxiety even before between age 6 and puberty [4]. That being said, school setting is unavoidable when talking about factors that support children and youth to thrive. It seems that students' feelings such as shy or withdrawn behavior, frequent worrying, fears, sadness, loneliness, hopelessness, and low sense of self-worth are unavoidable part of every classroom.

Newer American epidemiological studies state [4] that there is a prevalence of 32% of anxiety disorders and 14.3% mood disorders in the group of youth from 13 to 18 years old, while around 8% of American youth had a major depressive disorder. A British study included younger children, from 5 to 15, and found a prevalence of 3.7% for any anxiety disorder [4]. 1-year incidence rate for the first onset of major depression in adolescents is between 5.6 and 10%, while 17.9% of adolescents have a recurrent episode within a year [5–7]. Adolescent depression is associated with high rates of comorbid anxiety disorders, disruptive behavior disorders, and suicide attempts. It predicts future adjustment problems including marital difficulties, unemployment, and attachment problems in offspring [5–7]. By late adolescence, twice as many girls are depressed as boys, and 40% of those who experienced depression during youth end up with a diagnosis of major depression in adulthood [7]. After the first major depressive episode, the chance of recurrence and chronicity is very high [8]. Worldwide data shows that depression is a major public health problem that requires the development, implementation, and evaluation of interventions preventing its onset. The World Health Organization estimates that depression is the third leading cause of global disease with projections that it will rank first until 2030 [9]. There is also a great impact of depression on physical health: 40–60% of people who have experienced depression die prematurely [9], often show greater rates of smoking, and, as an aftermath of various circumstances affecting the quality of life, deal with heart disease [10]. When talking about the costs for adults, comprehensive European study estimates annual cost of mood disorders on 113. 4 billion Euros for 33.3 million affected people [11]. Burden is not only personal but also economic, affecting families, communities, and governments.

All this evidence shows that it is crucial to tackle emotional health problems early and shift focus from treatment to prevention and early intervention [4], enabling full potential for future adults. Emotional well-being has implications on children's and adolescent's self-esteem, prosocial behavior, school attendance, and success and increases risk of suicidal behavior, smoking, substance abuse, and delinquency [1, 12, 13] as well as choices of profession, directly leading to circumstances for adulthood [6] and future life chances [9]. Good sense of self in childhood is transferred to adulthood, together with good problem-solving skills, social competence, and feeling of purpose [13]. These resources vouch for good outcomes, serving as buffers in times of risks, stress, and hardship, and they are not only dependent upon child or a teen but also upon family characteristics and various environments in which they live [13, 14].

Many authors suggest that research of interventions for children and adolescents should be a priority since the first signs of disorder often happen in adolescence. Adolescence seems to be a crucial window for preventive interventions given the fact that rates of emotional ill health increase during this developmental stage. The 2009 Institute of Medicine report on prevention of mental, emotional, and behavioral disorders presented evidence that anxiety and mood disorders can be prevented [14]. Leaders in the field of mental health recommend further research on prevention and interventions for mental disorders of children and adolescents [1, 9, 15].

1.2. Risk and protective factors for internalized disorder trajectories

Risk and protective factors on individual, family, school, and community level help to understand the possibilities of organized support for sustaining a state of mental well-being and buffering possible adverse circumstances. Offering opportunities that support strengths should be planned within regular, already existent settings and systems supporting development of children and youth [13]. Program activities and interventions should be theory driven and science based, addressing well-known factors.

It is not surprising that research of developmental cascades implies crucial importance of family influences, early attachment, and parent-child relationship [16]. Transfer of emotional problems from parents to offspring is related both with shared genetic factors and vulnerability as well as with inadequate parenting [17]. It seems that maternal depression or existence of parental anxiety symptoms is a risk factor for elevated internalizing problems [17]. Parents' negative emotional expressiveness, including hostility and irritability, affect child's feeling of security [17, 18]: depressed mothers are less responsive to child's needs, more authoritarian, and rejecting, while anxious parents tend to be controlling and express less warmth. Additionally, internalized problems are related with family dynamics where emotion expression is quite restricted, i.e., both positive and negative emotions are suppressed, leading to heightened negativity and avoidance as a mean of regulation [17]. Children in such family context show less emotion recognition and lower emotion regulation strategies. Same authors explain risks specific to child's temperament, such as inhibition, fearfulness, shyness, and avoidance of new situations. Additionally, cognitive style characterized with pessimistic attributions, negative expectations, external locus of control, and rigidity is also a contributor.

One of few longitudinal studies [19] assessing internalized disorders has shown that academic problems, elevated parental stress, serious health issues, and social isolation strongly predict internalized symptomatology that lasts until early adulthood. Specifically, children with three or more negative life events were almost nine times likely to exhibit internalized problems. Such experiences were neglect, maltreatment, family violence, or sexual abuse, rarely found in sample, but also parental conflict and divorce which happen considerably more. Substantive influence on internalized problem development is reported upon peer victimization, rejection, and bullying [20] what stresses the need of school interventions once again.

The more opportunities young people have to accumulate protective factors that outweigh the influence of risks, the more likely they are to preserve their mental health well-being. Key protective factors for stable emotional development include a sense of family belonging as well as school attachment, i.e., caring and warm environments where both adults and peers are supportive [14]. Research shows that children who have a close emotional relationship with at least one peer have smaller chances to develop internalized problems than children who do not have such experience. Relationships with others are significant protective asset since they buffer negative experiences and low mood, symptoms often seen within children isolated by friends or by their own choice [20]. Active methods of coping such as problem-solving lessen the amount of negative feelings and improve functioning and regulation.

2. Interventions for prevention of internalized problems of children and youth

2.1. Changing role of schools in modern era

In the age of information, schools really have a duty to revise their mission: knowledge is available almost everywhere, but quality relationships are becoming quite rare. In order to prepare future adults for challenges in full scale, schools have to provide critical skills for future education, work, and life in general. Besides cognitive skills, to develop positively and be empowered and participating member of society, young people need social and emotional skills. Modern school has holistic focus and has to incorporate care for emotional and social well-being in their curricula [21–25]. Reduction of subjective distress as well as behavior problems is possible by implementing interventions and specific classroom-management practices that develop understanding of emotions, positive goal achievement, maintenance of positive relationships with others, and responsible decision-making. From preschool to middle school, those competencies are being taught within the process of socio-emotional learning and universal programs. International evidence strongly confirms that school interventions teaching socio-emotional learning advance mental health, social functioning, positive health behaviors, as well as academic success [21–25]. Cost benefit studies are also supporting the case: data from 2011 demonstrates that for every dollar invested in socio-emotional learning, average return is 11$ [26]. It is important to determine if universal evidence-based programs can respond to the needs of young people with different characteristics and if enhancement of young people's social and emotional skills and resilience building is sufficient strategy [24].

2.2. Evidence-based prevention programs for internalized problems

Since lots of evidence suggests that large proportion of children and young people with anxiety disorders and depression are not included in the treatment, universal prevention programs that promote well-being and preventative interventions are even more essential [27, 28]. Lack of effective treatment probably has a lot to do with problems in the provision of care and poor access to services but also has a cause in low symptom awareness, stigma, inadequate treatment, and available funding [29]. Comprehensive answer to the issue of internalized problems is slowly directing its aims to prevention since it could relieve the burden on health care and social services. When thinking about general evidence-based approach to internalized problems, findings from literature review [30] propose that effective strategy is using cognitive-behavioral therapy model, educating adolescents how to cope with negative thoughts, to solve problems more effectively and develop active coping strategies, as well as to support caring relationships and quality interactions with important others.

Terzian and colleagues have reviewed 37 programs [30] aiming at internalized problems in general, from depressive symptoms, suicidal thoughts or behaviors, anxious symptoms, PTSD, and shy/withdrawn behavior. Twenty-four out of thirty-seven programs had positive impact, three had mixed findings, and ten were not effective. Programs that were found to work were from either therapeutic approach (individual, family, and group) or skills training approach. Evidence suggest that good programs should teach children and youth to cope with negative thoughts and feelings through (1) building cognitive-behavioral skills such as thought monitoring, identification of triggers, and reframing of negative thoughts and (2) investment in coping skills such as relaxation, seeking help from others, and teaching participants to react adaptively on stress. When focusing only on prevention programs in this review: 10 out of 19 were found to have positive impact on at least one internalizing problem.

After 2010, several reviews and meta-analytic studies have considered effectiveness of various types of interventions, being universal or focused on specific populations in various levels of risk as well as for those with already diagnosable internalized problems [29–34]. Within Cochrane review [29], prevention studies were grouped in universal and targeted; targeted included both selective populations in higher risk and indicated programs focusing on signs suggesting the onset of disorder. Examples of population in higher risk are related with children of parents with diagnosable mental health issue; children with elevated family risks such as violence, neglect, and disputes; as well as children and youth with experience of trauma or bullying. Issue was raised [29] about the inclusion of secondary prevention studies, i.e., those that included children and youth with a history of anxiety or depression, but typically previous history is not described well. Preventive interventions aimed at internalized symptoms, especially those in school settings, need to be researched more thoroughly in the future. Findings are mixed or small to moderate, and it seems that the most problematic issue is that effects easily fade after the program completion. Universal prevention programs last for between 3 to 9 months. Evidence is promising in ways of reducing levels of depressive symptoms and only in some cases episodes of clinically significant depression [29].

Conclusions for internalized problems in general are even more difficult since studies are usually focused on specific problem, depression being most often nowadays, and not the whole group of issues. For example, Cochrane review of programs aiming at depression included 53 studies and more than 14,000 participants and concluded that both targeted and universal interventions are effective for prevention of depression although effects of selective interventions last longer. Also, it has been shown that psychological interventions are more effective than educational interventions since they do more than teach; they really change thinking strategies and skills. Secondary analysis of Cochrane trials [31] aimed at investigation whether specific therapeutic approach was more effective, indicating variation in outcomes across trials. There is some evidence that more consideration should be given to specific therapeutic approach since cognitive-behavioral interventions were more often proven effective. Also, that additional review showed that results were not moderated by the type of prevention. On the other hand, meta-analysis conducted by Horowitz and Garber [32] included 30 studies where prevention of depression of children and youth was in focus and their conclusion was that regarding depressive symptoms, selective and indicated interventions have larger effects than universal. Nevertheless, universal approach should not be neglected [33]: Australian examples show that universal programs involved less stigma and less attrition of participants.

Since the focus of this chapter is related to school context, choice of school preventive intervention programs is presented in **Table 1**. Current literature suggests those programs are either promising since they have mixed results in various evaluations or are still being adapted from more clinical interventions to preventive approach and school settings [30, 33–36]. Brunwasser, Gillham and Kim [34] looked at various studies of Penn Resiliency Program and highlighted promising results for more than eight-session program of longer duration, delivered by a healthcare professional. Generally, many school prevention programs for internalized problems tend to have cognitive-behavioral foundations, and it is notable that they incorporate optimism and hope as their values. Besides school, partners in prevention have to be parents, especially if parental style and parent–child relationship have its difficulties but also if they have anxiety or depression disorder as well. Parental part of the program is adjunct to program activities with youth, and it is implemented simultaneously [33–35].

It is important to emphasize that the use of online and computer delivery of interventions for internalized problems and their prevention is rapidly growing. For new generations of children and adolescents, usage of the Internet or their computer and cellphone seems easy and cost-effective, increases uptake, and secures anonymity that is often being an issue in help seeking. Description of new technology wave interventions is out of the scope of this chapter, but it is necessary to address numerous benefits such as instant availability (especially for mobile phones and apps) and less need for face-to-face professional or time-consuming

Name of the program.	Short description of the program
Mindfulness in Schools Programme (MISP)[1]	Universal, a set of nine scripted lessons tailored to secondary schools, supported by tailored teacher training; it involves learning to direct attention to immediate experience, moment by moment, with open-minded curiosity and acceptance
Learning to Breathe Mindfulness Curriculum[2]	Universal and selective, for adolescents, consists of six themes that may be delivered in 6, 12, 18, or more sessions; the six core lessons are body, reflection, emotions, attention, tenderness, and healthy mind habits
Mindfulness Group Program [53]	Universal, for students aged 13–20, includes eight weekly delivered 100-min sessions; it integrates elements of MBSR and mindfulness-based cognitive therapy (MBCT) [54]; students develop specific skills in their capacity to become nonjudgmentally aware of thoughts, feelings, and sensations and increase their capacity to replace automatic, habitual, and often judgmental reactions with more conscious and skillful responses
Mindfulness Training [42]	Universal, modified MBSR program, students aged 14–15, four 40-min group trainings one per week; training covers the concepts of awareness and acceptance, and practices include bodily awareness of contact points, mindfulness of breathing and finding an anchor point, awareness of sounds, understanding the transient nature of thoughts, and walking meditation

[1]https://mindfulnessinschools.org/what-is-b/b-curriculum/

[2]https://learning2breathe.org/

Table 1. Mindfulness school-based programs found promising/effective for internalized problem prevention.

teacher training [37]. There are several examples of promising interventions using the Internet, applied game or gamification interface for mental health, and meta-analysis shows a moderate effect of d = .55, favoring serious games over no intervention controls. Regarding the fact that this topic requires new chapter, just one illustration—excellent New Zealand example program, SPARX, interactive fantasy game using CBT approach—aims adolescents from 12 to 19 years with elevated depression symptoms, and it is goal-oriented and problem-solving. Each level module lasts 30 min and can be available online or at home computer [38]. Findings show positive impact on emotion regulation and depressive symptoms reduction, and there are several other international examples [37, 38].

2.3. Mindfulness interventions for internalized problem prevention

When thinking about new wave of approaches, mindfulness practice also enhances the very qualities and goals of education in the twenty-first century and is usually seen hand in hand with socio-emotional learning approach. Since of it focuses on the body and different approaches to mind, it is a good choice when addressing internalized problems. The application of mindfulness with children and adolescents has increased more recently. Regarding changing lifestyles and risks, it would be helpful if children could learn to stop their mind wandering and regulate attention and emotions, to deal with feelings of frustration, and to self-motivate. A review of the emerging body of research on mindfulness-based interventions with children and adolescents reveals that such interventions might be beneficial in many different ways [39]. Mindfulness is considered one of many contemplative practices and has become a very popular practice due to its various mental and physical health benefits [40]. It is said to have originated two and a half thousand years ago from the religious traditions of Buddhism. Around the late 1970s, Jon Kabat-Zinn introduced mindfulness to Western cultures as a secular health practice [41]. It is defined as the practice of "paying attention on purpose, in the present moment, and nonjudgmentally to the unfolding of experience moment by moment" ([42], p. 145). Mindfulness is considered as "the self-regulation of attention so that it is maintained on immediate experience… characterized by curiosity, openness, and acceptance" [43]. From this perspective, mindfulness practice can be understood as the foundation and basic precondition for education [44]. Modern education abilities embrace not only good attention skills and emotional competence but also prosocial abilities such as responsiveness, kindness, high ethics standards, sensitivity, imagination, and as well as good problem-solving. They allow children to face forthcoming challenges of the progressing environment, preferably becoming thoughtful, kind, and dedicated people [45, 46].

There are clear indications now that mindfulness-based programs with children and youth within school setting are feasible and acceptable [39]. Many of the existing school-based mindfulness programs for mental health have been adapted from Mindfulness Based Stress Reduction (MBSR) to meet children's and adolescents' developmental needs and shorter attention spans [47, 48]. These programs include a number of mindfulness-based activities such as breath awareness, psycho-education components, body scans, sitting meditations, and mindful movement, among others [44, 49]. Lately, scientists have initiated studies of various short mindfulness-based interventions, from 1 to 4 weeks long, including mindful eating, walking contemplation, and coloring, as well as combination of mindfulness and yoga activities. Findings suggest this is effective in diminishing emotional problems and problem behaviors in school settings [50–52]. Some of the promising/effective mindfulness school-based programs for internalized problems are presented in **Table 1**.

In terms of school-based mindfulness intervention effectiveness, these programs have been associated with decreases in stress levels [55–58], rumination, intrusive thoughts, emotional arousal [59, 60], and depression symptoms [53, 55, 57, 58, 61] along with increases in emotional well-being [62] and self-compassion among participants [57]. A study conducted by Britton et al. [47] on a sample of 100 elementary school students involved into Integrative Contemplative Pedagogy program has shown reduced suicidal ideations and affective disturbance among students after 6 weeks of everyday short meditation training (3–12 min per day). Studies have also confirmed that mindfulness-based interventions in schools lead to a reduction in symptoms of depression in minority children [63] and to a reduction in anxiety and increase of social skills in students with learning disorders [64].

Zenner and colleagues [44] have conducted a systematic review and meta-analysis to summarize data available on the effects of 24 studies of mindfulness-based trainings for children and youth in a school setting and report a significant medium effect size of $d = .40$ across all controlled studies and domains. In 2017, big meta-analysis of 24 studies (n = 3977) was led to examine specific moderators contributing to school-based mindfulness interventions for mental health in youth [65]. Overall, mindfulness interventions were found to be helpful, with small to moderate significant effects pre-post intervention compared to control groups; however, interventions that were delivered during late adolescence (15–18) and that consisted of combinations of various mindfulness activities had the largest effects on mental health and well-being outcomes.

3. Croatian example: Effects of socio-emotional learning on internalized problems

3.1. Research studies

The aim of this part of the chapter is to present two studies of empirical evaluation of social–emotional learning curriculum, Promoting Alternative Thinking Strategies (PATHS) [66], conducted in Croatian kindergartens [67] and elementary schools [68] in order to examine the effects on the level of internalized problems such as emotional withdrawal, depressive symptoms, and worry.

3.1.1. Preschool study

The preschool PATHS study involved a quasi-experimental design, evaluating the short-term outcomes of the preschool PATHS curriculum implemented in six buildings across three Croatian sites (Zagreb, the capital city of Rijeka, and the Region of Istria, Croatia). Within each building two groups were chosen, and twelve kindergarten groups were included in the study. The impact of the PATHS program was tested within the sample of 443 children (aged 3–6) for whom their preschool teachers collected data during three time points within a 2-year period. The first measurement was within the usual practices, before implementation, while second was at the start of the program and third in the end. Forty-five percent of children in the sample were girls.

3.1.2. School study

The study relied on a randomized controlled design to evaluate the impact of PATHS. Originally, 30 schools were recruited with the help of local authorities in three abovementioned implementation sites in Croatia. Within each region, equivalent pairs of schools were coordinated according to area features, household financial status, and proportion of pupils getting free-of-charge meals, number of pupils in school and classroom, as well as overall marks. Within each pair, one school was intervention and other continued typical program. Within each building, two first classrooms were chosen for the program. Only ten children from whole classroom were randomly nominated for assessment. Since some teachers failed to complete assessments, final sample consisted of 568 children and 546 children (96% of the sample) had complete post-intervention assessments. Forty-seven percent of the school children participants were girls. At the beginning of this study, all children were 7 years old in average and in the middle of the first grade. At the end of the study, children were near the end of the second grade.

3.1.3. Measures

Both preschool and schoolteachers were assessing children with the same battery. Among nine rated child behaviors, two of them are related with internalized symptoms:

3.1.3.1. Emotion regulation

Emotion regulation was measured with seven items from the *Social Competence Scale* from Fast Track Project (http://www.fasttrackproject.org/techrept/s/sct/). Sample item was "accepts things not going her/his way." All items were rated on a 6-point Likert scale with response options ranging from almost never to usually (α = .89) [68, 69].

3.1.3.2. Withdrawn/depressed behavior

Withdrawn/depressed behavior was assessed with six commonly used items compiled for Head Start REDI [28–30]. Sample items were "avoids playing with other children" and "sad, unhappy." All items were rated on a 6-point Likert scale, with response options ranging from almost never to usually (α = .81).

3.2. Paths

PATHS is one of the most effective socio-emotional learning programs for children from preschool to middle school worldwide. It has been tested in multiple randomized controlled trials and implemented in many different contexts with children of various backgrounds. Various research and independent studies show that PATHS program is a successful example of whole-school generalization, enhances classroom climate and significantly contributes to children's emotion recognition and self-regulation, improves relationships with others, and diminishes externalizing problems [70, 71].

3.3. Results in Croatia: effects of PATHS on internalized symptomatology

To test intervention effects, hierarchical linear models were estimated, nesting children within classrooms. In school study, analyses were conducted for subgroups of children within the sample. Each of the child behaviors included in this study was dichotomized to specify whether a child was above or below average in terms of her/his functioning at the pre-intervention assessment. Latent class analysis was applied to nine indicators to determine whether children were relatively high or low risk. In this analysis, 223 children had the highest probability of being in the most elevated risk group. Those children had highest likelihood for lower scores on prosocial behavior, control of emotions, and school-related performance. In the same time, the same kids had a highest chance for high results on problem list (inattentiveness, hyperactivity, opposition, aggression, difficulties with peers, and inhibited/sad behavior). Analysis showed that 335 children had maximum chance of being in the low-risk subclass, which was characterized by above average scores on the positive behaviors and below average scores on the negative behaviors.

In preschool study, analyses were done in two stages: the first stage aiming to see changes in intervention sample across time and the second stage to compare scores with comparison condition. The first stage of preschool analyses shows insignificant change score for emotional symptoms of −.14, $p < .0001$, $d = .41$; ICC = .02, p = ns. Second-stage analyses show differences among children who were in comparison and PATHS condition: there was statistically significant difference in rates of change for emotional symptoms, $\beta = -.33$, $p = < .05$, $d = .56$; ICC = .27, $p < .05$. The magnitude of this difference in rates of change was over one-half of one standard deviation. Results for school study are shown in **Table 2**.

In school study, the pre-intervention level of functioning on the outcome and child sex were included as covariates. Among the children who were relatively high risk, there were no statistically significant differences between intervention and control group children.

Among the children who were relatively low risk, there was a small to moderate effect for emotion regulation and a marginally statistically significant difference in withdrawn/depressed behavior but no changes for high-risk group. To examine the robustness of effects among the low-risk children, latent class analysis was used again to determine whether children exhibited any problems. In this analysis, 81 children had the highest probability of being in the low risk with social difficulties subgroup, which was characterized by below average scores on prosocial behavior and emotion regulation and above average scores on withdrawn/depressed behavior. The other 254 children had the highest probability of being in the low risk without social difficulties subgroup, which was characterized by above average scores on all the positive behaviors and below average scores on all the negative behaviors.

School study	Complete sample (N = 568)	High-risk children (n = 223)	All low-risk children (n = 335)	Low-risk children with social difficulties (n = 81)	Low-risk children without social difficulties (n = 254)
Emotion regulation	.18+	.06	.38**	.65**	.32*
Withdrawn behavior	−.09	.06	−.26+	−.52*	−.19

Legend:*level of significance* $p = <.05$;
***level of significance* $p = <.01$.

Table 2. School PATHS effects on emotion regulation and withdrawn behavior for the complete sample and subgroups of schoolchildren.

Problem in focus	Found to work	Short description of program
Depressive symptoms	Adolescents coping With stress	Fifteen sessions for group from three to ten participants, adapted from Coping with Depression Course[1], group CBT preventive intervention for adolescents in risk, managed by educated therapist
	Problem-solving for life	Universal, teacher-implemented classroom program[2], for 12–14 year olds, 8 sessions, focusing on life problem-solving skills, positive problem-solving orientation, and optimistic-thinking styles
	Penn Prevention Program/ Penn Resiliency Program	School based, facilitated by school counselor[3], 12 sessions, aimed at depression and anxiety symptom reduction, special accent on optimism, coping strategies and perspective taking, one of the most widely disseminated
Anxiety symptoms	FRIENDS Program/Friends for Life Program	Cognitive-behavioral approach for adolescents, delivered by school staff supported by trained graduate psychology student, 10 one and half hour sessions, teaching coping skills and problem-solving + parallel parent intervention, four sessions
Suicidal thoughts or behaviors	Signs of Suicide Prevention Program	Universal, school-based program for middle school and high school; central activities are raising awareness for depression and suicide signs and help seeking behavior[4]

[1]https://www.childtrends.org/programs/adolescent-coping-with-stress/
[2]https://www.childtrends.org/programs/problem-solving-for-life/
[3]https://ppc.sas.upenn.edu/research/resilience-children
[4]https://nrepp.samhsa.gov/ProgramProfile.aspx?id=85

Table 3. Prevention programs found promising/effective for internalized problems prevention.

Among the children who were relatively low risk with social difficulties, there were statistically significant differences on emotion regulation and withdrawn/depressed behavior. Intervention effects of this magnitude shown in **Table 3** would be considered moderate to large. Among the children who were low risk without social difficulties, there was a small effect on emotion regulation but no effect on withdrawn behavior.

3.4. Discussion of results

Both of the presented studies of PATHS curriculum in Croatia indicate participation of children in universal, social-emotional curriculum that promotes emotion recognition and relationships with others and self-esteem and self-control can diminish emotional symptoms, withdrawal, depressed symptoms, and worry, even for young children from 3 to 6. Also, data clearly shows that the decrease of risks for development of internalized problems is not uniform for all children: benefits vary depending upon sets of negative behaviors or lack in social or learning skills.

Analyses conducted for subgroups of children show that effectiveness depends upon child's capacity and needs. For children that are low risk but seem to have smaller issues in relating to others and lower social skills as well as lower learning behaviors, it is plausible to conclude that mental health promotion intervention like PATHS is very useful. For that group of children that need additional but not clinical support, improvement of classroom climate, boost of social competencies, and focus on feelings, such classroom intervention gives promising results. For that subgroup, improvement of emotion regulation and decline in withdrawal happened within a year of program implementation. Our results for high-risk children subsample show that they need additional care and support, probably more attention within indicated prevention approach or even clinical support. Nevertheless, within comprehensive policy addressing mental and emotional well-being of children, Croatian example shows that universal strategies are helpful and should be considered when planning prevention of internalized symptoms.

4. Conclusion

This chapter focused on internalized problem prevention in academic setting, since they are integral part of every classroom. Teachers and even parents do not recognize them in exact amount; children and youth tend to hide them and avoid reporting they need help. Findings from literature clearly accent that schools have an important role in reducing internalized problems, starting early on with emotional well-being promotion and responding to first symptoms. Comprehensive whole-school approach to mental health and internalized problems could serve as a climate change since research shows that besides supporting relationships, skill-building approach is most promising. Effects of school prevention programs are small to moderate, but thinking strategically, comprehensive planning of interventions on all levels could relieve the burden on health care and social services.

More research is needed to identify effectiveness of various types of programs, but it seems that universal school prevention programs have small to moderate effects and there is evidence that mindfulness programs also reduce internalizing symptoms. Conclusions for internalized problem selective and indicated prevention are still mixed, some studies showing effects in reducing depressive symptoms and enhancing emotional regulation and coping skills, but other studies show effect only for some measures. Making general conclusions is hard since studies are usually focused on specific internalized problem, depression being most often nowadays. Answer to a public health problem has to be comprehensive. Combination of investments from early years, coming from universal approach such as socio-emotional learning and mindfulness-based programs, and then being followed with selective programs for those in elevated risk and indicated interventions for those showing first symptoms, seems promising public health strategy and a way forward.

Acknowledgements

Studies mentioned in this chapter were financed by the Unity through Knowledge Fund, Republic of Croatia, and the local authorities of three Croatian regions. Josipa Basic, retired full professor of Faculty of Education and Rehabilitation Sciences, University of Zagreb, Croatia, was the project leader; Celene Domitrovich, now at Department of Psychiatry, Georgetown University, USA, was the coleader. Robert L. Nix, University of Wisconsin, Madison, USA, contributed to the chapter by conducting analyses.

Conflict of interest

Authors certify they have no financial or nonfinancial interest in the subject matter of this manuscript.

Author details

Miranda Novak* and Josipa Mihić

*Address all correspondence to: miranda.novak@erf.hr

Department of Behavioral Disorders, Prevention Research Laboratory, Faculty of Education and Rehabilitation Sciences, University of Zagreb, Croatia

References

[1] World Health Organization. Adolescent's Mental Health: Mapping Actions of Non-Governmental Organizations and Other International Development Organizations. Geneva: World Health Organization; 2012

[2] Lack CW, Green AL. Mood disorders in children and adolescents. Journal of Pediatric Nursing: Nursing Care of Children and Families. 2009;**24**(1):13-25. DOI: 10.1016/j.pedn.2008.04.007

[3] Jane Costello E, Erkanli A, Angold A. Is there an epidemic of child or adolescent depression? Journal of Child Psychology and Psychiatry. 2006;**47**(12):1263-1271. DOI: 10.1111/j.1469-7610.2006.01682.x

[4] Merikangas KR, He JP, Burstein M, Swanson SA, Avenevoli S, Cui L, Benjet C, Georgiades K, Swendsen J. Lifetime prevalence of mental disorders in US adolescents: Results from the National Comorbidity Survey Replication–Adolescent Supplement (NCS-A). Journal of the American Academy of Child & Adolescent Psychiatry. 2010;**49**(10):980-989. DOI: 10.1016/j.jaac.2010.05.017

[5] Barrera AZ, Torres LD, Muñoz RF. Prevention of depression: The state of the science at the beginning of the 21st century. International Review of Psychiatry. 2007;**19**(6): 655-670. DOI: 10.1080/09540260701797894

[6] Seeley JR, Rohde P, Lewinsohn PM, Clarke GN. Depression in youth: Epidemiology, identification, and intervention. In: Interventions for Academic and Behavior Problems II: Preventive and Remedial Approaches. Washington, DC, US: National Association of School Psychologists; 2002. pp. 885-911

[7] Lewinsohn PM, Hops H, Roberts RE, Seeley JR, Andrews JA. Adolescent psychopathology: I. Prevalence and incidence of depression and other DSM-III—R disorders in high school students. Journal of Abnormal Psychology. 1993;**102**(1):133. DOI: 10.1037/0021-843X.102.1.133

[8] Lewinsohn PM, Allen NB, Seeley JR, Gotlib IH. First onset versus recurrence of depression: Differential processes of psychosocial risk. Journal of Abnormal Psychology. 1999; **108**(3):483. DOI: 10.1037/0021-843X.108.3.483

[9] World Health Organization. Mental Health Action Plan 2013-2020. 2013. WHO web site: http://scholar.google.com/scholar. 2017

[10] Sher Y, Lolak S, Maldonado JR. The impact of depression in heart disease. Current Psychiatry Reports. 2010;**12**(3):255-264. DOI: 10.1007/s11920-010-0116-8

[11] Gustavsson A, Svensson M, Jacobi F, Allgulander C, Alonso J, Beghi E, Dodel R, Ekman M, Faravelli C, Fratiglioni L, Gannon B. Cost of disorders of the brain in Europe 2010. European Neuropsychopharmacology. 2011;**21**(10):718-779. DOI: 10.1016/j.euroneuro.2011.08.008

[12] Ford T, Goodman R, Meltzer H. The British child and adolescent mental health survey 1999: The prevalence of DSM-IV disorders. Journal of the American Academy of Child and Adolescent Psychiatry. 2003;**42**(10):1203-1211. DOI: 10.1111/j.1469-7610.2006.01682.x

[13] Morgan A, Currie C, Due P, Gabhain SN, Rasmussen M, Samdal O, Smith R. Mental well-being in school-aged children in Europe: Associations with social cohesion and socioeconomic circumstances. In: Social Cohesion for Mental Well-Being Among Adolescents. WHO/HBSC Forum: Copenhagen; 2008

[14] National Research Council. Preventing Mental, Emotional, and Behavioral Disorders Among Young People: Progress and Possibilities. Washington DC: National Academies Press; 2009

[15] Wykes T, Haro JM, Belli SR, Obradors-Tarragó C, Arango C, Ayuso-Mateos JL, Bitter I, Brunn M, Chevreul K, Demotes-Mainard J, Elfeddali I. Mental health research priorities for Europe. The Lancet Psychiatry. 2015;**2**(11):1036-1042

[16] Bornstein MH, Hahn CS, Haynes OM. Social competence, externalizing, and internalizing behavioral adjustment from early childhood through early adolescence: Developmental cascades. Development and Psychopathology. 2010;**22**(4):717-735

[17] Marakovitz SE, Wagmiller RL, Mian ND, Briggs-Gowan MJ, Carter AS. Lost toy? Monsters under the bed? Contributions of temperament and family factors to early internalizing

problems in boys and girls. Journal of Clinical Child and Adolescent Psychology. 2011;**40**(2):233-244

[18] Cummings EM, Cheung RY, Davies PT. Prospective relations between parental depression, negative expressiveness, emotional insecurity, and children's internalizing symptoms. Child Psychiatry and Human Development. 2013;**44**(6):698-708

[19] Melchior M, Touchette É, Prokofyeva E, Chollet A, Fombonne E, Elidemir G, Galéra C. Negative events in childhood predict trajectories of internalizing symptoms up to young adulthood: An 18-year longitudinal study. PLoS One. 2014;**9**(12):e114526

[20] Yeung Thompson RS, Leadbeater BJ. Peer victimization and internalizing symptoms from adolescence into young adulthood: Building strength through emotional support. Journal of Research on Adolescence. 2013;**23**(2):290-303

[21] Durlak JA, Weissberg RP, Dymnicki AB, Taylor RD, Schellinger KB. Enhancing students' social and emotional development promotes success in school: Results of a meta-analysis. Child Development. 2011;**82**(1):405-432

[22] Weare K, Nind M. Mental health promotion and problem prevention in schools: What does the evidence say? Health Promotion International. 2011;**26**(Suppl_1):i29-i69

[23] Weissberg RP, Goren P, Domitrovich C, Dusenbury L. CASEL Guide Effective Social and Emotional Learning Programs: Preschool and Elementary School Edition. Chicago, IL: CASEL; 2013

[24] Barry MM, Clarke AM, Dowling K. Promoting social and emotional well-being in schools. Health Education. 2017;**117**(5):434-451

[25] Clarke AM, Hussein Y, Morreale S, Field CA, Barry MM. What Works in Enhancing Social and Emotional Skills Development During Childhood and Adolescence? A Review of the Evidence on the Effectiveness of School-Based and Out-of-School Programmes in the UK. National University of Ireland Galway: WHO Collaborating Centre for Health Promotion Research; 2015

[26] Belfield C, Bowden AB, Klapp A, Levin H, Shand R, Zander S. The economic value of social and emotional learning. Journal of Benefit-Cost Analysis. 2015;**6**(3):508-544

[27] Beardslee WR, Brent DA, Weersing VR, Clarke GN, Porta G, Hollon SD, Gladstone TR, Gallop R, Lynch FL, Iyengar S, DeBar L. Prevention of depression in at-risk adolescents: Longer-term effects. JAMA Psychiatry. 2013;**70**(11):1161-1170. DOI: 10.1001/jamapsychiatry.2013.295

[28] Pennant ME, Loucas CE, Whittington C, Creswell C, Fonagy P, Fuggle P, Kelvin R, Naqvi S, Stockton S, Kendall T. Computerised therapies for anxiety and depression in children and young people: A systematic review and meta-analysis. Behaviour Research and Therapy. 2015;**67**:1-8

[29] Merry SN, Hetrick SE, Cox GR, Brudevold-Iversen T, Bir JJ, McDowell H. Cochrane review: Psychological and educational interventions for preventing depression in children and ado-

lescents. Evidence-Based Child Health: A Cochrane Review Journal. 2012;7(5):1409-1685

[30] Terzian M, Hamilton K, Ericson S. What Works to Prevent or Reduce Internalizing Problems or Socio-Emotional Difficulties in Adolescents: Lessons from Experimental Evaluations of Social Interventions. Washington DC: Fact Sheet. Child Trends; 2011. Publication# 2011-34

[31] Hetrick SE, Cox GR, Merry SN. Where to go from here? An exploratory meta-analysis of the most promising approaches to depression prevention programs for children and adolescents. International Journal of Environmental Research and Public Health. 2015;**12**(5):4758-4795. DOI: 10.3390/ijerph120504758

[32] Horowitz JL, Garber J. The prevention of depressive symptoms in children and adolescents: A meta-analytic review. Journal of Consulting and Clinical Psychology. 2006; **74**(3):401

[33] Spence SH, Sheffield JK, Donovan CL. Preventing adolescent depression: An evaluation of the problem solving for life program. Journal of Consulting and Clinical Psychology. 2003;**71**(1):3

[34] Garber J, Clarke GN, Weersing VR, Beardslee WR, Brent DA, Gladstone TR, DeBar LL, Lynch FL, D'Angelo E, Hollon SD, Shamseddeen W. Prevention of depression in at-risk adolescents: A randomized controlled trial. Journal of the American Medical Association. 2009;**301**(21):2215-2224

[35] Brunwasser SM, Gillham JE, Kim ES. A meta-analytic review of the Penn resiliency Program's effect on depressive symptoms. Journal of Consulting and Clinical Psychology. 2009;**77**(6):1042

[36] Schilling EA, Aseltine RH, James A. The SOS suicide prevention program: Further evidence of efficacy and effectiveness. Prevention Science. 2016;**17**(2):157-166

[37] Lau HM, Smit JH, Fleming TM, Riper H. Serious games for mental health: Are they accessible, feasible, and effective? A systematic review and meta-analysis. Frontiers in Psychiatry. 2017;**7**:209. DOI: 10.3389/fpsyt.2016.00209

[38] Merry SN, Stasiak K, Shepherd M, Frampton C, Fleming T, Lucassen MF. The effectiveness of SPARX, a computerised self help intervention for adolescents seeking help for depression: Randomised controlled non-inferiority trial. BMJ. 2012;**344**:e2598. DOI: 10.1136/bmj.e2598

[39] Burke CA. Mindfulness-based approaches with children and adolescents: A preliminary review of current research in an emergent field. Journal of Child and Family Studies. 2010;**19**(2):133-144. DOI: 10.1002/14651858.CD012518

[40] Meiklejohn J, Phillips C, Freedman ML, Griffin ML, Biegel G, Roach A, Frank J, Burke C, Pinger L, Soloway G, Isberg R. Integrating mindfulness training into K-12 education: Fostering the resilience of teachers and students. Mindfulness. 2012;**3**(4):291-307. DOI: 10.1007/s12671-012-0094-5

[41] Burke AL, Hawkins K. Mindfulness in education: Wellness from the inside out. Encounter: Education for Meaning and Social Justice. 2012;**25**(4):36-40

[42] Kabat-Zinn J. Mindfulness-based interventions in context: Past, present, and future. Clinical Psychology: Science and Practice. 2003;**10**(2):144-156. DOI: 10.1093/clipsy.bpg016

[43] Bishop SR, Lau M, Shapiro S, Carlson L, Anderson ND, Carmody J, Segal ZV, Abbey S, Speca M, Velting D, Devins G. Mindfulness: A proposed operational definition. Clinical Psychology: Science and Practice. 2004;**11**(3):230-241

[44] Zenner C, Herrnleben-Kurz S, Walach H. Mindfulness-based interventions in schools—A systematic review and meta-analysis. Frontiers in Psychology. 2014;**30**(5):603. DOI: 10.3389/fpsyg.2014.00603

[45] Shapiro SL, Brown KW, Astin JA. Toward the Integration of Meditation Into Higher Education: A Review of Research. The Center for Contemplative Mind in Society. 2008. Retrieved from: http://www.contemplativemind.org/admin/wp-content/uploads/2012/09/MedandHigherEd.pdf

[46] Davidson RJ, Dunne J, Eccles JS, Engle A, Greenberg M, Jennings P, Vago D, Mind and Life Education Research Network (MLERN). Contemplative practices and mental training: Prospects for American education. Child Development Perspectives. 2012;**6**(2):146-153

[47] Britton WB, Lepp NE, Niles HF, Rocha T, Fisher NE, Gold JS. A randomized controlled pilot trial of classroom-based mindfulness meditation compared to an active control condition in sixth-grade children. Journal of School Psychology. 2014;**52**(3):263-278

[48] Zoogman S, Goldberg SB, Hoyt WT, Miller L. Mindfulness interventions with youth: A meta-analysis. Mindfulness. 2015;**6**(2):290-302

[49] Kabat-Zinn J, Hanh TN. Full Catastrophe Living: Using the Wisdom of your Body and Mind to Face Stress, Pain, and Illness. Delta Trade Paperbacks, New York: Delta; 2009

[50] Atkinson MJ, Wade TD. Mindfulness-based prevention for eating disorders: A school-based cluster randomized controlled study. International Journal of Eating Disorders. 2015;**48**(7):1024-1037

[51] Parker AE, Kupersmidt JB, Mathis ET, Scull TM, Sims C. The impact of mindfulness education on elementary school students: Evaluation of the master mind program. Advances in School Mental Health Promotion. 2014;**7**(3):184-204

[52] Carsley D, Heath NL, Fajnerova S. Effectiveness of a classroom mindfulness coloring activity for test anxiety in children. Journal of Applied School Psychology. 2015;**31**(3):239-255

[53] Raes F, Griffith JW, Van der Gucht K, Williams JM. School-based prevention and reduction of depression in adolescents: A cluster-randomized controlled trial of a mindfulness group program. Mindfulness. 2014;**5**(5):477-486

[54] Segal ZV, Williams JM, Teasdale JD. Mindfulness-Based Cognitive Therapy for Depression. New York: Guilford Press; 2012

[55] Bluth K, Campo RA, Pruteanu-Malinici S, Reams A, Mullarkey M, Broderick PC. A school-based mindfulness pilot study for ethnically diverse at-risk adolescents. Mindfulness. 2016;**7**(1):90-104

[56] Costello E, Lawler M. An exploratory study of the effects of mindfulness on perceived levels of stress among school-children from lower socioeconomic backgrounds. The International Journal of Emotional Education. 2014;**6**(2):21

[57] Edwards M, Adams EM, Waldo M, Hadfield OD, Biegel GM. Effects of a mindfulness group on Latino adolescent students: Examining levels of perceived stress, mindfulness, self-compassion, and psychological symptoms. The Journal for Specialists in Group Work. 2014;**39**(2):145-163

[58] Kuyken W, Weare K, Ukoumunne OC, Vicary R, Motton N, Burnett R, Cullen C, Hennelly S, Huppert F. Effectiveness of the Mindfulness in Schools Programme: Non-randomised controlled feasibility study. The British Journal of Psychiatry. 2013;**203**(2):126-131

[59] Mendelson T, Greenberg MT, Dariotis JK, Gould LF, Rhoades BL, Leaf PJ. Feasibility and preliminary outcomes of a school-based mindfulness intervention for urban youth. Journal of Abnormal Child Psychology. 2010;**38**(7):985-994

[60] Sibinga EM, Perry-Parrish C, Chung SE, Johnson SB, Smith M, Ellen JM. School-based mindfulness instruction for urban male youth: A small randomized controlled trial. Preventive Medicine. 2013;**57**(6):799-801

[61] Lau NS, Hue MT. Preliminary outcomes of a mindfulness-based programme for Hong Kong adolescents in schools: Well-being, stress and depressive symptoms. International Journal of Children's Spirituality. 2011;**16**(4):315-330

[62] Viafora DP, Mathiesen SG, Unsworth SJ. Teaching mindfulness to middle school students and homeless youth in school classrooms. Journal of Child and Family Studies. 2015;**24**(5):1179-1191

[63] Liehr P, Diaz N. A pilot study examining the effect of mindfulness on depression and anxiety for minority children. Archives of Psychiatric Nursing. 2010;**24**(1):69-71

[64] Beauchemin J, Hutchins TL, Patterson F. Mindfulness meditation may lessen anxiety, promote social skills, and improve academic performance among adolescents with learning disabilities. Complementary Health Practice Review. 2008;**13**(1):34-45

[65] Carsley D, Khoury B, Heath NL. Effectiveness of mindfulness interventions for mental health in schools: A comprehensive meta-analysis. Mindfulness. 2017:1-5. DOI: 10.1007/s12671-017-0839-2

[66] Kusché CA, Greenberg MT. The PATHS Curriculum. Seattle: Developmental Research and Programs; 1994

[67] Mihic J, Novak M, Basic J, Nix RL. Promoting social and emotional competencies among young children in Croatia with preschool PATHS. The International Journal of Emotional Education. 2016;**8**(2):45

[68] Novak M, Mihić J, Bašić J, Nix RL. PATHS in Croatia: A school-based randomised-controlled trial of a social and emotional learning curriculum. International Journal of Psychology. 2017;**52**(2):87-95

[69] Bierman KL, Coie JD, Dodge KA, Greenberg MT, Lochman JE, McMahon RJ, Pinderhughes E. The effects of a multiyear universal social–emotional learning program: The role of student and school characteristics. Journal of Consulting and Clinical Psychology. 2010;**78**(2):156. DOI: 10.1037/a0018607

[70] Crean HF, Johnson DB. Promoting alternative thinking strategies (PATHS) and elementary school aged children's aggression: Results from a cluster randomized trial. American Journal of Community Psychology. 2013;**52**(1-2):56-72. DOI: 10.1007/s10464-013-9576-4

[71] Greenberg MT, Kusche CA, Cook ET, Quamma JP. Promoting emotional competence in school-aged children: The effects of the PATHS curriculum. Development and Psychopathology. 1995;**7**(1):117-136. DOI: 10.1017/S0954579400006374

3

A Qualitative Tool for Detecting and Approaching Psychological Trauma in Children Victims of the 2009 Italian Earthquake

Francesca Giordano

Abstract

Expressive therapies are considered effective intervention modalities with children who have experienced traumatic events such as natural disasters. Particularly, drawing consent to trauma affected children to convey the complexity of traumatic feelings by giving them a shape and a sense. But the efficacy of art therapies with children exposed to natural disasters, has not been research proved. This chapter present an exploratory and pilot study on the use of the specific technique "Test de trois dessins: avant, pendant et avenir" (Three Pictures Test: Past, Present, and Future), which may accomplish the double function of diagnostic instrument, for detecting the presence of psychological trauma, and therapeutic technique, for facilitating recovery from psychological distress, with children exposed to natural disasters. The graphic tool has been employed with children victims of the Italian earthquake which affected the region of Abruzzi, on the 6th April 2009. The case studies analysis illustrates the efficacy of the test in both detecting the presence and the extent of the psychological trauma, and in enhancing the trauma recovery process. Further researches need to be done in order to validate the use of the "Three Pictures Test: Past, Present, and Future" as a validated technique with children experiencing disasters.

Keywords: trauma, child, earthquake, drawing test, test de trois dessins

1. Introduction

The Centre for Research on Epidemiology of Disasters (CRED) [1] defines disaster as "a situation or event which overwhelms local capacity, necessitating a request to a national or international level for external assistance; an unforeseen and often sudden event that causes great damage, destruction and human suffering." Disasters can be caused by nature or by men's action. The transdisciplinary nature of disasters has given different perspectives to their study. In particular, engineers and physicians observe the structural proprieties, economists estimate the direct and indirect economic damages, sociologists investigate their impact on the social organization, doctors examine their consequences on the population health, and psychologists study the emotional, cognitive, and behavioral dynamics.

Through the psychological studies, a special attention has been given to the traumatic effects of disasters. Psychological trauma occurs as a response to a threatening event, such as natural disasters, in which the psyche surrenders to a situation of terror and of personal death perception [2]. In order to preserve a sense of safety, control, and gratification linked to the self, the parts of the self associated with the trauma are encapsulated and segregated out of the consciousness [2]. Emotions, feelings, and perceptions, which constitute the memory of the traumatic event, assume the form of a "corps étranger (…) qui menace le système dans son ensemble" [3], as they may suddenly break through the consciousness in the forms of nightmares, flashbacks, hallucinations, and unconscious trauma reenactments [4, 5]. The segregation of the traumatic memory out of the consciousness and its threatening nature block the process of symbolization, as cognition linking affects may lead to re-experiencing the trauma [2, 6]. Crocq [7] has defined the main effect of a psychological trauma as a "trou noir où un panne psychique par défaut de parole et de pensée."

Children exposed to disasters are considered a particularly vulnerable group for developing psychiatric disorders [8–11]. In particular, several studies have been reported in youth who have experienced natural disasters; negative outcomes, such as anxiety and depression [12, 13]; and posttraumatic stress disorder (PTSD) symptoms [14, 15], which include re-experiencing, avoidance, emotional numbing, and hyperarousal [16]. The reason is that the energy that is supposed to be used for accomplishing the developmental tasks is employed by the child for defending the self against recurring threatening thoughts [2, 17]. Therefore, it is important to develop appropriate and effective interventions aimed at helping children to recovery from trauma and preventing the development of posttraumatic pathologies.

1.1. The use of drawing technique following traumatic events

Following the rise of experimental psychology between the end of the nineteenth century and the beginning of the twentieth century, several psychologists and scholars in Europe and in North America started to explore the relationship between children's drawing and their own emotional, social and cognitive functioning, as a result of which children's drawings ended up to be used as a tool for projective testing. The first graphical tests were aimed to measure child's intelligence, assuming that the graphical acts develop in parallel with the cognitive development [18]. Gradually, authors started considering drawings as precious informants on the child's personality and his internal world [19].

House [20–22], family [23], and self [24–27] have been considered the main objects of analysis in projective drawing tests. They have been largely employed even in the specific kinetic drawing approaches, such as Burns and Kaufman's [28] research on the Kinetic Family Drawing, the Kinetic House-Tree-Person [29], the Kinetic School Drawings [30], House-Tree-Person-Test [31], and the Draw-a-Person-Test [32].

In scientific literature, drawing techniques appeared to be employed with children victims of traumatic experiences, in double functions: as therapeutic techniques that lead to overpass the defensive mechanisms and to promote the symbolization process and as diagnostic tools that provide traumatic contents with representations.

Projective tests are based on the idea of the presence of structural and symbolical elements that illustrate psychological sufferance [33]. Drawing gives a way to express needs, thoughts, and feelings that are hardly communicable because of their traumatic nature. Children victims of traumatic experiences often do not manage to express their internal feelings through verbal communication. Therefore, projective tests may represent a way to understand and diagnose childrens' internal world [34]. Drake et al. [35] affirm that through the information transmitted by the projective tool, it is possible to evaluate the anxiety not expressed and not elaborated, the child's coping style, and the presence of traumatic issue that influence on his/her self-image and on relations.

Concerning therapeutic value, several scholars affirm that art therapy is a successful technique for treating children who have experienced trauma [36–42]. In particular, expressive therapies:

- Provide a means of communication by which the child can express grief, loss, feelings, perceptions, thoughts, and memories linked to traumatic events and, as a result, succeed in bridging language barriers [6, 43, 44].
- Offer a "protected environment," within the external and internal chaos, where the child can take distance from the intense affect associated with the disaster, funnel his energy into the art by examining, exploring and giving meaning to threatening thoughts, and, consequently, interrupt the cycle of disruptive thinking, acting out, and symptoms [17];
- Present a way for children to become active participants in their own healing process and to see themselves as "survivors," rather than "victims" [6, 45]
- Bring to the surface, through the employing of drawings, issues relevant to treatment and accelerate, as a result, the capacity of helping professionals to intervene and assist traumatized children [26]. Furthermore, drawing is considered a useful tool in trauma debriefing as it provides sensory-based methods, which have been proved to be helpful in disclosure and crisis resolution [46–48].
- Stimulate the resilience process by promoting internal resources, such as creativity, self-reliance, and problem-solving, and external resources, such as the client-therapist relationship, which is one of the most important predictors of traumatized client outcomes [6, 43, 45, 49]

Even though art therapy is widely used as a treatment regimen for traumatized children, its efficacy has not been scientifically demonstrated. Researches that have been conducted on this theme turn out to have several limits [43]: lack of precision on the nature of the psychosocial symptoms and on the diagnosis of the sample who took part in the research; lack of methodological specificity of the type of art therapy employed; mostly limited on the qualitative outcome, which do not permit empirical inquiry. Notwithstanding these limitations, scholars [6, 43, 50] agree to encouraging further investigation that may establish and validate art therapy as an effective interventions modality in disaster situations.

The aim of this research is to present an exploratory and pilot study on the use of the specific technique "Three Pictures Test: Past, Present, and Future," which may accomplish the functions of *diagnostic instrument*, for detecting the presence of psychological trauma, and of *therapeutic technique*, for facilitating recovery from psychological distress, with children exposed to natural disasters.

2. Methods

The sample is composed of 14 children (seven boys and seven girls), aged between 8 and 12, who have experienced directly the earthquake, measuring 5.8 on the Richter scale, which took place on 6 April 2009, in the Italian Region of Abruzzi, and killed 300 civilians. All of them have been living most of their life in the affected area. Six of them were born in Macedonia, one comes from Morocco, and the other seven are Italians. Since the day after the earthquake, all of them had to leave their houses, which have been partly or completely destroyed by the seism, and they have been hosted in the two refugee camps "Monticchio1" and "Paganica5" set up by the Italian Civil Protection in the two provinces of L'Aquila: Monticchio and Paganica. None of the children suffered any family losses or serious injury after the earthquake.

Since the beginning of May 2009, the children have been attending the psycho-social intervention, conducted by a team of psychologists and educators from the Resilience Research Unit of the Catholic University of Milan. The objective of the intervention was to provide them with a temporary protection and structured setting, in contrast with the chaos and the fragility of the external environments, where resilience processes may be enhanced and stimulated by several actions, based on the use of creative-expressive languages. Consequently, creative expressive languages became familiar to children.

The test was administered on August 2009, after two months of psycho-social activities by the psychologists who have conducted most of the activities since the beginning of the project. There by, the interviewers have already built a trusting relation with each child. Furthermore, the test has been administered individually in the tent where all the other psychosocial activities took place.

The tool that has been used is a drawing test named "test de trois dessins: avant, pendant et avenir" (Three Pictures Test: Past, Present, and Future). It has been developed by the psychiatry Crocq [51], following the interventions conducted with child victims of war and natural catastrophes. The test is composed by three tasks:

1. Draw your house, your family, and yourself before the earthquake.
2. Draw your house, your family, and yourself during the earthquake.
3. Draw your house, your family, and yourself how you would like them to be in the future.

The first drawing illustrates the representation of the child's life before the earthquake. The second drawing is aimed at tackling the block in the expression of traumatic thoughts and emotions by promoting the sense-making process of the experience lived. The third drawing invites the child to detach from the traumatic event and to project himself/herself in a desired future.

Each drawing is followed by an interview, where the interviewer encourages the child to talk about what he/she has drawn. The data analysis is based on a nonstatistical qualitative observation and takes into consideration both the graphical and the verbal levels. The test has not been standardized by the author.

This research is a study pilot, aimed at validating the two hypothesis speculated by Crocq [52], on the possible functions of the Three Pictures Test: Past, Present, and Future.

The first one considers it as a *diagnostic technique* for detecting the presence and the impact of the psychological trauma. Particularly, the administration of the test may permit to examine whether the traumatic event has distorted the mental representations of the three significant objects, house, family, and self, in the three temporal phases, before and during the traumatic event, and in the future, when it will be over.

The second hypothesis affirms that the tool may be employed as a *therapeutic technique*, with traumatized children. Drawing and talking about thoughts, perceptions, feelings, and emotions directly or indirectly linked to the traumatic event, with the guide and the support of the interviewer, may contrast the expressive block, caused by the absence of symbolic representations referred to the event, and, at the same time, it may facilitate the sense-making process.

3. Results and discussion

In order to answer the first hypothesis on the tool efficacy in detecting the presence and the level of psychological trauma, we tried to identify any traumatic mark in each one of the three tasks. No case study has been diagnosed with PTSD, as the test has been administered only few (two to three) months after the earthquake. But some children exhibited symptoms linked to the posttraumatic stress disorder (PTSD) or comorbidity, as described in the following case study presentations.

3.1. Draw your family, your house, and yourself before the earthquake

Case study No.1: Francesco is a 9-year-old boy. He has been hosted in the camp since the day after the earthquake, with his family: mother, father, and elder sister. His academic performance used to be good, but since the earthquake, he has shown difficulties in listening, concentrating, and a low motivation in accomplishing any task. He often exhibits hyperactive behaviors, attitudes of defiance, and difficulties in respecting rules.

In **Figure 1**, Francesco draws as house details, the door and the window, which are very much related to the traumatic event: both of them are the ways out that lead to run away from a house during the earthquake. After having drawn the door, he affirms that it was made by iron, and that during the earthquake it was blocked, therefore, they did not manage to open it. The door occupies a lot of space in the drawing; it is seen from the front and has iron bars, which manages to transmit the idea of closure and imprisonment.

Case study No. 2: Alessio is a 12-year-old boy. He often shows a hyperactive and exuberant behavior. But at the same time, he takes part in the activities proposed by educators and collaborates well in team works. He is very much engaged in the tasks that stimulate his fantasy and creativity such as artistic workshops. His family consists of father, mother, and little four-year-old brother. He lives with his mother, brother, and paternal grandmother since the day of the earthquake (6 April 2009).

In Alessio's drawing (**Figure 2**), the house becomes the only protagonist of the past before the earthquake. The empty space at the right side of the house was probably supposed to be used by the family members, but in the end, he did not draw them. The boy decided to reformulate the task in "My house before the earthquake" and wrote it on the top of the sheet.

Case study No. 3: Giada is an ethnic Macedonian 9-year-old girl. She lived through a very hard experience during the earthquake night: she was exposed to death as her room floor fell on the ground floor and she has been staying under rubbles for few hours before fireman came to save her. Since then, her finger has been permanently injured as she could not bend it anymore. Giada shows several difficulties in elaborating the traumatic memories, especially

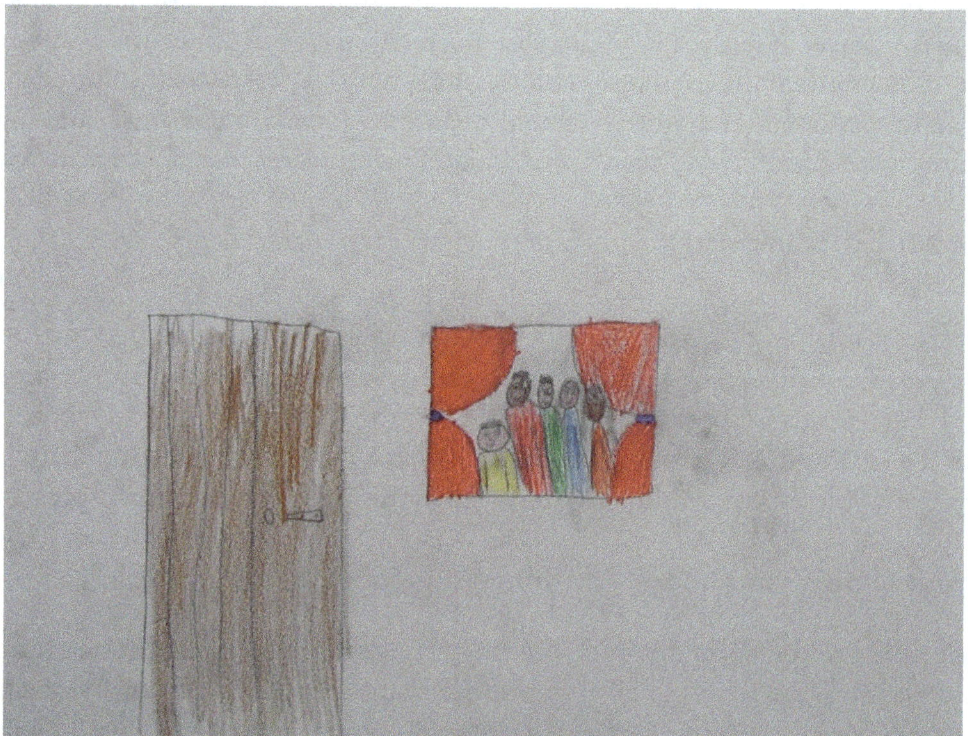

Figure 1. Draw your house, your family, and yourself before the earthquake—Francesco, 9 year old.

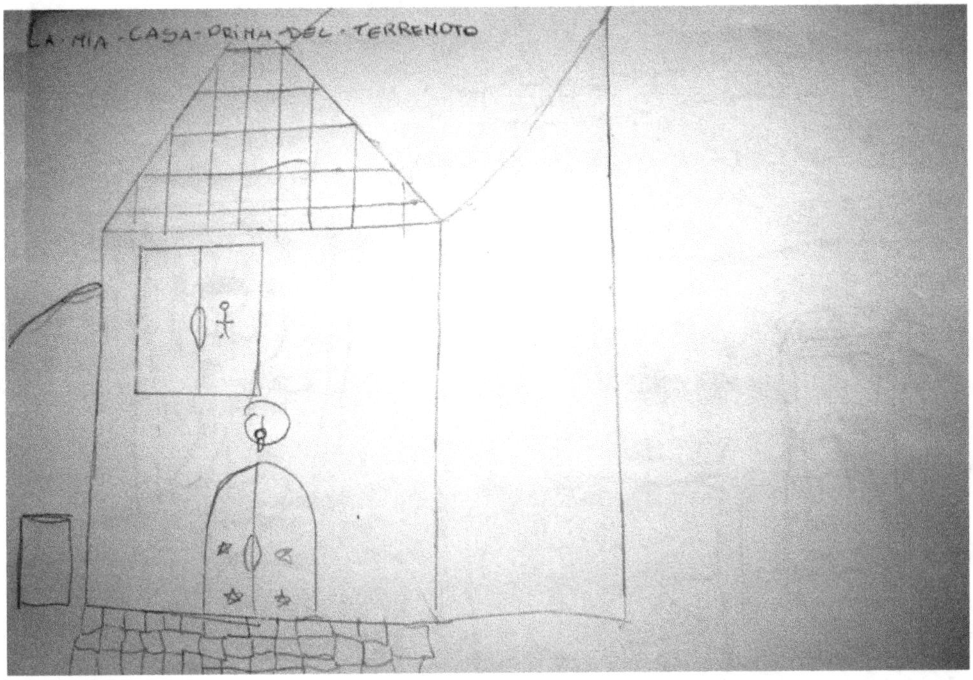

Figure 2. Draw your house, your family, and yourself before the earthquake—Alessio, 12 year old.

in accepting the loss of her house. She has struggled during several workshops that she has been doing in the camp. In particular, during the house thematic workshops, Giada could not draw a house spontaneously, but she copied the castle image represented on the colors pencils box. When educators asked her the reason why she decided to draw the castle, she said that its her dream house, where she would like to live forever.

Furthermore, she showed difficulties in joining sport activities, in particular volleyball: when the ball goes toward her instead of playing, she immediately tries to protect herself from it. It seems that the image of the ball coming toward her is a kind of traumatic reviviscence related to rubbles which fell on her, during the earthquake.

For Giada (9 year old) (**Figure 3**), the past memory is inaccessible: the house is installed in an empty space, without any context detail that could situate it in a temporal and spatial setting. The window and the door are closed and the handles are very prominent, it reinforces the idea of lack of access. The sidewalk around the house is sharply interrupted by the outline of the house: it is not supposed to lead anywhere.

3.2. Draw your family, your house, and yourself during the earthquake

In the second task, Giada (**Figure 4**) expressed the confrontation with the reality of death. The child kept on repeating that if she had fallen asleep in front of the television, like she used to, now she would be dead. During the earthquake, her room floor fell onto the ground floor, where the sitting room and the television were located. The child spent several hours under the rubbles, until firemen managed to get her out. The only object that she managed to draw while she was speaking was the television, but then she tried to erase it as if it was too complicated to access the memory.

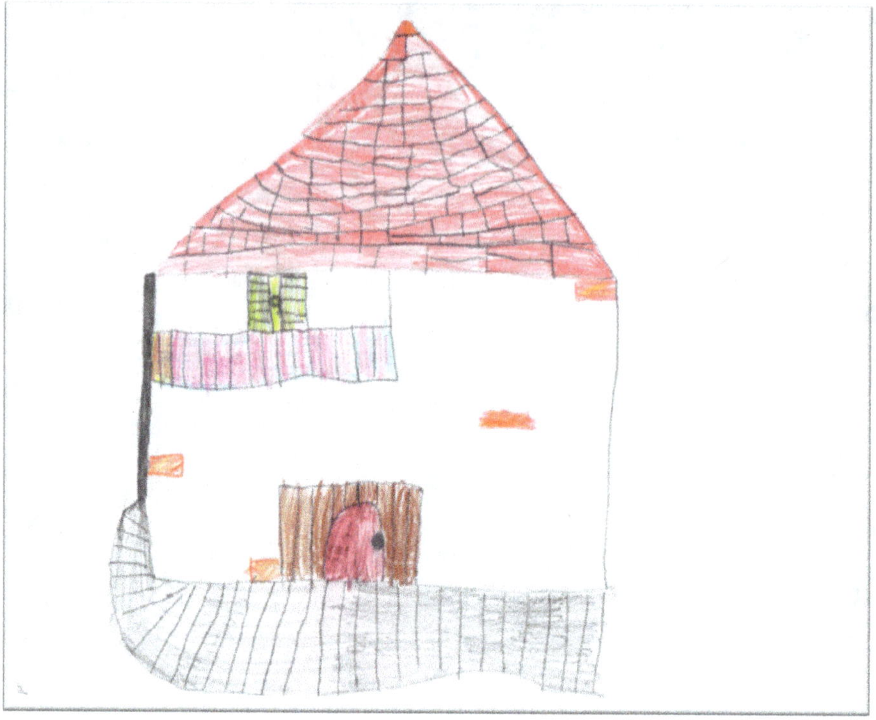

Figure 3. Draw your house, your family, and yourself before the earthquake—Francesco, 9 year old.

Case study No. 4: Rebecca is a cheerful, bright 9-year-old girl. She enjoys taking part in educational activities and collaborating with other kids. She behaves in an appropriate way in different situations. Her family, composed of her parents, a 10-year-old sister, and a 5-year-old brother, is Muslim Macedonian, but she was born in Italy. Her father risked dying because of a work accident, happened after the earthquake. But fortunately during the test administration, he was no more at risk of death. She did not exhibit specific psychological difficulties following the earthquake. She used to spend most of the time playing with her sisters and with the other kids from the camp.

Rebecca made three drawings for the second task. In the first two (**Figures 5** and **6**), she drew her parents' bedroom and the bedroom she shares with her sister. The black color occupies the whole paper and seems to invade both bedrooms, and all objects look as if they are floating in the terrifying blackness.

Figure 4. Draw your house, your family, and yourself during the earthquake—Giada, 9 year old.

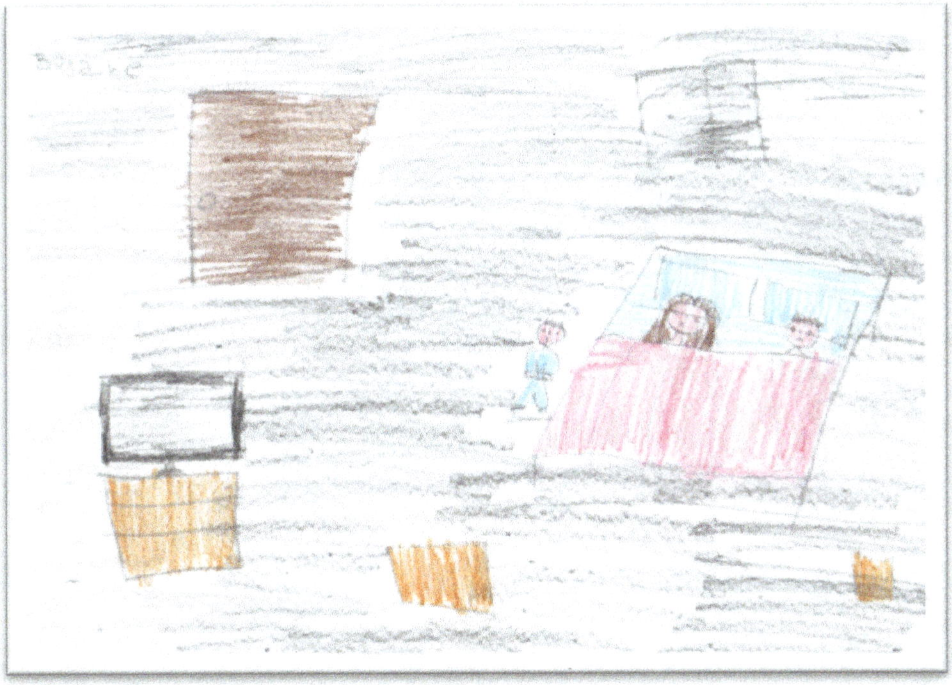

Figure 5. Draw your house, your family, and yourself during the earthquake—Rebecca, 10 year old, first drawing.

In the third drawing (**Figure 7**), the floor line divides it in two parts: the upper part still invaded by the terrifying blackness and the lower part which is left completely white. She could not find any way to represent what was happening in the earth. The lack of symbolic representations of the traumatic event of the earthquake leads Rebecca to leave the half of the draw uncolored.

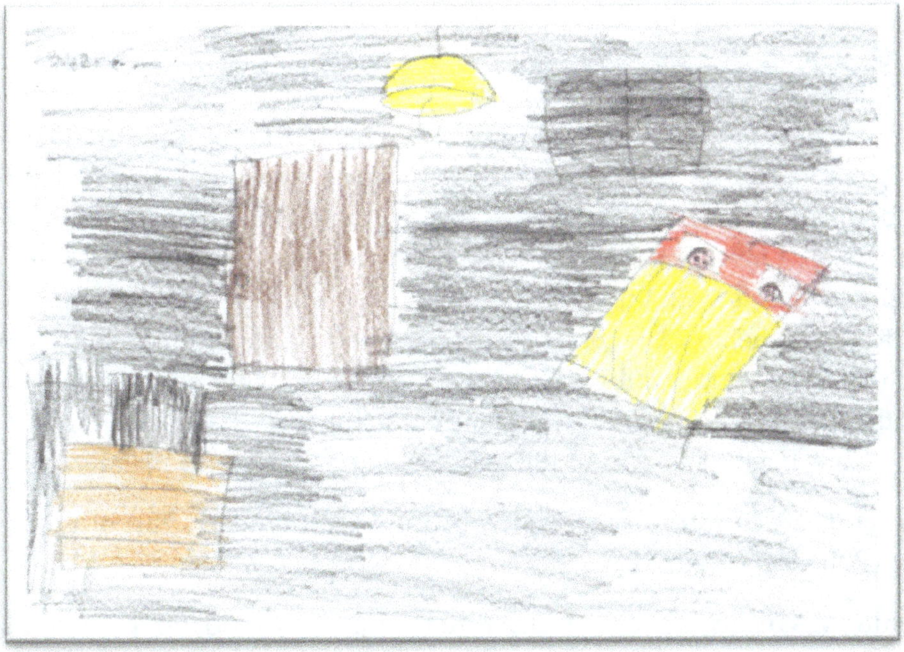

Figure 6. Draw your house, your family, and yourself during the earthquake—Rebecca, 10 year old, second drawing.

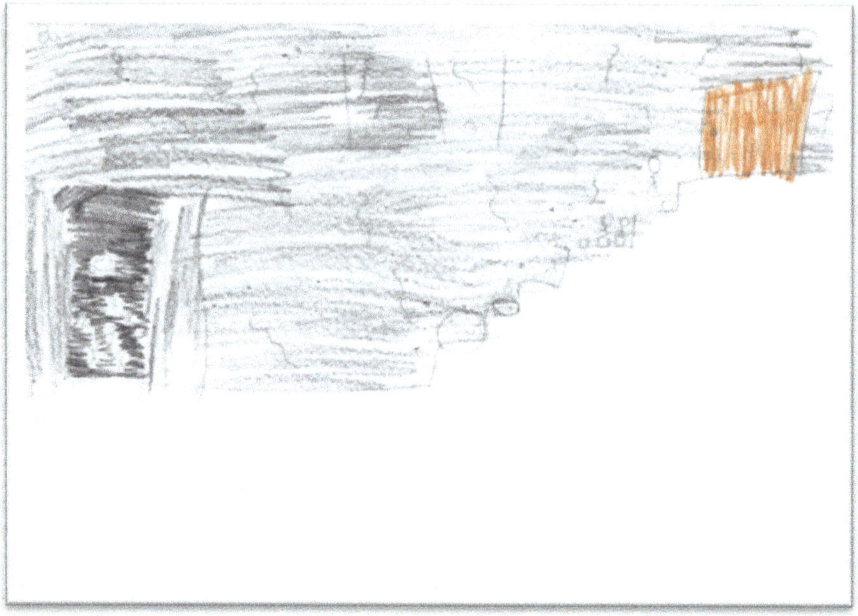

Figure 7. Draw your house, your family, and yourself during the earthquake—Rebecca, 10 year old, third drawing.

3.3. Draw your family, your house, and yourself, how you would like them to be in future

Two of the sample children did not manage to accomplish the third task. The lack of the third drawing can be due to the fixation on the traumatic moment, which does not let the children detach from it and figure out a positive future.

In other cases, the need for security prevailed and seemed to be the unavoidable/essential base for building up a future. Several children have figured out different solutions for a safe future. In particular:

1. A five-floor house drawn by Giacomo (**Figure 8**).

Case study No. 5: Giacomo is a 9-year-old boy. He lives in the camp with his mother, his two aunts, and his grandmother. He exhibits an aggressive attitude, with low frustration tolerance and frequent bouts of anger that lead him assuming rough and sometimes violent behaviors against the others. His mother says that those behaviors have increased following the earthquake. The frequent fights with the other children lead him to get away from the educational activities and to cry alone, in a corner. If someone tries to comfort him, Giacomo says that he would have rather died under rubbles. During the earthquake, he got trapped in his bunk bed; his parents took his brother, who was sleeping in the upper bed, and ran out of the house, without him. He has been taken out of the rubbles by his uncle and firemen, few hours later.

2. A house in another country, far away from the earthquake threat, but still without any inhabitants (Rebecca) (**Figure 9**)
3. A magic solution as reality is still too much threatening and cannot offer any safe solution. Luca (8 years old) (**Figure 10**) left the drawing pencil, took the gray-colored pencil and started drawing all objects « made of iron » : the house with nails strengthening the wall, himself, and his mother. At the end of the task he added: "She wont like the dress, but at least we will all be safe."

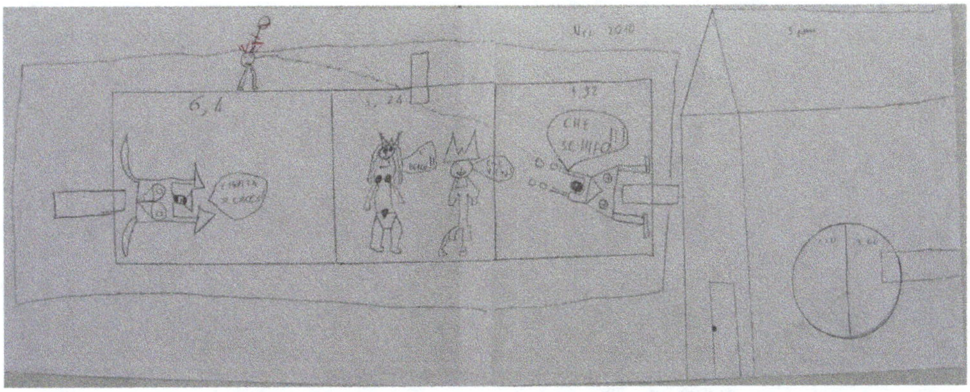

Figure 8. Draw your house, your family, and yourself how you would like them to be in the future—Giacomo, 9 year old.

Case study No. 6: Luca is a 8-year-old boy. His father was alcohol addicted and died one year before the earthquake due to a serious illness linked to his addiction. He lives with his mother, his grandmother, and his uncle. Luca was really attached to his father and he suffered a lot because of his death. He still shows several difficulties in facing this sufferance: if a child teases him mentioning his father, he exhibits bursts of uncontrollable rage and can become very violent. He manages to calm down only with the help of the educator. Since the earthquake he moved to the camp with his grandmother and his uncle, as his mother did not accept to live in the tent because of the multiethnic population that live in the camp. She keeps on living in her house, despite the danger. Luca is very attached to his mother. Since the earthquake anxious attitudes have increased: if his mother or his grandmother do not answer the mobile, he gets worried very quickly and does not manage to go on with the activity. But in general, he enjoys taking part in the educational workshops, where he shows independency in the individual task and collaborating skills in team works.

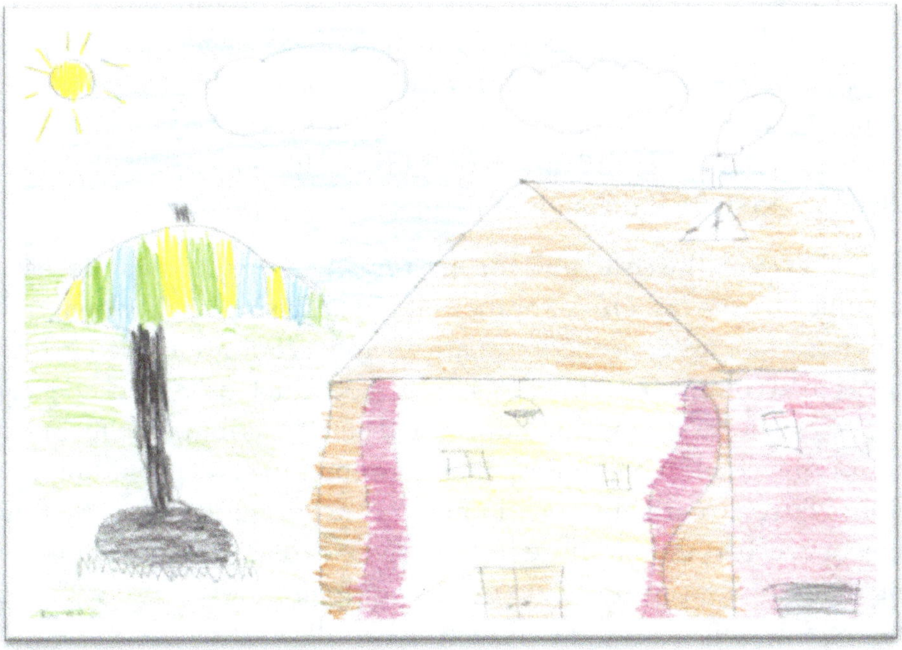

Figure 9. Draw your house, your family, and yourself how you would like them to be in the future—Rebecca, 10 year old.

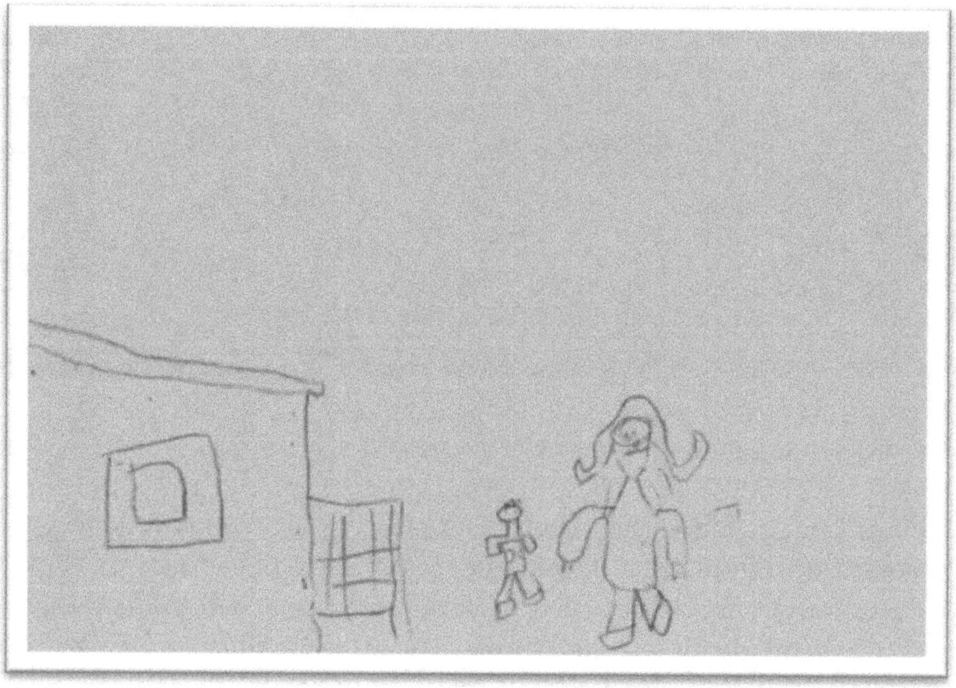

Figure 10. Draw your house, your family, and yourself how you would like them to be in the future—Luca, 8 year old.

Concerning the second hypothesis, on the "Three Pictures Test: Past, Present, and Future" capacity of promoting meaning attribution process to the traumatic event, two main functions assumed by the test have been identified:

1. **Mediating role between child's conscious and unconscious mind**: drawing has assumed the role of prelanguage, as it allowed the child to access the traumatic memory and to share it with the interviewer. The graphical language difficulty in following the rhythm of narration, which appeared to be very rich and full of details, has generated in some children a sort of frustration that annoyed them and provided them with several self-critics on their own tasks. Therefore, we can affirm that the test has allowed the child to get in contact and explore the raw traumatic memory and to provide it with both a verbal and graphical form that permitted him to share it through drawings and narration.
2. **Mediating role between the child and the interviewer**: In particular, the test has let the interviewer assume the role of a guide for the child in accessing his/her own traumatic memory and in giving a first order to the traumatic memory. Some children exhibited defenses and resistances in accomplishing the tasks, which obstructed or blocked expressive channels. In those cases, the task reformulation, aimed at re-inscribing the memory in a defined moment, helped the child to break it up and therefore, to start providing it with a sort of order and form. Furthermore, the containing and encouraging role of the interviewer has been fundamental, especially for those children who experienced loneliness and abandonment during the traumatic event due to the lack of their parents' protecting role. Building up a trusting relationship with the interviewer has allowed them to face the loss of trust on the protecting solidity of external world and on the illusion of the other's capability to

provide him with the sense of safety [53]. The inter-relation with the interviewer led him to co-create a new image of himself and of the external world. In the second task, several children demanded for more papers, in order to represent the complexity of the memories that little by little came to their mind, in a crescendo of emotionality. The protecting frame offered by the interviewer has allowed to embrace and answer to this need.

Finally, the test structure, divided into the "before," "during," and "after" the earthquake, has allowed a gradual access to the memories of the event and has stimulated the integration process of the traumatic experience in the childrens' life story.

4. Conclusion

This pilot study has succeeded in investigating the two functions of diagnostic tool and therapeutic technique of the "Three Pictures Test: Past, Present, and Future", through a non-statistical qualitative observation, which has taken into consideration a small group of participants. The results that have been brought out through the case study analyses encourage further researches, which may validate scientifically the efficacy of this technique through the employment of both qualitative and quantitative methodology. The use of standardize questionnaires would allow to collect statistical findings, which may be generalized and adopted in different contexts. Particularly, the scientific validation of the tool may provide art therapists with standard criteria that can be employed for detecting the presence of psychological trauma in both the graphical and the verbal data, and with instructions on the most appropriate and effective practices that should be adopted for promoting the uncovering of traumatic memories and for fostering reintegration of the traumatic event in the childrens' life story.

Author details

Francesca Giordano

Address all correspondence to: francesca.giordano@unicatt.it

Department of Psychology, Resilience Research Unit, Università Cattolica del Sacro Cuore, Milan, Italy

References

[1] EM-DAT. The OFDA/CRED International Disaster Database [Internet]. Available from http://www.emdat.be/. [Accessed 2016-10-23]

[2] Johnson D.R. The role of the creative arts therapies in the diagnosis and treatment of psychological trauma. The Arts in Psychotherapy. 1987; 14: 7–13. Doi: 10.1016/0197-4556(87)90030-X

[3] Braunstein N. La jouissance. Un concept Lacanien (The jouissance. A Lacanien concept). Paris: Ed. Point Hors Ligne; 1992. 18 p.

[4] Horowitz M. Stress Reponses Syndromes. New York: Jason Aronson; 1993. Doi: 10.1007/978-1-4615-2820-3_4

[5] Van der Kolk B. Psychological Trauma. Washington DC: American Psychiatric Press; 1987.

[6] Orr P. Art therapy with children after a disaster: a content analysis. The Arts in Psychotherapy. 2007; 34,4: 350–361. Doi: 10.1016/j.aip.2007.07.002

[7] Crocq L. Le traumatisme psychique chez l'enfant (The psychological trauma in children). *Actes des journées d'études et de réflexion de l'Unité de Formation et de Recherche de la Fondation pour l'Enfance: Des lieux de soins et de réparations pour les enfants victimes d'agressions sexuelles* (Acts of the seminar of the "Unité de Formation et de Recherche de la Fondation pour l'enfance": Context of caring and reparation for victims of sexual abuse); Paris, 1997. p. 10.

[8] Papageorgiou V., Frangou-Garunovic A., Iordanidou R., Yule, W., Smith P., Vostanis P. War trauma and psychopathology in Bosnian refugee children. European Child and Adolescent Psychiatry. 2000; 9: 84–90. Doi: 10.1007/s007870050002

[9] Pfefferbaum B., Nixon S.J., Krug R.S., Tivis R.D., Moore V.L. & Brown I.M. Clinical needs assessment of middle and high school students following the 1995 Oklahoma City bombing. American Journal of Psychiatry. 1999; 156: 1069–1074.

[10] Rome E.M., Lewis J., Castillo-Matos H., Martinez O., Busquets R., Martinez I. Posttraumatic stress disorder among Cuban children and adolescents after release from a refugee camp. Psychiatric Services. 2002; 53: 970–976. Doi: 10.1176/appi.ps.53 .8.970

[11] Vizek-Vidovic V., Kuterovac-Jagodic G., Arambasic L. Posttraumatic symptomatology in children exposed to war. Scandinavian Journal of Psychology. 2000; 41: 297–306. Doi: 10.1111/1467-9450.00202

[12] Groome D., Soureti A. Post-traumatic stress disorder and anxiety symptoms in children exposed to the 1999 Greek earthquake. British Journal of Psychology. 2004; 95: 387–397. Doi: 10.1348/0007126041528149

[13] McDermott B.M., Palmer L.J. Postdisaster emotional distress, depression, and event-related variables: Findings across child and adolescent developmental stage. Australian and New Zealand Journal of Psychiatry. 2002; 36: 754–761.

[14] Garrison C.Z., Bryant E.S., Addy C.L., Spurrier P.G., Freedy J.R., Kilpatrick D.G. Posttraumatic stress disorder in adolescents after Hurricane Andrew. Journal of the American Academy of Child and Adolescent Psychiatry. 1995; 34: 1193–1201. Doi: 10.1097/00004583-199509000-00017

[15] Shaw J.A., Applegate B., Tanner S., Perez D., Rothe E., Campo-Bowen A.E., et al. Psychological effects of Hurricane Andrew on an elementary school population. Journal of the Academy of Child and Adolescent Psychiatry. 1995; 34: 1185–1192. Doi: 10.1097/00004583-199509000-00016

[16] American Psychiatric Association. Diagnostic and Statistical Manual of Mental Disorders, 4th ed. Washington DC: Text Revision; 2000.

[17] Howard R. Art therapy as an isomorphic intervention in the treatment of a client with post-traumatic stress disorder. American Journal of Art Therapy. 1990; 28: 79–86.

[18] Prudhommeau M. Le dessin de l'enfant. Paris: P.U.F.; 1947.

[19] Liebert P. Aider l'enfant à dire par le dessin: les apports diagnostics du dessin chez l'enfant victime d'agression sexuelle. Publications de l'Université de Rouen; 1998.

[20] Minkowska F. De Van Gogh et Seurat aux dessins d'enfants : à la recherche du monde des formes (Rorschach) (From Van Gogh and Seraut to children drawings: searching for a world of shapes (Rorschach). Beresniak, Paris - Guide catalogue illustré et commenté par F. Minkowska, préface par Raymond Bayer - Exposition au Musée Pédagogique du 20 avril au 14 mai 1949 (Catalogue guide illustrated and commented by F. Minkiwska, preface by Raymond Bayer – Exposed in Musée Pédagogique from 20th of April, untill 14th may 1949.

[21] Royer J. Le dessin d'une maison: Image de l'adaptation sociale de l'enfant (The house drawing: an image of the child social adaptation). Issy-Les-Moulineaux : E.A.P.; 1989.

[22] Kim-Chi, N. La Personnalité et l'épreuve de dessins multiples :maison, arbre, deux personnes, d'après le test house, tree, person. (Personality and multiple drawings test: house, tree, person, according to the test house, tree, person). Paris : Presses Universitaires De France; 1989.

[23] Corman L. Le test du dessin de famille dans la pratique médico-pédagogique (Family drawing test in the medical-pedagogical practice). Paris : P.U.F.; 1964.

[24] Machover K. ì Personality projection in the drawing of the human figure. Springfield: Charles C. Thomas; 1978.

[25] Abraham A. Le dessin d'une personne : Le Test de Machover (Person drawing: the Machover test). Paris : Delachaux&Niestlé ; 1963.

[26] Royer J. Dessin du bonhomme, la personnalité de l'enfant dans tous ses états (Human figure drawing, the child personality as it is). Bruxelles: Editest ; 1977.

[27] Koppitz E. Psychological evaluation of children's human figure drawings. New York: Grune & Stratton; 1968.

[28] Burns R.C. & Kaufman S.H. Action, Styles and Symbols in Kinetic Family Drawings (K-F-D). An interpretation Manual. New York: Brunner/Mazel; 1972.

[29] Burns R.C. Kinetic-House-Tree-Person Drawings (K-H-T-P). Paris: Taylor & Francis; 1987.

[30] Knoff M. & Prout T. The Kinetic Drawing System for Family and School. Log Angeles: Western Psychological Services; 1985.

[31] Buck J.N. The H-T-P test. Journal of Clinical Psychology. 1948; 4: 151–159.

[32] Naglieri J.A. McNeish T.J. & Bardos A.N. Draw a Person: Screening Procedure for Emotional Disturbance. Austin, TX: Pro-Ed; 1991.

[33] Malchiodi C. Handbook of Art Therapy, 2nd edition. New-York: The Guilford Press; 1998.

[34] Nader K. Understanding and Assessing Trauma in Children and Adolescents: Measures, Methods and Youth Context. New York: Routledge; 2007.

[35] Drake E.B, Bush S., Van Corp W. Evaluation and Assessment of PTSD in Children and Adolescents, Washington D.C: American Psychiatric Association; 2001.

[36] Avidar A. Art therapy and pervasive trauma: Working with children in violent communities. Pratt Institute Creative Arts Therapy Review. 1995; 16: 10–16.

[37] Clements K. The use of art therapy with abused children. Clinical Child Psychology and Psychiatry. 1996; 1: 181–198. Doi: 10.1177/1359104596012002

[38] Davis C. The use of art therapy and group process with grieving children. Issues in Comprehensive Pediatric Nursing. 1989; 12: 269–280. Doi: 10.3109/01460868909026834

[39] Kozlowska K., Hanney L. An art therapy group for children traumatized by parental violence and separation. Clinical Child Psychology and Psychiatry. 2001; 6: 49–78. Doi: 10.1177/1359104501006001006

[40] Pifalo T. Pulling out the thorns: Art therapy with sexually abused children and adolescents. Art Therapy. 2002; 19: 12–22. Doi: 10.1080/07421656.2002.10129724

[41] Prager A. Pediatric art therapy: Strategies and applications. Art Therapy. 1995; 12: 32–38. Doi: 10.1080/07421656.1995.10759121

[42] St. Thomas B., Johnson P. In their own voices: Play activities and art with traumatized children. Groupwork. 2002; 13: 34–48.

[43] Eaton L.G., Doherty K.L., Widrick R.M. A review of research and methods used to establish art therapy as an effective treatment method for traumatized children. The Art in Psychotherapy. 2007; 34: 256–262. Doi: 10.1016/j.aip.2007.03.001

[44] EM-DAT. American Art Therapy Association. Using art in trauma recovery with children. 2003.[Internet]. Available from http://assets1.mytrainsite.com/500051/arttx_traumacm.pdf. [Accessed 2016-10-23]

[45] Malchiodi C.A. Using drawing as intervention with traumatized children. TLC's Journal, TRAUMA AND LOSS: Research and Interventions. 2001; 1, 1.

[46] Malchiodi C.A. Breaking the silence: Art therapy with children from violent homes. Rev. ed. New York: Brunner/Mazel; 1997.

[47] Pynoos R., Eth S. Developmental perspective on psychic trauma in childhood. In Figley C.R. editor. Trauma and its Wake. New York: Brunner/Mazel; 1985. pp. 193–216.

[48] Steele W. Using drawing in short-term trauma resolution. In Malchiodi C.A. editor. The Clinical Handbook of Art Therapy. New York: The Guilford Press; 2001.

[49] Asay T.P., Lambert M.J. The empirical case for the common factors in therapy: Quantitative findings. In Hubble M.A., Duncan B.L. editors. The heart and soul of change: What works in therapy. Washington, DC: American Psychological Association; 1999. pp. 23–55. Doi: 10.1037/11132-001

[50] Reynolds M., Brewin C.R. Intrusive cognitions, coping strategies and emotional responses in depression, post-traumatic stress disorder, and a non-clinical population. Behaviour Research and Therapy. 1998; 36: 135–147. Doi: 10.1016/S0005-7967(98)00013-8.

[51] Crocq L. Les traumatismes psychiques de guerre. 1er vol. Paris: Odile Jacob; 1999.

[52] Crocq L., Hariki S., Gandelet J.P., Lançon J.M., Passamr M. Se reconstruire après le séisme: le test des trois dessins "avant," "pendant" et "avenir". Journal des Professionnels de l'Enfance. 2005; 5: 17–23.

[53] Janoff-Bulman R. Shattered Assumptions: Towards a New Psychology of Trauma. New York: The Free Press; 1992.

4

Use of Antidepressants in Children and Adolescents

Isabel Hernández-Otero,
Carlos Gómez Sánchez-Lafuente and
Cecilia Hernández González

Abstract

Depression is a serious disorder that can cause significant problems in mood, thinking, and behavior at home, in school, and with peers. It is estimated that major depressive disorder (MDD) affects about 5% of adolescents. Research has shown that, as in adults, depression in children and adolescents is treatable. Certain antidepressant medications, called selective serotonin reuptake inhibitors (SSRIs), can be beneficial to children and adolescents with MDD. Certain types of psychological therapies also have been shown to be effective. However, our knowledge of antidepressant treatments in youth, though growing substantially, is limited compared to what we know about treating depression in adults. The U.S. Food and Drug Administration (FDA) issued a public warning in October 2004 about an increased risk of suicidal thoughts or behavior (suicidality) in children and adolescents treated with SSRI antidepressant medications. However, SSRI medications are considered to have an improvement over older antidepressant medications and they have been shown to be safe and effective for adults. In this chapter we provide an updated and well-documented review of the current scientific evidence on this topic.

Keywords: antidepressants, children, adolescents

1. Overview

Major depressive disorder (MDD) is one of the most common mental disorders in children and adolescents [1, 2]. Although the estimated prevalence is 5–6% in adolescents aged 13–18 years and 5–6% in children aged 6–12 years, there are fewer studies to understand how antidepressants work in this age group [1]. Children and adolescents present with undifferentiated depressive symptoms, like irritability, school refusal, and aggressive behavior [3], which is possible the main reason why major depressive disorder is still under diagnosed and untreated comparing to adults. Depression often impaired social functioning and it may cause suicidal ideation and attempts as a symptom of low mood [4]. Use of antidepressants is wide, in spite of the recommendations of psychotherapy as first-line treatment in most clinical trials [5]. In 2004, the US Food and Drug Administration (FDA) practitioners set a black-box warning relating the use of antidepressants in children and adolescents to an increased risk of suicide [7]. Since then, the use of antidepressants in this group of age remains controversial [3].

The European Medicines Agency has completed its review of two classes of antidepressants and concluded that they should not be used in children and adolescents except in their approved indications [4, 6]. The review of serotonin-selective reuptake inhibitor (SSRI) and serotonin-norepinephrine reuptake inhibitor (SNRI) medicines looked at the potential risk of suicidal behavior in children and adolescents treated with these products [13].

The Agency's scientific committee, the Committee for Medicinal Products for Human Use (CHMP), concluded at its April 19–22, 2005 meeting that suicide-related behavior (suicide attempt and suicidal thoughts) and hostility (predominantly aggression, oppositional behavior, and anger) were more frequently observed in clinical trials among children and adolescents treated with these antidepressants compared to those treated with placebo [13].

The Agency's committee is therefore recommending the inclusion of strong warnings across the whole of the European Union to doctors and parents about these risks. Doctors and parents will also be advised that these products should not be used in children and adolescents except in their approved indications [13].

Most of these products are approved for the treatment of depression and anxiety in adults in the European Union, but are not licensed Europe-wide for the treatment of these conditions in children or adolescents. Some of these products are however licensed for pediatric use for the treatment of obsessive-compulsive disorder and one of them for the treatment of attention deficit/hyperactivity disorder [13].

The efficacy of antidepressants is well documented among adults with major depressive disorder, however, in children and adolescents there are fewer studies and they tend to have worse methodology and more risk of bias [8, 9]. Randomized controlled trials (RCT) have shown that antidepressants agents have positive risk-benefit ratio in children and adolescents, but their clinical use should balance the potential risk and the clinical need. Young people should be closely monitored for suicidal ideation and behaviors, especially when starting an antidepressant and at dosage adjustments [7].

A recent network meta-analysis has proved antidepressants to be well-tolerated in major depressive disorder in children and adolescents [9], although they do not seem to offer a clear advantage against psychotherapeutic interventions. These trials include use of amitriptyline, citalopram, clomipramine, desipramine, duloxetine, escitalopram, fluoxetine, imipramine, mirtazapine, nefazodone, nortriptyline, paroxetine, sertraline, and venlafaxine [8]. Only fluoxetine showed statistically significant differences with placebo. In terms of tolerability, fluoxetine was better than duloxetine and imipramine. According to these results, fluoxetine should be considered the best option when considering medication to treat moderate-to-severe depression in children and adolescents, when they do not have access to psychotherapy or have not responded to nonpharmacological interventions. Evidence suggests a significantly increased risk for suicidality (suicidal behavior or ideation) in young people given venlafaxine for the treatment of major depressive disorder [10].

2. Selective serotonin reuptake inhibitors (SSRIs)

2.1. Fluoxetine

2.1.1. Pharmacodynamics

- Action mechanism: fluoxetine increases the release of serotonin (5-HT) and inhibits reuptake pump. Possibly increases serotonergic neurotransmission.
- A receptor affinity: receptors desensitize 5-HT, especially 5-HT1A autoreceptors. It also has antagonist properties on 5-HT2C (serotonin) receptors, which could increase the release of norepinephrine and dopamine.

2.1.2. Pharmacokinetics

Fluoxetine is absorbed in gastrointestinal tract and metabolized by the liver. The active metabolite, norfluoxetine, has a half-life of 2 weeks. The original drug has a half-life of 2–3 days. Inhibits cytochrome P450 2D6 (CYP2D6) and cytochrome P450 3A (CYP3A).

2.1.3. Drug and food interactions

- Fluoxetine can increase tricyclic antidepressants concentrations.
- It can cause a fatal serotonin syndrome when combined with monoamine oxidase inhibitors (MAOIs), so it should be used only after 14 days of treatment with this group of drugs.
- It can displace other drugs with high protein binding (warfarin).
- It can cause weakness, hyperreflexia, and incoordination when combined with sumatriptan and other triptans.
- It can cause bleeding, especially when combined with other blood thinners.
- It may interfere with the analgesic actions of codeine (by inhibiting CYP2D6). By the same route could increase the concentration of atomoxetine and some beta-blockers. It could increase concentrations of thioridazine and cause heart arrhythmias.
- It can reduce the clearance of trazodone and diazepam, increasing their concentrations.
- By inhibiting cytochrome CYP3A4 may increase concentrations of alprazolam, buspirone, and triazolam as well as the concentration of some cholesterol-lowering HMG Coa (3-hidroxi-3-metilglutaril-coenzima A o β-hidroxi-β-metilglutaril-coenzima A) (e.g., simvastatin, atorvastatin, and lovastatin).

- It could increase concentrations of pimozide and produce dangerous QTc prolongation and cardiac arrhythmias.
- Tramadol increases the convulsion risk in patients taking antidepressants.

2.1.4. *Side effects and toxicology*

- Sexual dysfunction.
- Decreased appetite, nausea, diarrhea, constipation, and dry mouth.
- Insomnia, sedation, agitation, tremors, headache, and dizziness.
- Sweating.
- Hematomas and rarely bleeds.
- Patients diagnosed with bipolar disorder, psychotic disorder, or bipolar or psychotic disorder undiagnosed may be more vulnerable to the pharmacological actions of SSRIs on the central nervous system (CNS).

The appearance of these side effects by itself does not need the withdrawal of the drug, but the decision should be individualized. Sometimes these adverse effects could be very disturbing por the patient, so if this happens we recommend to decrease the dose and wait, being able to rise again progressively in case of improving the symptoms. In case of persistent effects despite decreasing the dose, consider withdrawing the drug.

In high risk bleeding patients, consider prescribing another antidepressants (nonSSRIs). In patients taking antidepressants with high affinity for serotonin receptors, it is advised to avoid or decrease the use of nonsteroidal anti-inflammatory drugs or aspirin.

2.1.5. *Use in children and adolescents*

- Posology: fluoxetine has been approved for depression and obsessive-compulsive disorder (OCD). Teens usually receive the same dose as adults, children receive slightly lower dose. They should be administered in a single dose, usually in the morning. The liquid solution facilitates management in children.
- How to start treatment: you have to gradually increase the drug. The starting dose is 10 mg/day for anxiety disorders and depressive disorders; gradually increase the dose to achieve therapeutic range (usually 20 mg/day). In bulimia nervosa, the dose is 60–80 mg/day in adolescents and in children slightly lower.
- Phase maintenance dose should be carefully adjusted: it is recommended that treatment should be maintained between 6–12 months after reaching the clinical improvement.
- For long-term use: it is safe for an extended period.
- Treatment withdrawal: no need to taper the dosage as fluoxetine alone is removed gradually due to the long half-life that has and shares with its active metabolites.

2.2. Sertraline

2.2.1. *Pharmacodynamics*

- Action mechanism: potentiates the action of 5-HT by blocking the reuptake pump. Increases 5-HT neurotransmission.
- Pharmacological profile: has an affinity for the receptors. Desensitizes especially 5HT-1A. It has slight antagonistic actions in the sigma receptors.

2.2.2. *Pharmacokinetics*

The original drug has a half-life of 22–36 hours. The half-life of the metabolite is from 62 to 104 hours. Also, inhibits CYP2D6 and CYP3A4 (weakly).

2.2.3. *Drug and food interactions*

- Sertraline may increase concentrations of tricyclic antidepressants (TCA).
- It can cause a fatal serotonin syndrome when combined with MAOIs.
- It can displace protein-based drugs (e.g., warfarin).
- It can increase the risk of bleeding when combined with anticoagulant.
- It can produce boxes infrequently weakness, hyperreflexia, and incoordination when combined with sumatriptan and other triptans, requiring close monitoring of the patient.
- By inhibition of CYP2D6 could interfere with the analgesic action of codeine, increasing concentrations of thioridazine, and cause dangerous cardiac arrhythmias.
- By inhibiting CYP3A4 could increase the concentrations of alprazolam, buspirone, and triazolam, and the concentrations of certain hypolipidemic inhibitors HMG CoA reduced (particularly simvastatin, atorvastatin, and lovastatin).
- It could increase concentrations of pimozide and prolong the QTc interval and dangerous cardiac arrhythmias.
- Tramadol increases the convulsion risk in patients taking antidepressants.

2.2.4. *Side effects and toxicology*

- Sexual dysfunction.
- Gastrointestinal: nausea, decreased appetite, diarrhea, constipation, dry mouth.
- CNS: insomnia or sedation, agitation, tremor, headache, and dizziness.
- Autonomic: sweating.
- Haemorrhaging is rare.

- Hyponatremia is rare.
- Hypotension is rare.

As we discuss with fluoxetine, the appearance of these adverse effects alone does not need withdrawal of the drug, but the decision should be individualized. If these adverse effects are very annoying to the child, we recommend decreasing the dose and wait, being able to rise again progressively in case of improving the side effects. In case of persistent effects despite decreasing the dose, consider withdrawing the drug.

Note: Patients with diagnosed or bipolar disorder or psychotic disorders may be more vulnerable to the pharmacological actions of SSRIs.

Toxicology: It is rare to be lethal in overdose alone; vomiting, sedation, abnormal heart rhythm, mydriasis, agitation; deaths have been reported with overdoses of sertraline, in combination with other drugs or alcohol.

2.2.5. Use in children and adolescents

- Posology: for children aged 6–12 years, the initial dose is 25 mg/day. From the age of 13, one can start the adult dose of 50 mg daily.
- How to start treatment: gradual increase in dose, 25 mg/7 days to reach the minimum effective dose.
- Maintenance phase: the dose should be carefully adjusted and maintain the drug for 6–12 months after clinical improvement.
- Long-term use: it is safe for an extended period.
- Treatment withdrawal: the dose should be gradually reduced to avoid withdrawal symptoms (dizziness, nausea, stomach cramps, sweating, tingling, and dysesthesia). Some patients tolerate a decrease of 50% of the dose in 3 days, another 50% over the next 3 days to complete withdrawal.

2.3. Citalopram

2.3.1. Pharmacodynamics

- Action mechanism: blocking reuptake pump 5-HT, serotonin neurotransmission increasing.
- Pharmacological profile: receptor affinity. Increases concentration of 5-HT receptors and desensitizes, especially, 5-HT1A.

2.3.2. Pharmacokinetics

The original drug has a half-life of 23–45 hours. It is a weak inhibitor of CYP2D6.

2.3.3. *Drug and food interactions*

- Citalopram can increase tricyclic antidepressants concentrations.
- It can cause a fatal "serotonin syndrome" when combined with MAOIs. One should not start treatment with citalopram at least until two weeks after stopping the MAOI.
- It can displace drugs with strong protein (e.g., warfarin) union.
- Once can cause weakness, hyperreflexia, and incoordination when combined with sumatriptan or other triptans, requiring careful monitoring of the patient.
- Possibly increases the risk of bleeding when combined with anticoagulant.
- By inhibition of CYP2D6 pathway could interfere with codeine analgesic and increases plasma concentrations of some beta-blockers and atomoxetine.
- By the same route could increase concentrations of thioridazine and causes dangerous cardiac arrhythmias.

2.3.4. *Side effects*

- Sexual dysfunction.
- Gastrointestinal: decreased appetite, nausea, diarrhea, constipation, and dry mouth.
- On CNS: insomnia, sedation, agitation, tremors, headache, and dizziness.
- Autonomic: sweating.
- Hematomas and bleeding (rare).
- Hyponatremia (rare).
- Syndrome of inappropriate secretion antidiuretic hormone (SIADH).

The advice for action in case of appearance of side effects is the same as that discussed in previous SSRIs.

2.3.5. *Toxicology*

- Citalopram overdose death can occur rarely.
- Can cause vomiting, sedation, heart rhythm disturbances, dizziness, sweating, nausea, and trembling.
- Rarely produces amnesia, confusion, coma, and convulsions.

2.3.6. *Use in children and adolescents*

- Posology: the right dose in children is 5–10 mg/day. In adolescents it may be administered to 10–20 mg/day.
- Phase maintenance: carefully adjust the dose. You can increase the dose to 5 mg/day after one or two weeks. In adolescents it can be increased to 10 mg/day after one or more weeks until the desired effectiveness. The maximum is 60 mg/day. It can be administered as a single dose in the morning or evening.
- For long-term use: it is safe for an extended period.
- Treatment withdrawal: no progressive reduction of the drug is needed. However, it is advisable to avoid potential withdrawal symptoms. Most patients tolerate doses decreased 50% in 3 days; another 50% reduction in 3 days, and then the dose may be suspended. If withdrawal symptoms appear during reduction, the dose should be increased to stop symptoms. Restart the reduction more progressively.

2.4. Escitalopram

2.4.1. *Pharmacodynamics*

- Action mechanism: enhanced release of 5-HT reuptake inhibiting pump.
- Pharmacological profile: receptor affinity. Desensitize 5-HT receptors, especially 1A autoreceptors.

2.4.2. *Pharmacokinetics*

The elimination half-life is 27–36 hours. Stable mean plasma concentrations are reached within weeks. It has no effect on the CYP450.

2.4.3. *Drug and food interactions*

- Tramadol increases the risk of convulsion in patients taking antidepressants.
- Can cause a fatal "serotonin syndrome" when combined with MAOIs; not starting an MAOI up to 14 days after it is suspended.
- It could theoretically cause weakness, incoordination hyperreflexia, and when combined with sumatriptan or other triptans, so careful monitoring of the patient is necessary.
- It can increase the risk of bleeding, especially when combined with anticoagulants.

2.4.4. *Side effects*

- Sexual dysfunction.
- Gastrointestinal (decreased appetite, nausea, diarrhea, constipation, and dry mouth).

- On CNS (insomnia, sedation, agitation, tremors, headache, and dizziness).
- Autonomic (Sweating).
- Hematomas and bleeding (rare).
- Hyponatremia (rare).

The advice for action in case of appearance of side effects is the same as that discussed in previous SSRIs.

2.4.5. Toxicology

Mortality is rare to the overdose of escitalopram alone or in combination with other drugs. Symptoms associated with overdose are nausea, vomiting, sedation, sweating, tremor, and rarely amnesia, coma, and convulsions.

2.4.6. Use in children and adolescents

- Dosage: recommended for children 5–10 mg/day and for adolescents 10–15 mg/day.
- Home treatment: gradual dose escalation. In children, we must start at a dose of 5 mg/day, reaching up to 10 mg/day. In adolescents, we will start with a dose of 10 mg/day, increasing the dose to 15–20 mg/day.
- Maintenance phase: the dose should be carefully adjusted. Maintaining treatment is recommended 6–12 months produced clinical improvement.
- Long-term use: it is safe for an extended period.
- Treatment withdrawal: no need to make a gradual decline but it is wise to carry it out to avoid a withdrawal syndrome. Many patients tolerate a decrease of 50% of the dose in 3 days, and then the other 50%. If withdrawal symptoms appear during the gradual decline of the drug, the dose can be increased until they disappear. Restart the reduction more progressively.

There are other antidepressants such as paroxetine and fluvoxamine that have not demonstrated superior efficacy to placebo in children and adolescents with depression.

3. Serotonin and norepinephrine reuptake inhibitors (SNRIs)

Although none of them is approved by European Medicines Agency or US FDA, some antidepressants not related with SSRI have also been used to children and adolescents for childhood and juvenile depression and anxiety disorders.

3.1. Venlafaxine

3.1.1. Pharmacodynamics

Venlafaxine is a selective serotonin and norepinephrine reuptake inhibitors (SSNRIs). Although, the exact mechanism of action is not well known, venlafaxine and its metabolite,

O-desmethylvenlafaxine (ODV) inhibit the reuptake of serotonin at low doses, serotonin and norepinephrine (NE) at higher doses, and have a weak inhibitory effect on the reuptake of dopamine at even higher doses. Venlafaxine has little affinity for histaminergic, cholinergic, and alpha-adrenergic receptors, not clinically significant.

3.1.2. Pharmacokinetics

Venlafaxine is well absorbed. Food does not affect the absorption of venlafaxine. Bioavailability is 45% following oral administration. Venlafaxine is metabolized by cytochrome P450 2D6 and cytochrome P450 2C19 to ODV, the major metabolite, which is clinically active. Renal elimination is the main route of excretion. The half-life is about 5–11 hours.

3.1.3. Drug and food interactions

Venlafaxine is a moderate inhibitor of cytochrome P450 2D6. Tramadol increases the risk of seizures in patients taking antidepressants. Venlafaxine could inhibit the metabolism of tramadol, reducing his analgesic efficacy and increasing the risk of serotonin syndrome.

3.1.4. Side effects and toxicology

- Sustained elevation of blood pressure is dose-dependent (rarely occurs below 255 mg/day doses) related to inhibition of NE reuptake. In patients with sustained blood pressure raises during venlafaxine therapy, dose reduction, or discontinuation should be considered. Monitoring blood pressure and heart rate is recommended when using venlafaxine.
- Sexual dysfunction, especially abnormal ejaculation and orgasm.
- Gastrointestinal: nausea, dry mouth, constipation. Consider reducing the dose if these symptoms are annoying.
- Central nervous system: sedation, dizziness, nervousness, anxiety, insomnia, somnolence, and tremor. Consider reducing the dose if these symptoms are annoying.
- Mydriasis: patients at risk of angle-closure glaucoma should be monitored.
- In young people, venlafaxine could lead to decrease appetite and weight loss.
- While all antidepressants have the black-box warning about increased suicidal behaviors, venlafaxine is the only one that have demonstrated in RCT and meta-analysis to be associated with higher rates of self-harm events in patients with higher levels of suicidal thoughts. Close monitoring of suicidal ideation and behaviors is necessary during treatment with this drug.

3.1.5. Use in children and adolescents

Venlafaxine is FDA approved for major anti-inflammatory in adults; meanwhile extended-release venlafaxine is approved for the treatment of adults with generalized anxiety disorder, panic disorder, and social phobia besides major depressive disorder.

Two multicenter, randomized, double-blind, and placebo-controlled trials have evaluated the efficacy and tolerability of venlafaxine extended release (ER) for children and adolescents with major depressive disorder. The primary main outcome was the Children's Depression Rating Scale-Revised (CDRS-R) total score. Analysis of each trial independently showed no statically significance between venlafaxine ER and placebo. In the age subgroup analysis, the pooled data showed greater improvement with venlafaxine ER among adolescents (ages 12–17) but not among children (ages 7–11). This study also found that hostility and suicide-related events were more common in venlafaxine ER-treated participants than in placebo-treated participants. There were no completed suicides.

The treatment of resistant depression in adolescents (TORDIA) study was a RCT of treatment resistant adolescents (ages 12–18) with major depressive disorder, who had not responded to a 2-month treatment with an SSRI. Then they were randomized to another SSRI alone, alternate SSRI plus cognitive behavioral therapy (CBT), venlafaxine alone, or venlafaxine plus CBT. Combination of CBT and a switch to another antidepressant had a higher rate of clinical response than medication alone. Changing to an alternate SSRI or venlafaxine had no different response rates. Venlafaxine groups have shown increase in blood pressure and frequency rate, rarely of clinical impact.

Venlafaxine ER has been also studied for anxiety disorders. An RCT of 320 youth (ages 6–17) diagnosed with generalized anxiety disorder shown statistically significant improvement in both the primary outcome and the response rate compared to placebo. Statistically significant changes in weight, blood pressure, pulse, and cholesterol levels were observed in the venlafaxine ER group.

3.1.6. Dosage and administration in children and adolescents

- Venlafaxine dosing schedule among children is similar to adults.
- Home treatment: the recommended initial dosage is 37.5 or 75 mg daily administered in 2 or 3 doses or as a single dose daily when using extended-release capsules. To minimize nausea and other gastrointestinal symptoms, venlafaxine should be taken with food.
- Maintenance phase: the dosage can be increased by 75 mg daily every 4–7 days. A total of 225 mg daily is the maximum dose recommended. Maintaining treatment is recommended 6–12 months produced clinical improvement.
- Long-term use: it is safe for an extended period.
- Treatment withdrawal: no need to make a gradual decline but it is wise to carry out to avoid a withdrawal syndrome. We advise to a decrease of 37.5 mg every 6 days. If withdrawal symptoms appear during the gradual decline of the drug, the dose should be increased until they disappear and then start the reduction again.

3.2. Desvenlafaxine

3.2.1. Pharmacodynamics

Desvenlafaxine (O-desmethylvenlafaxine), the major metabolite of venlafaxine, is a selective serotonin and norepinephrine reuptake inhibitor. As venlafaxine and desvenlafaxine inhibit the reuptake of serotonin at low doses, serotonin and norepinephrine at higher doses, and have a weak inhibitory effect on the reuptake of dopamine at even greater doses. Desvenlafaxine has no clinically significant affinity for histaminergic, cholinergic and alpha-adrenergic receptors.

3.2.2. Pharmacokinetics

Bioavailability is approximately 80% and is unaffected by food. Desvenlafaxine undergoes simple metabolism via conjugation mediated by UGT isoforms and oxidative N-demethylation via cytochrome P450 3A4 to a minor extent. CYP2D6 is not involved. Approximately 45% of the total oral dose is excreted by urine as unchanged desvenlafaxine. The half-life is about 11 hours.

3.2.3. Drug and food interactions

Compared to other SSNRIs, desvenlafaxine has a low risk of drug-drug interactions since there is minimal metabolization by cytochrome P450 pathway.

3.2.4. Side effects and toxicology

- Sustained elevation of blood pressure, dose-dependent, related to inhibition of NE reuptake. Monitoring blood pressure and heart rate is recommended when using desvenlafaxine. In patients with sustained blood pressure raises during desvenlafaxine therapy, dose reduction or discontinuation should be considered.
- Sexual dysfunction, especially abnormal ejaculation and orgasm.
- Gastrointestinal: nausea, dry mouth, constipation.
- Central nervous system: sedation, dizziness, nervousness, anxiety, insomnia, somnolence, and tremor.
- Mydriasis: patients at risk of angle-closure glaucoma should be monitored.

3.2.5. Use in children and adolescents

Desvenlafaxine is FDA approved for the treatment of major depressive disorder in adults. There is no clinical study in the literature about the use of desvenlafaxine in the pediatric population.

3.2.6. Dosage and administration in children and adolescents

- Desvenlafaxine is presented in 50 and 100 mg extended-release tablets.
- Home treatment: the recommended initial dosage is 50 mg as a single dose daily.
- Maintenance phase: the dosage can be increased by 50 mg daily every 4–7 days. Clinical studies have not observed additional efficacy with dosages greater than 50 mg but side effects were more common. A total of 200 mg daily is the maximum dose recommended. Maintaining treatment is recommended 6–12 months produced clinical improvement.

- Long-term use: it is safe for an extended period.
- Treatment withdrawal: the dosage should be decreased gradually to prevent withdrawal symptoms like dizziness, gastrointestinal discomfort, headache, nervousness, or agitation. Many patients tolerate a decrease of 50% of the dose in 3–7 days and then the other 50%. If withdrawal symptoms appear during the gradual decline of the drug, the dose should be increased until they disappear and then start the reduction again.

3.3. Duloxetine

3.3.1. Pharmacodynamics

Duloxetine is another selective serotonin and norepinephrine reuptake inhibitor (SSNRIs). The major difference to venlafaxine is that duloxetine has comparable binding affinity to both norepinephrine and serotonin transport sites. Duloxetine has no significant affinity for dopaminergic, histaminergic, cholinergic, and alpha-adrenergic receptors.

3.3.2. Pharmacokinetics

Duloxetine is well absorbed and unaffected by food. Protein binding is greater than 90%. Duloxetine is metabolized by cytochrome P450 2D6 and 1A2 to the metabolites, which are not active. Renal elimination is the main route of excretion (70%) followed by fecal excretion (20%). The half-life is about 12 hours [8–17].

3.3.3. Drug and food interactions

Duloxetine is a moderate inhibitor of cytochrome P450 2D6. Tramadol increases the risk of seizures in patients taking antidepressants. As result of a pharmacokinetic interaction, duloxetine could increase plasma levels of thioridazine, which may result in increased risk of ventricular arrhythmias.

3.3.4. Side effects and toxicology

- Increase of heart frequency, dose-dependent. Monitoring blood pressure and heart rate is recommended when using duloxetine. In patients with sustained effects, dose reduction or discontinuation should be considered.
- Sexual dysfunction especially decreased sexual desire and problems with erection.
- Gastrointestinal: nausea, dry mouth, constipation, decreased appetite.
- Central nervous system: fatigue, sedation, dizziness, somnolence.

3.3.5. Use in children and adolescents

Among adults, duloxetine is usually used for the acute and maintained treatment of major depressive disorder, acute treatment of anxiety disorders, fibromyalgia, and neuropathic pain, especially when is associated with peripheral neuropathy.

Two multicenter, randomized, double-blind, and placebo-controlled trials have evaluated the efficacy and safety of duloxetine for children and adolescents with major depressive disorder and compared to fluoxetine. The primary main outcome was the Children's Depression Rating Scale-Revised (CDRS-R) total score. In these studies, neither duloxetine nor fluoxetine demonstrated a statistically significant improvement compared with placebo. Headache and nausea were the main treatment-emergent adverse events. Weight decrease was more common among duloxetine and fluoxetine groups compared to placebo. Suicidal behavior did not occur in acute treatment, while seven cases occurred during extended treatment. There were no completed suicides. No patients had sustained elevation in systolic or diastolic blood pressure during the 36-week study.

Another randomized, double-blind, and placebo-controlled trials have evaluated duloxetine for children and adolescents with generalized anxiety disorder. They found that duloxetine was statistically better than placebo on Pediatric Anxiety Rating Scale (PARS).

3.3.6. Dosage and administration in children and adolescents

- Duloxetine is presented in 20, 30, and 60 mg capsules.
- Home treatment: the recommended initial dosage is 30 mg as a single dose daily in the morning.
- Maintenance phase: the target dose is 30–60 mg in both adolescents and children. Clinical studies have not observed additional efficacy with dosages greater than 60 mg but side effects were more common. A total of 120 mg once a day is the maximum dose recommended. Maintaining treatment is recommended 6–12 months produced clinical improvement.
- Long-term use: it is safe for an extended period.
- Treatment withdrawal: the dosage should be gradually decreased over at least 2 weeks to prevent withdrawal symptoms like gastrointestinal discomfort, headache, nervousness, or agitation. If withdrawal symptoms appear during the gradual decline of the drug, the dose should be increased until they disappear and then start the reduction again.

4. NaSSRI

4.1. Mirtazapine

4.1.1. Pharmacodynamics

Mirtazapine is a piperazinoazepine with an anxiolytic effect. Mirtazapine acts as an antagonist at central presynaptic alpha-2-receptors. This antagonism inhibits negative feedback to the presynaptic nerve and enhances the release of both norepinephrine and serotonin. Mirtazapine is also a weak antagonist of 5-HT1 receptors and a potent antagonist of 5-HT2 (particularly subtypes 2A and 2C) and 5-HT3 receptors. Mirtazapine could also cause sedation through H1 receptor antagonism. It has minimal activity at dopaminergic and muscarinic receptors and NE and 5-HT reuptake are not affected.

4.1.2. Pharmacokinetics

Mirtazapine is completely absorbed but, due to first-pass metabolism, bioavailability is about 50%. Protein binding is about 85%. Duloxetine is metabolized by cytochrome P450 3A4, 2D6 and to a lesser extent by 1A2 to many different metabolites, several of whom are active, but plasma levels are low. Kidneys excrete about 75% of mirtazapine. Half-life is about 20–40 hours.

4.1.3. Drug and food interactions

Mirtazapine is a weak CYP2D6 inhibitor. CYP3A4 potent inhibitors could increase plasma levels of mirtazapine. Adding another serotonin antidepressant may produce serotonin syndrome

4.1.4. Side effects and toxicology

- Mirtazapine is usually well-tolerated.
- The most common adverse effects are sedation and weight gain due to increased appetite.
- Gastrointestinal: dry mouth, constipation.
- Central nervous system: dizziness.

4.1.5. Use in children and adolescents

Mirtazapine is an FDA approved for the acute and maintenance treatment of major depressive disorder in adults.

Few studies till date have evaluated mirtazapine in children and adolescents. There is not strong data with double-blind and placebo-controlled trials. In a recent network meta-analysis, Cipriani and colleagues reported two randomized, placebo-controlled trials funded by a pharmaceutical company in 170 patients aged 7–17. Mirtazapine was not significantly different to placebo on any outcome rating.

4.1.6. Dosage and administration in children and adolescents

- Mirtazapine is available in 15, 30, and 45 mg tablets.
- Home treatment: the recommended initial dosage is 15 mg as a single dose daily at night before bedtime, due to its sedative effects.
- Maintenance phase: the target dose is 30–45 mg in both adolescents and children. 45 mg daily is the maximum dose recommended.

- Long-term use: it is safe for an extended period.
- Treatment withdrawal: the dosage should be gradually decreased over at least 2 weeks to prevent withdrawal symptoms like gastrointestinal discomfort, headache, nervousness, or agitation. If withdrawal symptoms appear during the gradual decline of the drug, the dose should be increased until they disappear and then start the reduction again.

5. MAOI

5.1. Nonselective

5.1.1. Tranylcypromine

5.1.1.1. Pharmacodynamics

5.1.1.1.1. Action mechanism

Tranylcypromine irreversibly blocks monoamine oxidase (MAO) from breaking norepinephrine, serotonin, and dopamine. This presumably boosts noradrenergic, serotonergic, and dopaminergic neurotransmission. As the drug is structurally related to amphetaine, it may have some stimulant-like actions due to monoamine release and reuptake inhibition [14].

5.1.1.1.2. Pharmacological profile

Tranylcypromine is a nonhydrazine monoamine oxidase inhibitor with a rapid onset of activity. It increases the concentration of epinephrine, norepinephrine, and serotonin in storage sites throughout the nervous system and, in theory, this increased concentration of monoamines in the brain stem is the basis for its antidepressant activity [14].

5.1.1.1.3. Pharmacokinetics

Tranylcypromine achieves an initial peak within approximately 1 hour and a secondary peak within 2–3 hours. It has been suggested that this apparent biphasic absorption in some individuals may represent different absorption rates. Following discontinuance of tranylcypromine, the drug is excreted within 24 hours. On withdrawal of tranylcypromine, MAO activity is recovered in 3–5 days (possibly in up to 10 days). Concentration of urinary tryptamine, an indicator of MAO-A inhibition return to normal, however, within 72–120 hours [14].

5.2. Selective

5.2.1. Moclobemide

Moclobemide is a reversible inhibitor of monoamine-oxidase-A (RIMA) and has been extensively evaluated in the treatment of a wide spectrum of depressive disorders and less extensively studied in anxiety disorders.

There is a growing evidence that moclobemide is not inferior to other antidepressants in the treatment of subtypes of depression, such as dysthymia, endogenous (unipolar and bipolar), reactive, atypical, agitated, and retarded depression as with other antidepressants limited evidence suggests that moclobemide has consistent long-term efficacy.

5.2.1.1. Pharmacodynamics

5.2.1.1.1. Action mechanism

Moclobemide is a substrate of CYP2C19. Few clinically significant drug interactions between moclobemide and teother drugs have been reported in spite of the fact that it acts as an inhibitor of CYP1A2, CYP2C19, and CYP2D6. Switch to another antidepressants could be quick as its half-life in plasma is short, 24 hours. As it is well-tolerated, therapeutic doses can be reached rapidly upon onset of treatment. After one week following dose adjustment plasma levels are reached. Patients with severe hepatic impairment require dose adjustment, not those with renal dysfunction.

5.2.1.1.2. Pharmacological profile and pharmacokinetics

A positive correlation between the plasma concentration of moclobemide and its therapeutic efficacy has been found. Due to negligible anticholinergic and antihistaminic actions, moclobemide has been better tolerated than tri or heterocyclic antidepressants.

5.2.1.1.3. Side effects and toxicology

Side effects such as dizziness, nausea, and insomnia were more frequent with moclobemide than with placebo. Sexual dysfunction and gastrointestinal side effects are much less frequent with moclobemide than with SSRIs. Gastrointestinal side effects and, especially, sexual dysfunction were much less frequent with moclobemide than with SSRIs. After multiple dosing the oral bioavailability of moclobemide reaches almost 100% [15].

5.2.1.1.4. Drug and food interactions

Moclobemide has propensity to induce hypertensive crisis after ingestion of tyramine-rich food like cheese, so dietary restrictions are mandatory.

5.2.1.1.5. Use in children and adolescents

No use in children and adolescent has been reported in clinical trials.

5.2.1.1.6. Tricyclic antidepressants

Tricyclic antidepressants (TCAs) have had a substantial role in the pharmacotherapy of children and adolescents over the past three decades. However its efficacy has been unproven in major depression. Considering the current epidemiologic estimates of the prevalence of child and adolescent mental disorders, as many as 10% of children in the USA, may have a potentially TCA-responsive disorder [12]

Most common tryciclic antidepressants are: Amitriptyline, clomipramine, doxepin, opipramol, trimipramine, imipramine and nortriptyline.

5.3. Amitriptyline

5.3.1. Pharmacodynamics

Amitriptyline is a tricyclic agent with sedative effects. Amitriptyline is thought to be a potent inhibitor of noradrenergic reuptake at the adrenergic nerve endings [17].

5.3.2. Pharmacokinetics

Amitriptyline is completely but slowly absorbed by the gastrointestinal tract after oral administration, and peak plasma concentration are usually reached within 4–8 hours. Amitriptyline has hepatic extensive elimination, and its systemic bioavailability ranges from 33 to 66% after oral administration [18]. In 24 hours, about one-third to one-half of the drug will be excreted. The plasma half-life ranges from 10 to 28 hours.

5.3.3. Drug and food interactions

Amitriptyline is widely distributed throughout the body and extensively bound to plasma and tissue proteins. It has got a highly lipophilic compound [17].

5.3.4. Side effects and toxicology

Amitriptyline most common side effects are blurred vision, constipation, and dry mouth which are due to anticholinergic effects. Due to the blockage of histamine receptors, it may cause sedation. In high doses, amitriptyline has cardiac effects such as dysrhythmia, prolonged conduction time, and sinus tachycardia [18].

5.3.5. Use in children and adolescents

No clinical trials on children and adolescents have been conducted with this drug.

5.4. Clomipramine

Clomipramine (Anafranil) was the first drug to obtain Food and Drug Administration (FDA) approval for treating OCD. It is a tricyclic antidepressant (TCA) with a potent ability to inhibit serotonin reuptake; it also inhibits the reuptake of norepinephrine, and has dopamine-blocking effects [19].

5.4.1. Pharmacokinetics

Clomipramine is completely but slowly absorbed by the gastrointestinal tract after oral administration, and peak plasma concentration are usually reached within 4–8 hours. It has hepatic extensive elimination, and its systemic bioavailability ranges from 33 to 66% after oral administration [18]. In 24 hours about one-third to one-half of the drug will be excreted. The plasma half-life ranges from 10 to 28 hours.

5.4.2. Side effects and toxicology

The most common side effects of clomipramine are blurred vision, constipation, and dry mouth which are due to anticholinergic effects. It may cause sedation. In high doses, clomipramine has cardiac effects such as dysrhythmias, prolonged conduction time, and sinus tachycardia [18].

5.4.3. Use in children and adolescents

No clinical trials have been conducted in children and adolescents.

6. Other antidepressants

6.1. Vortioxetine

6.1.1. Pharmacodynamics

Vortioxetine has a dual mechanism for depression. First, it inhibits serotonin reuptake by inhibition of serotonin transporter. Second, Vortioxetine is a partial agonist of 5-HT_{1B}, 5-HT_{3}, 5-HT_{7}, 5-HT_{1D}, and HT_{1A}.

These actions modulate serotonin neurotransmitter system and, to a lesser extent, in other systems like dopamine, norepinephrine, histamine, gamma amino butiric acid (GABA) and glutamate.

6.1.2. Pharmacokinetics

Vortioxetine is well absorbed and unaffected by food. Bioavailability is about 75%. It is mainly metabolized by cytochrome P450 2D6 to two metabolites, which are not active. Renal elimination is the main route of excretion (59%) followed by fecal excretion (26%). The half-life is about 66 hours.

6.1.3. Drug and food interactions

- Tramadol increases the risk of seizures in patients taking antidepressants.
- It can cause a fatal "serotonin syndrome" when combined with MAOIs. One should not start treatment with vortioxetine at least until two weeks after stopping the MAOI.
- It can displace drugs with strong protein (e.g., warfarin) union.
- CYP450 2D6 potent inhibitors like bupropion or quinidine could increase plasma concentrations of vortioxetine.

6.1.4. *Side effects and toxicology*

- Gastrointestinal: nausea is the most common side effect. Other effects like decreased appetite, diarrhea, constipation, and dry mouth could also occur.
- Central nervous system: dizziness, bruxism and abnormal dreams.
- Skin: itching and, rarely, night sweats.
- Flushing (rare).
- Vortioxetine has no sexual side effects.

6.1.5. *Use in children and adolescents*

At this moment, some phase II clinical trials are being developed to test efficacy and tolerability of vortioxetine in pediatric patients.

6.2. Bupropion

Bupropion is a dopamine and norepinephrine reuptake inhibitor that belongs to a second-generation group of antidepressants. Bupropion has shown good results for treating major depressive disorder according to measures like the Hamilton Depression Rating Scale, and the Clinical Global Impression Severity and Impairment Scales. Its efficacy is similar to most other common antidepressants and it has an acceptable profile and good tolerability. Bupropion has shown to have a minimal effect on sexual function, and similar or even lower rates of somnolence than placebo, and it has shown lower rates of weight gain and sedation than some other commonly used antidepressants. Bupropion has indication to treat MDD in the USA, Canada, and many countries in Europe, although none of the studies has been conducted to address its safety and effectiveess in children and adolescents [11].

6.2.1. *Pharmacodynamics*

Chemically, bupropion is a **monocyclic phenylbutylamine** of the **aminoketone group**, which could be associated with an effect of profile different from that of other antidepressant drugs. It is also known as amfebutamone. Its primary action mechanism is neuronal reuptake inhibition of norepinephrine and dopamine without significant serotonergic effects. Bupropion lacked anticholinergic and direct sympathomimetic activity and its cardiac depressant activity is at least 10 times lower than that shown with tricyclic antidepressants.

6.2.2. *Pharmacokinetics*

Administration of bupropion is oral and it has been absorbed by the intestine. It has got a low molecular weight and a good liposolubility. Its half-life, in the modified release formulation, is 21 hours. The drug is metabolized in the liver and it is excreted through the kidney. The stale plasma concentration of the drug and its active metabolites are reached at 5–7 days after initiation of its administration. It is metabolized in the liver by the cytochrome P450

(CYP) 2B6, that catalyzes the hydroxylation of the side chain to form an active metabolism, the hydroxybupropion. It is excreted through the kidney.

6.2.3. Drug and food interactions

Drugs that inhibit the CYP450 2B6 such as clopidogrel and ticlopidine (antiplatelet) and valproate may have an effect of reducing the proportion between hydroxybupropion and bupropion, observing up to 68% reduction in the case of clopidogrel and up to 90% in the case of ticlopidine. Due to the important contribution of hydroxybupropion in the clinical efficacy of bupropion, it may be affected by this interaction. Concurrent use of bupropion with tobacco, alcohol, phenobarbital, and carbamazepine, furthermore, could induce the production of its active metabolite, the hydroxybupropion.

6.2.4. Use in children and adolescents

No use in children and adolescent has been reported in clinical trials.

6.3. Reboxetine

6.3.1. Pharmacodynamics

Reboxetine is a selective norepinephrine (noradrenaline) reuptake inhibitor with indication to treat depression in many European countries, but the application of approval was rejected in the USA. Reboxetine mainly acts by binding to the norepinephrine transporter and blocking reuptake of extracellular norepinephrine. The drug is indicated for the acute treatment of depressive illness or major depression and for maintaining the clinical improvement in patients initially responding to treatment [16].

6.3.2. Pharmacokinetics

Reboxetine has potent antidepressant activity, low affinity for alpha-adrenergic and muscarinic receptors, and low toxicity in animals. Humans rapidly absorb reboxetine (tmax about 2 hours) with a terminal half-life of elimination (t1/2) of 13 hours, allowing twice-daily administration. Food does not affect bioavailability. Elimination is principally renal of therapeutic actions and is usually not immediate, but often delayed 2–4 weeks. If it is not working within 6–8 weeks for depression it may require a dosage increase or it may not work at all [16].

6.3.3. Drug and food interactions

Multiple dosing, gender, or liver insufficiency had no significant effects on the pharmacokinetics. Elderly (particularly frail elderly) patients and patients with severe renal impairment may need dose reduction. Reboxetine shows no clinically relevant interaction with lorazepam and has no inhibitory effects on the major enzymes involved in drug metabolism [16].

6.3.4. Use in children and adolescents

No use in children and adolescents has been reported in clinical trials.

7. Conclusions

Fluoxetine has shown reduced depressive symptoms in young people under 18 in randomized clinical trials, although the extent up to this reduction is clinically significant and remains uncertain. In spite of this, fluoxetine is still considered the best option when a pharmacological treatment is indicated. In the therapeutic plan of young people with major depressive disorder, clinical guidelines recommend psychotherapy (especially cognitive-Behavioral therapy or interpersonal therapy) as the first-line intervention, and fluoxetine only in moderate-to-severe depressed patients who cannot access psychotherapy or have not responded to nonpharmacological approaches. Antidepressants are not well studied in this population, and further research is needed on antidepressants in young people. In all cases when a patient is started on antidepressants, he/she should be carefully monitored in prevention of risk of suicidal thoughts or attempts [10].

Author details

Isabel Hernández-Otero[1*], Carlos Gómez Sánchez-Lafuente[2] and Cecilia Hernández González[2]

*Address all correspondence to: isabelhotero@hotmail.com

1 Department of Child and Adolescent Psychiatry, University Hospital Virgen de la Victoria, Málaga, Spain

2 University Hospital Virgen de la Victoria, Málaga, Spain

References

[1] Costello JE, Erkanli A, Angold A. Is there an epidemic of child or adolescent depression?. Journal of Child Psychology and Psychiatry. 2006;**47**:1263–1271

[2] Olfson M, Blanco C, Wang S, Laje G, Correll CU. National trends in the mental health care of children, adolescents and adults by office-based physicians. Journal of the American Medical Association Psychiatry. 2014;**71**:81–90

[3] Thapar A, Colishaw S, Pine DS, Thapar AK. Depression in adolescence. Lancet. 2012;**379**: 1056–1067

[4] Hopkins K, Crosland P, Elliott N, Bewley S. Diagnosis and management of depression in children and young people: Summary of updated NICE guidelines. British Medical Journal. 2015;**350**:h824

[5] Malhi GS, Bassett D, Boyce P, et al. Royal Australian and New Zealand College of Psychiatrists clinical practice guidelines for mood disorders. The Australian and New Zealand Journal of Psychiatry. 2015;**49**:1087–1206

[6] Bachmann CJ, Aagaard L, Burcu M, et al. Trends and patterns of antidepressant use in children and adolescents from five western countries, 2005-2012. European Neuropsychopharmacology. 2016;**26**:411–119

[7] US Food and Drug Administration. Suicidality in Children and Adolescents Being Treated with Antidepressant Medications [Internet]. Available from: www.fa.gov/safety/medwatch/safetyinformation/safetyalertsforhumanmedicalproducts/ucm155488.htm, [Accessed 18-10-2015]

[8] Hertrick SE, McKenzie JE, Cox GR, Simmons MB, Merry SN. Newer generation antiderpessants for depressive disorders in children and adolescents. The Cochrane Database of Systematic Reviews. 2012;**11**:CD004851

[9] Whittington CJ, Kendall T, Fonagy P, Cottrell D, Cotgrove A, Boddington E. Selective serotonin reuptake inhibitors in childhood depression: Systematic review of published versus unpublished data. Lancet. 2004;**363**:1341–1345

[10] Cipriani A, Zhou X, Del Giovane C, Hetrick S, Qin B, Whittigton C, Coghill D, Zhang Y, Hazell P, Leucht S, Cujpers P, Pu J, Cohen D, Ravindran AV, Liu Y, Michael K, Yang L, Liu L, Xie P. Comparative efficacy and tolerability of antidepressants for major depressive disorder in children and adolescents: A network meta-analysis. Lancet. 2016;**S0140-6736** (16) 30385–3

[11] Saiz-Ruiz J, Gibert-Rahola J, Gutiérrez-Fraile M. Bupropion: Efficacy and safety in the treatment of depression. Actas españolas de Psiquiatría. 2011;**39**(suppl 1):1–25

[12] Daly J, Wilens T. The use of Tricyclic Antidepressants in children and adolescents. Pediatric Clinics. 2011;**45**(5):1123–1135

[13] European Medicines Agency website. www.ma.europa.eu. Serotonine-specific reuptake inhibitors. European Commission Final Decision. Doc. Ref. EMEA/CHMP/128918/2005 corr. London, 25 April 2005

[14] Foye I, et al. Foye´s Principles of Medicinal Chemistry. 6th ed. Lippicot Williams & Wilkins. p. 38. ISBN: 978-0-7817-6879-5.

[15] Bonnet U. Moclobemide: therapeutic use and clinical studies. CNS Drug Reviews. 2003;**9**(1):97–140. https://www.ncbi.nlm.nih.gov/pubmed/12595913

[16] Eyding D, et al. Reboxetine for Acute Treatment of Major Depression: Systematic Review and Meta-Analysis of Published and Unpublished Placebo and Selective Serotonin Reuptake Inhibitor Controlled Trials. BMJ online FIRST. BMJ.com

[17] Sir Colin D, Churchill, editors. Therapeutic Drugs. Edinburgh: Livingstone; 1991.p. A95-A100

[18] Schultz P, et al. Amitryptiline disposition in youth and elderly men. Clinical Pharmacology and Therapeutics. 1983b;**33**:360–366

[19] Bokor Gand Anderson PD. Obsessive-Compulsive disorder. Journal of Pharmacy Practice. 2014;**27**(2):116–130

5

Draw, Write, Speak, Play: The Role of Projection in Diagnosis and Therapy of Children and Adolescents

Martin H. Maurer

Abstract

In this chapter, I will (1) review the concept and function of projective mechanisms on a psychodynamic basis. In this section, I will outline the relation of projection to the unconscious, its use in innerpsychic dynamics, and the underlying mechanisms for its use in psychotherapy like creativity, imagination, and symbolization; (2) give an overview over the use of projective methods for testing and diagnosis in the psychological sciences; and (3) exemplify the use of projective methods in diagnostics and psychotherapy of children and adolescents. I will present current methods based on drawing, verbally describing and imaginating, and playing arts, focusing on sand play therapy and miniature figure play.

Keywords: projective methodology, object relation theory, sandplay therapy, figure play, operationalized psychodynamic diagnostics in children and adolescents (OPD-CA-2), thematic apperception tests, narrative

1. Concept and function of projective mechanisms

1.1. The relation of projections to the unconscious

The Latin word "proiectus" means "to throw forth," or "to cast forward," and with regard to psychological sciences, several definitions have been provided. First of all, Sigmund Freud [1] described the "classical" projection as defense mechanism when the *ego* is threatened and refuses to acknowledge the trait, it attributes the trait to the outside world [2]. Later on, Freud broadened his view of projective mechanisms and refers the term projection to a general primitive mechanism, not only a defense mechanism, implying that projection may also be present when there is no conflict [3].

In this sense, the attributive projection can be understood as "ascribing one's own motivations, feelings, and behavior to other persons" [2]. This definition seems to be the most common, but also the most (over-)simplified one. There seem to be no relations to psychoanalytical concepts of the self, or the unconscious. Most authors use this term to describe "any kind of externalization" [2] with a correlation between characteristics of the proband and predictions or statements issued. The attributive projection is mostly similar what Horney called the "naïve" projection, which means that the subject assumes that others think, feel and behave in the same way as oneself [4]. Today, this view can be integrated into the concept of mentalization.

In a third view, Murstein introduced the autistic projection as "perceived aspects of another person which are modified to accomplish own needs [2]."

In the fourth mode of rationalized projection, the process of projection lies in the unconscious, but the projector is conscious of his/her behavior. In this context, the rationalized projection can be understood as "defence against guilt [2]," and is a special subtype of the classical projection.

In a critique of projective methods, Lilienfeld et al. describe the aim of projective testing as a method to "circumvent the conscious defenses of respondents" and to "gain privileged access to … psychological information … of which respondents are not consciously aware [5]." This caused a discussion about the mechanisms and function of projection and projective testing [6]. This seems to be a misconception of what projective mechanisms are capable of, since it is not an aim to circumvent defense mechanisms but to elucidate them and to work on them in a clinical setting. Freud lists the free association and the interpretation of dreams as two possible ways to access the unconscious, or at least, processes of the unconscious [7]. Later, parapraxis [8], hypnosis [9], and play [10] added additional access ways.

Thus, in the present chapter, the term projection is used to describe a transfer mechanism of intrapsychic elements called "representations of objects" either to other intrapsychic elements, or external elements (**Figure 1**). Of note, here only the mechanism is connoted, its presumable function is regarded as a secondary aspect.

1.2. The function of projections in innerpsychic dynamics

For diagnostic purposes and the planning of therapy, an elaborated system for operationalized psychodynamic diagnostics in children and adolescents (OPD-CA-2) has been established [11]. This system is a multiaxial diagnostic and classification system, including psychodynamic, developmental, and clinical aspects. The axes comprehend interpersonal relations, conflicts, structure, prerequisites for treatment, and the ICD-10 classification. The axes have been aligned to the DSM-5 system [12].

Currently, no studies have been published evaluating the usefulness of projective techniques with regard to the OPD-CA-2. On the other hand, the psychoanalytic theoretical background of projective techniques proposes a close relationship of the both [13–15].

What can be the functions of projections in intrapsychic dynamics? Besides the above-mentioned functions as defense mechanism, and developmental characteristic, projections may be used as a translator and connector of distinct and separate representation of objects. With regard to the object-relations theory [16–18], aspects the self and its conceptualization

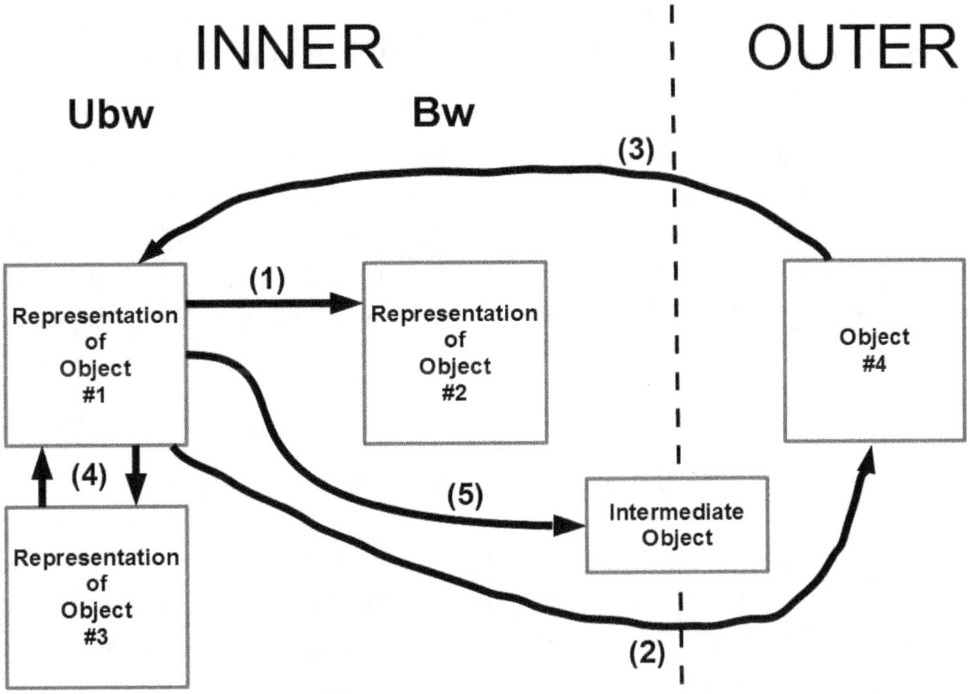

Figure 1. Depiction of projective pathways of objects or their representations, respectively. Inner unconscious objects can either project onto objects in the conscious which are also intrapsychic objects (1) or they can project onto objects in the outer world (2). In reverse, outer objects can project onto inner objects via internatization (3). Moreover, intrapsychic unconscious objects can project onto other intrapsychic onconscious objects (4). Finally, objects can project onto intermediate objects (5), a preferential way in children. (Ubw = the unconscious, Bw = the conscious).

contributed largely to an expanded understanding of projective mechanisms. A translating function of projections may be that characteristics of objects, for example, moral attributions such as "good", "bad," or "angry" can be transferred to another object, which seems to be less dangerous for the stability of the psychic system. Moreover, the connector function might be a possibility to link not closely related objects, or objects of diametrical attributes without generating internal psychological conflicts.

The main prerequisites for the application of projective techniques seem to be creativity, imagination, and the capability of symbolization [19, p. 27]. Of note, these prerequisites depend on the respective developmental level and are influenced by other steps in development, such as speech, conceptualization, abstractive ability, fine and gross motor skills, as well as the level of intelligence. Moreover, the influence of culture, descent and origin, religious belief, moral values, and educational history may strongly contribute to the usefulness of the application of projective techniques in children and adolescents. For example, in the author's clinical experience with children and adolescents with an Islamic background originating from Syria, Iraq, and Afghanistan, these children do not easily use drawing or graphic techniques as means of expression. Thus, projective techniques such as human figure drawings may not be valid tools of assessment.

Another field of special care compromises the child's cultural experiences with magic. For example, in cultures where witchcraft and magical forces are present in every-day life, for example in West-African or indigenous cultures of the Americas, deliberate use of the respective test which is to be applied should be made, since these tests may be threatening to the child, or nonprojective mechanisms come into the foreground, diminishing the validity of the test result.

A third aspect is, for example, the connotation of specific animals, such as pigs, as impure. Then the application of the Patte Noire test [20] may be difficult for children with Islamic or Jewish background. Thus the child cannot identify with the hero of the story, and the validity of the test is severely restricted. On the other hand, the connotation of specific animals, for example, snakes or rats, in the occidental world is strongly different from the oriental connotations.

2. Projective methods for testing, diagnosis, and therapy

A wealth of projective methods has been developed for clinical and nonclinical use, for diagnostics, therapy and personality assessment, and for decision processes in human resource management. Several approaches to classify projective methods have been proposed, and in this chapter, I will follow the taxonomy of Lindzey [21], suggesting five groups of projective techniques based on the handling of the material. This classification is also reflected in the title of the present chapter.

First, *construction techniques* provide the material for creative processes such as drawing or writing, for example, pencil and paper for the various drawing tasks.

Second, *association techniques* involve the presentation of a stimulus, may it be verbal (like the wordlist in the C. G. Jung experiment of 1908 [22]) or nonverbal (such as an inkblot). The proband is then asked to provide verbal associations, or a narrative.

Third, *completion methods* provide stimulus material containing blanks, for example incomplete sentences such as in the Washington University Sentence Completion Test (SCT) [23], or incomplete stories [24–26]. Additionally, combined material such as comic-like pictures with an empty speech bubble has been used [27].

Fourth, *arrangement or selection methods* are based on picture material or building bricks and block, such as the Lowenfeld Mosaic Test [28].

Fifth, *expression techniques* involve playful arts material, such as miniature figures as in doll or figurine play [29, 30], or expressive sandplay [31–33].

There is no strict separation of these fields, and mostly combined methodologies seem to be in use in the clinical practice.

A similar classification has been proposed by Frank [34, 35], with constitutive, constructive, interpretive, carthartic, and refractive techniques. A discussion of both classifications is provided by Semeonoff [36]. Of note, there is a certain overlap between the different categories as well as the different categorization systems. In general, a three-dimensional model of classification systems has been proposed, containing the various aspects of stimulus, response, and intention (**Figure 2**).

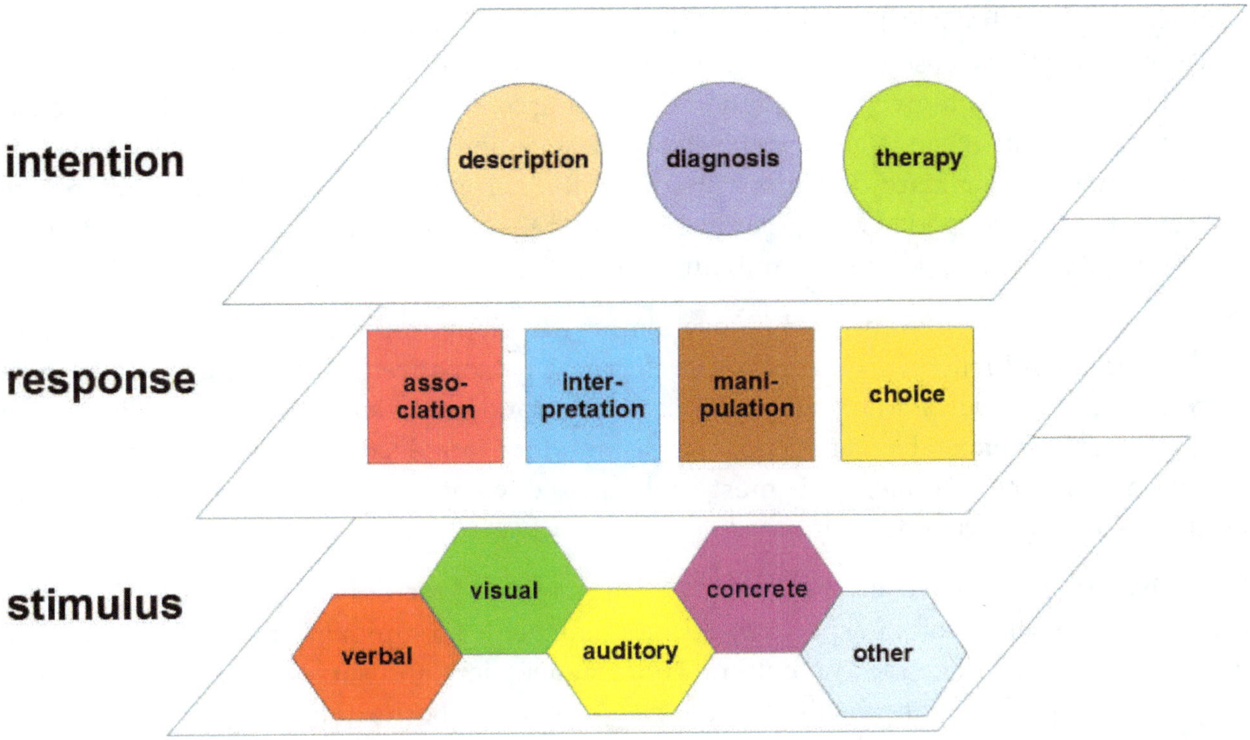

Figure 2. Multidimensional classification system of projective methods. Projective techniques can be classified according to the sensual quality of the stimulus (verbal, visual, auditory, etc.), the category of response (e.g., association, interpretation, manipulation as in play or construction, or choice and ordering), and the intention or purpose, may it be diagnostic, may it be therapeutic, or may it be for the description of personality traits.

With regard to the nomenclature, the term "apperceptive" means that the proband is asked for a projective response to visual stimuli, for example in the TAT [37] and the variants derived from this test. The term "thematic" means in this context that a narrative, or a story is created, not only short response, or value on a rating scale.

The term "semiprojective" means that a test provides operant, or projective, stimuli and records the answers in a respondent way, such as with a questionnaire [38]. Another definition of "semiprojective" describes the creation of a real-world scene by symbolic, or transformed, means, such as figurines, drawings etc. [39].

There has been a debate on the psychometric properties of diagnostic tests, criteria including norms, reliability, objectivity, validity and incremental validity, and its utility for treatment purposes [5, 6], but in the current chapter, I will not add to this debate. In the literature review for this chapter, there has been numerous doubtful and dubious "tests," which seem to be based on individual ideology, not scientific scholarship. Moreover, the terms "test," "technique," and "method" are often used interchangeably, but in the light of the current literature, a "test" is related to a clinical diagnostic purpose, and it can be judged and challenged by the above-mentioned psychometric criteria. For a "technique" or "method" lesser demands are necessary with regard to the latter, and it seems that "techniques" / "methods" mainly serve the therapeutic objectives. In this case, their clinical use can be assessed by means of the methods of evidence-based medicine, which for example include the evaluation of clinical studies with regard to randomization, blinding, and the description of withdrawals or drop-outs [40, 41].

Standardized psychological diagnostics relying on clinical interviews, questionnaires, rating scales, etc., which are based on normalization of samples, will result in the relative position of an individual within a given distribution. For example, the standard normal distribution is characterized by its mean value and the standard deviation. Thus, all values obtained smaller or larger than two standard deviations are out of the normal range. An individual taking the test can hence be grouped in categories like "meeting the criteria" or "not meeting the criteria" or will result in the position of the individual in a percentile rank (PR).

On the other hand, projective techniques aim at describing an individual not relatively to others, but individually. With regard to developing a personalized medicine, this will become more and more important. Psychometric data like standardization, objectivity, validity, and reliability can be obtained using adequate measures, for example, the OPD-CA. Normalization of data may not be sensible, since most of the projective methods do not aim at placing an individual in a relative order compared to others (such as percentile ranks).

Projective techniques have also been used in anthropology for cross-cultural studies [15], with the background that verbal aspects could be eliminated. In summary, the use of projective techniques strongly depended on cultural conceptualization, and surprising results for example with regard to drawing methods have been observed. For example, in the past, human figure drawings like the Machover Draw-a-Person test [42] have been applied for the intelligence and developmental measures. Administered in field studies in Inuit and Cree children, it revealed that the Western conceptualization of intelligence cannot be measured using this task [15, p. 294]. In conclusion, a projective test should test projective mechanisms, and not be used for other variables, such as intelligence measures, motor skills, speech development, or questions of child custody, since the validity of this approach is not guaranteed.

3. Clinically used projective tests, methods, and techniques: an overview

In the following section, I will give an overview over the most commonly used projective tests, methods, and techniques applied to children and adolescents. The following descriptions are neither complete nor representative, but they may give a fast first glance on the available techniques.

Table 1 gives an overview of available projective tests, methods, and techniques. (Data and tests compiled from [15, 19, 36, 43–48].)

3.1. Drawing

3.1.1. Human figure drawings: Machover Draw-A-Person Test (DAP); Goodenough-Harris Drawing Test; Goodenough Draw-a-Man (DAM) Test

Description: In the original version of Goodenough [49] and also later by Ziler [50], the child is instructed to draw a man (today: person), "as good as you can." Later, the instruction was extended to "draw a man, a woman, and yourself." Additional modifications involve the drawing of "a man, a woman, and yourself [42]."

1. Association

1.1. Verbal

Word Association Technique (Jung 1910)

Brook Reaction Test (Brook & Heim 1960)

Adjective Generation Technique (AGT) (Allen & Potkay 1973)

Kent-Rosanoff Free Association Test (Kent & Rosanoff 1910)

Composite Free Association (Wells 1928)

Polygraph Test (Larson 1921)

1.2. Visual

Rorschach Inkblot Technique [Psychodiagnostics Plates] (Rorschach 1921)

(Derivatives:)

Behn-Rorschach Test (Bero) (Zulliger 1941)

Fuchs-Rorschach-Test (Fu-Ro-Test) (Drey-Fuchs 1958)

Zullinger Test (originally Z Test) (Zulliger 1951)

Harrower Blots (Harrower-Erickson 1945)

Kataguchi-Rorschach Test (Ka-Ro) (Kataguchi & Shobo 1970)

Structured-Objective Rorschach Test (SORT) (Stone 1958)

Baughman's New Method of Rorschach Inquiry (Baughman 1958)

Barron's Movement Blots (Barron 1955)

(Non-Rorschach inkblot techniques:)

Holtzman Inkblot Technique (HIT) (Holtzman 1958)

Howard Ink Blot Test (Howard 1953)

Helsingfors Test (Bruhns c1963)

Somatic Inkblot Series (SIS) (Cassell 1980)

Cloud Picture Method (Stern 1937)

Hand Test (HT) (Wagner 1962; revision 1983)

Paired Hands Test (PHT) (Zucker 1968)

[Apperceptive Situations Test] (A-S-T) [German version only] (Laufs 1990)

Columbus Test (Langeveld 1969)

1.3. Auditory

Verbal Summator (=Recorded Auditory Apperception Test) (Skinner 1936)

Tautophone Technique (Rosenzweig 1942)

Auditory Projective Technique (=Azzageddi Test) (Davids & Murray 1955)

Auditory Apperception Test (AAT) (Stone 1953)

2. Construction

2.1. Pictorial stimulus

Thematic Apperception Test (TAT) (Murray 1935)

Children's Apperception Test (C.A.T.) (Bellak & Bellak 1949)

Thompson Modification of the Thematic Apperception Test (T-TAT) (Thompson 1949)

Picture Impressions Test (Libo 1957)

South African Picture Analysis Test (SAPAT) (Nel & Pelser 1960)

Bender Visual Motor Gestalt Test (Bender 1938)

Blacky Pictures (Blum 1947)

Patte Noire (PN) Test (Corman 1961)

Object Relations Technique (ORT) (Phillipson 1955)

Children's Object Relations Technique (CORT) (Wilkinson 1975)

Pickford Projective Pictures (Pickford 1963)

Jackson's Test of Family Attitudes (TFA) (Jackson 1952)

Family Relations Indicator (FRI) (Howells & Lickorish 1962)

Family Story Technique (FST) (Kadushina, Cutlera, Waxenberga & Sagera 1969)

Interpersonal Perception Method (IPM) (Laing, Phillipson & Lee 1966)

Children's Apperceptive Story-Telling Test (CAST) (Schneider 1989)

Children's Hospital Apperception Test (no reference found)

Tell-Me-A-Story (TEMAS) (Costantino Malgady & Rogler 1988)

Make-A-Picture Story Test (MAPS) (Shneidman 1948)

Themes Concerning Blacks (TCB) (Williams 1972)

Visual Apperception Test (VAT) (Khan 1960)

Roberts Apperception Test for Children Test (RATC) (Roberts 1982; revised 2001)

School Apperception Method (S.A.M.) (Solomon & Starr 1968)

School Apperception Story Procedure (SASP) (Jones 2001)

Senior Apperception Technique (S.A.T.) (Bellak & Abrams 1998)

Educational Apperception Test (EAT) (Thompson & Sones 1975)

Pediatric Pain Inventory (Lollar, Smits & Patterson 1982)

Indian Modification of the Thematic Apperception Test (Chowdhury 1967)

Social-Situation Pictures (Schwarz 1932)

Family Apperception Test (FAT) (Sotile, Julian, Henry & Sotile 1988)

Adolescent Apperception Cards (AAC) (Silverton 1993)

Waechter Picture Test (Waechter 1982)

Fairy Tale Test (FTT) (Coulacoglou 1995)

Homosexual Apperception Test (HAT) (Rosenzweig 1940)

Symonds Picture-Story Test (PST) (Symonds 1948)

Tasks of Emotional Development Test (TED Test) (Cohen & Weil 1971)

Michigan Picture Test (MPT) (Andrew, Hartwell, Hutt & Walton 1953; revised 1980)

Adolescent Separation Anxiety Test (Hansburg 1972; modified by Klagsbrun & Bowlby 1976; modified by Main, Kaplan & Cassidy 1985)

Test Filmique Thématique (Cohen-Séat & Rébeillard 1955)

Adoption Story Cards (Gardner 1978)

Projective Story Telling Cards (Caruso 1993)

[Geschichten-Erzähl-Test projektiv (GETp)] (German adaptation of the Projective Story Telling Cards) (Preuß & Landsberg 1996)

Four Picture Test (FPT) (van Lennep 1930)

Symbol Elaboration Test (S.E.T.) (Krout 1950)

Thurston-Cradock Test of Shame (TCTS) (Thurston & Cradock 2009)

Children's Self-Report and Projective Inventory (CSRPI) (Ziffer & Shapiro 1992)

IES (Id, Ego, Super-Ego) Test (Dombrose & Slobin 1958)

Group Personality Projective Test (GPPT) (Cassell & Kahn 1958)

Adult Attachment Projective (AAP) (George, West & Pattem 1997)

2.2. Verbal stimulus

The Insight Test (Sargent 1953)

Schulangst-Test (SAT) (Husslein 1978)

[Fairy Tale Dialogs with Children] (Available in German as: Märchendialoge mit Kindern) (Simon-Wundt 2004)

[Wish Test] (Wilde 1950)

[Ten Wishes Phantasy Game] (available in German as: 10-Wünsche-Phanstasie-Spiel) (Klosinski 1988)

2.3. Computer-based

Self-Administered Global Apperception Scales (SAGAS) (Volcani 2000)

Parent Administered Child Test (PACT) (Volcani 2000)

Multi-person Administered Child Test (M-PACT) (Volcani 2000)

3. Completion

3.1. Verbal or Narrative

Sentence Completion Test (Sachs & Levy 1950)

Washington University Sentence Completion Test (WUSCT) (Loevinger 1948)

Rotter Incomplete Sentences Blank (RISB) (Rotter & Rafferty 1950)

Düss Fable Method (Despert Fables) (Düss 1940; English version Despert 1946; revised and enlarged by Fine 1948)

Madeleine Thomas Completion Stories Test (Thomas 1937; English version Mills 1953)

Munsterburg Incomplete Stories (Munsterberg-Koppitz 1955)

MacArthur Story Stem Battery (MSSB) (Bretherton, Oppenheim, Buchsbaum, Emde & the MacArthur Narrative Work Group 1990)

Rosenzweig Picture Frustration Test (P-F Study) (Rosenzweig 1948)

Punishment Situation Index (PSI) (Morgan & Geier 1957)

Rock-a-bye-Baby (Haworth 1957) [Film]

3.2. Graphic or Drawing

Incomplete Man Test (Gesell 1925)

Drawing Completion Test (Kinget 1952)

Healy Pictorial Completion Test (Healy 1918)

4. Choice or Ordering

4.1. Pictures

Szondi Test (Szondi 1935)

Radke Projective Pictures (Radke 1946)

Iowa Picture Interpretation Test (IPIT) (Hurley 1955)

Tomkins-Horn Picture Arrangement Test (Tomkins 1952)

Welsh Figure Preference Test (WFPT) (=Barron-Welsh Art Scales (BWAS)) (Welsh 1949)

MARI Card Test (Kellogg 1980)

Arrington Visual Preference Test (AVPT) (Arrington 1986)

Full-Range Picture Vocabulary Test (Ammons 1948)

4.2. Human Figures

Family Relations Test (FRT) (Bene-Anthony 1957)

4.3. Symbols

Lüscher Color Test (Lüscher 1947)

Color Pyramid Test (CPT) (Pfister 1950)

Kahn Test of Symbol Arrangement (KTSA) (Kahn 1949)

Design Judgment Test (Graves 1948)

Meier Art Tests I, Art Jugdement (Meier 1942)

Meier Art Tests II, Aesthetic Perception (Meier 1963)

5. Expression

5.1. Drawing

5.1.1. Individual tasks

Draw-a-Man Test (D-A-M) (Goodenough-Harris Drawing Test) (Goodenough 1926)

Draw-A-Person Test (D-A-P) (Machover 1949)

[Man Drawing Test] (German version available as: Mann-Zeichen-Test) (MZT) (Ziler 1949)

House-Tree-Person Projective Drawing Technique (H-T-P) (Buck 1948)

Chromatic House-Tree-Person Drawing Test (Payne 1948)

Kinetic House-Tree-Person Test (Burns 1967)

Kinetic Family Drawing (K-F-D) (Burns & Kaufman 1970)

Kinetic School Drawing (KSD) (Prout and Phillips 1974)

Kinetic Kindergarten Drawing (KKD)

Kinetic Nursery Drawing (KND)

Kinetic Hospital Drawing (KHD) (Dóra 2010)

Kinetic Business Drawing (KBD) (Burns 1987)

Kinetic Political Drawing (KPD) (Burns 1987)

Kinetic Religious Drawing (KRD) (Burn 1987)

Kinetic House-Tree-Person Drawings (K-H-T-P) (Burns 1986)

Family Centered Circle Drawings (F-C-C-D) (Burns 1991)

Kinetic Shop Window Drawing (Burns 1991)

Parent's Self-Centered Circle Drawing (Burns 1990)

Mother-and-Child Drawing (Dewdney & Dewdney 1970)

Family Circles Method (Geddes & Medqay 1977)

Five Step Intervention Method (Vass 2011)

Prospective Kinetic Family Drawing (Kymissis 1992)

Draw-a-Classroom (DAC) (Kutnick 1978)

Draw-a-Group Test (Hare & Hare 1956)

Teacher, Doctor, Policeman (Klepsch 1980)

Human Figure Drawings (HFD) (Klepsch & Logie 1982)

Draw-a-Dog Scale (Levinson & Mezei 1973)

Draw-a-Family (DAF) Test (Hulse 1951)

Corman's Family Drawing (Corman 1964)

Sun Family Drawing (Iten 1980)

Draw-a-Member of a Minority Test (Hammer 1958)

Draw-a-Person in the Rain Test (DAPR) (Abrams in: Hammer 1958)

Most Unpleasant Concept Test (Harrower 1950)

Family Drawing (Appel 1931; Hulse 1952)

Draw-a-Story (DAS) (Silver 1983)

Silver Drawing Test (SDT) (Silver 1983)

Childhood Hand That Disturbs Test (CHaD) (Davido 1994)

Dot-to-Dot (Hays 1979)

Eight card redrawing test (8CRT) (Caligor 1957)

Two Houses Technique (2HT) (Szyrynski 1949)

Star Wave Test (SWT) (Avé-Lallament 1979; English 1984)

Enchanted Family Drawing Test (Kos & Biermann 1973)

Animal Family Drawing (AFD) (Brem-Gräser 1957)

Animal Kinetic Family Drawing (AKFD) (Niesenbaum Jones 1985)

Bird's Nest Drawing (BND) (Kaiser 1996)

Regressed Kinetic Family Drawing (RKFD) (Fürth 1988)

Tree Test (Koch 1952)

Bolander's Tree Drawing Test (Bolander 1977)

Stora's Tree Drawing Test (Stora 1963)

Four Trees Test (undocumented: in Vass 2011)

Three Trees Test (Corboz, Gygax& Helfenstein 1962; Waser 1986)

Tree Family Drawing (Feuer 2005)

Projective Tree Drawing before, during and after a Storm (Miller 1997)

Wartegg Drawing Test (WZT) (Wartegg 1939)

Eight Frame Colored Squiggle Technique (McKim & Steinhardt 1983)

Social Atom (Moreno 1921)

Sociogram (Moreno 1921)

Draw-a-Group Test (Hares 1956)

Dynamic Examination of Drawings (Hárdy 1956)

Rosenberg's Draw-a-Person Technique (Levy 1950)

Projective Road Drawing (Hanes 1995)

Multi-Dimensional Drawing Task (MDDT) (Bloch 1968)

Personal Sphere Model (Schmiedek 1973)

Finger Painting (Kadis 1950)

5.1.2. Squiggles

Squiggle Technique / Game (Winnicott 1971)

Scribble Test (Winnicott 1971; Cane 1983)

Meurisse Scribble Test (Meurisse 1948)

Grätz Scribble Test (Grätz 1978)

Vass Scribble Test (Vass 2008)

Kutasch and Gehl Scribble Test (Graphomotor Projection Technique) (

5.1.3. Group drawings

Collaborative Drawing Technique (CDT) (Smith 1985)

Joint Family Holiday Drawing Technique (Jordan 2001)

Drawing Together Method (DTM) (Nagy 2007)

5.2. Blocks and bricks

Lowenfeld Mosaic Test (LMT) (Lowenfeld 1951)

Manikin Construction Task (Cox & Parkin 1986)

5.3. Theater/Play/Psychodrama

Psychodrama (Moreno 1930s)

5.4. Figurine Positioning

World Technique (Lowenfeld 1929)

World Test (=Toy World Test) (Bühler 1936)

Picture World Test (PWT) (Bühler & Manson 1956)

Bolgar-Fischer Little World Test (Bolgar & Fischer 1940)

Village Test (Arthus 1949)

Imaginary Village (Mucchielli 1960)

Dramatic Productions Test (DPT) (Homberger [=Erikson] 1938)

Erica Method (Harding & Danielson c1934)

Sandplay Therapy (Kalff 1950s, published 1966)
Expressive Sandwork (Pattis Zoja, Lan, Shen & Thom 2002)
Sceno Test (von Staabs 1938, published 1964)
5.5. Playing arts
Floor Games (Wells 1911)
Little Wars (Wells 1913)
[Children's World Test] (German version only available as: Kinder-Welt-Test) (KWT) (Baulig & Baulig 2006)
Miniature figure play with the PlaymoCase (Plämokasten) (Ärztliche Akademie für Psychotherapie von Kindern und Jugendlichen, Munich, 2013; revision 2015)
Structured Doll Play Test (SDT) (Lynn 1957)

Table 1. Overview of projective methods.

Aim: The test aims at detecting the level of intellectual abilities, and was intended as test for school entry qualification. It gives information about the developmental status and the self-esteem of a child. The DAP depends on visual perception, the spatial organization of apperception and the coordination of visual and motor skills.

Age: not limited, best from 3 to 14, but it is advisable not to use the test on children 11+.

Time: not specified, but 10–15 min seem to be sufficient

Scores/norms: 1651 drawings from children [50], in the revised edition, 1125 children aged 3–14 [51].

Only a poor correlation has been found to intelligence tests [52, 53], thus the DAP should *not* be used instead of an intelligence test.

Publication date: 1926 (revised 1963).

References: [42, 49, 51, 54].

3.1.2. House-Tree-Person projective drawing technique (H-T-P)

Description: The child is instructed to draw "a house, a tree, and a person" without further specification which house, which tree, or which person is meant. Then the child is invited to explain the drawings.

Aim: The test aims at measuring personality traits, brain damage and general mental functioning, and developmental psychopathology.

Age: 3+.

Time: Not specified, but 10–15 min should be sufficient.

Scores/norms: N/A.

Publication date: 1970.

References: [55].

3.1.3. Kinetic Family Drawing (K-F-D)

Description: The child is asked to draw a picture of its family, including themselves, "doing something," which is meant to give the kinetic aspect.

Aim: The test intends to describe the child's attitudes toward the family members and the family dynamics.

Ages: Not specified.

Time: Not specified, but mostly, 15 min seem sufficient.

Scores/norms: N/A.

Publication date: 1987.

References: [56].

3.1.4. Star Wave Test (SWT)

Description: The child is instructed to "draw a starry sky above sea waves."

Aim: The test aims at detecting developmental retardation and psychopathology. It can be applied in children with various cultural backgrounds.

Age: 3+.

Time: Not specified, but 10–15 min seem to be sufficient.

Scores/norms: N/A.

Publication date: 1994.

References: [57].

3.1.5. Enchanted family drawing test

Description: The child is asked "to put the members of a family under the spell of a magician, without any limits being set on the child's imagination in the choice of objects to be drawn [58]." Then the child is invited to tell a story about the spell and its casting.

Aim: The test aims at describing the family system and revealing psychic conflicts of the child.

Age: 3+.

Time: Not specified, but 15–20 min should be sufficient.

Scores/norms: Statistical data are available on 4000 drawings from children and adolescents, of which 1562 had behavioral, neurotic, or psychosomatic issues [58].

Publication date: 1973.

References: [58, 59].

Note: Care should be taken with regard to the cultural background of the child with regard to magical experiences (see Section 1).

3.1.6. Tree test

Description: The child is instructed to "draw a tree" without further specifications.

Aim: The test aims at detecting personality traits. It is linked to intelligence and developmental status.

Age: 6+.

Time: 5–10 min.

Scores/norms: Formal aspects of the tree like root, trunk, branches, and treetop. Additional features like fruit, leaves, or fauna (bird, squirrels) are noted.

There are quantitative and qualitative valid data available, based on 1800 tree drawings [60].

Publication date: 1952.

References: [61, 62].

3.1.7. Wartegg drawing test (WZT)

Description: The proband is given a standardized sheet containing eight square fields with a stimulus in each of the squares (lines, dots). The proband is instructed to complete the stimuli to drawings. The proband is asked to describe each drawing and give a title to each square.

Aim: The test aims at discovering "innerpsychic layers," which are thought to constitute a person's character and to describe the proband's personality structure.

Age: Not specified.

Time: 20–30 min.

Scores/norms: Sequence of drawings and time used, "profile of [innerpsychic] layers," "profile of qualities," "quantitative dominant feature," "qualitative relation of poles," "structure of the picture," "characterologic projection."

Publication date: 1939.

References: [63–65].

Note: The test is not based on a common theoretical basis and does show several critical issues [66, 67].

3.1.8. Winnicott's squiggle technique

Description: The therapist begins with drawing a squiggle (any abstract figure, line, scheme, or pictorial element) on a sheet of paper. Then the child is asked to "make a picture out of it." The picture should be a drawing and should not contain numbers or letters, but there is no strict interdiction. Then roles are reversed and the child starts with a squiggle, which the therapist completes. Both can give verbal comments about the drawing.

It is useful to use two different colors for the child and the therapist, respectively, to discriminate between the contributions.

Aim: The test aims at enhancing in-depth communication between the child and therapist and access unconscious parts of the proband.

Age: 7+ (or earlier).

Time: not limited.

Scores/norms: None.

Publication date: 1971.

References: [68, 69].

3.2. Verbal description and imagination

3.2.1. Thematic Apperception Test (TAT)

Description: The proband is presented 8–12 black-and-white picture cards out of a set of 32 cards, 31 of these showing various persons in ambiguous situations, one card is completely blank. The cards are numbered and some contain letters for presenting these cards only to specific subgroups: B for boys, G for girls, M for male (14+), and F for female (14+). The proband is asked to create "dramatic" story for the pictures shown with regard to the story shown, the depicted persons' feelings and thoughts, and the possible solution of the story.

Aim: This test aims at describing personality traits and neurotic personalities.

Age: 4+.

Time: Not specified.

Scores/norms: There are several scoring systems available for the TAT, including the analysis of defense mechanisms [70, 71].

Scoring systems have been proposed like SCORs [72] and SCORS-Q [73].

Murray [37] suggested the following six aspects: Who is the main person of the story? What are the motives, aspirations, and emotions of the main person ("needs" in the original)? What is the influence of the social environment on the main person ("presses" in the original)? What is the solution, or the ending, of the story? What is the theme with regard of the "needs," "presses," and the ending of the story? Which interests and emotions are expressed by the narrator?

Publication date: 1943.

References: [37].

3.2.2. Children's Apperception Test (CAT)

Description: Based on the Thematic Apperception Test (TAT), the CAT adapts the pictures presented. The child is presented 10 pictures of social scenes, where the figures are represented as animals. The child is asked to create a narrative out of each picture.

Aim: The test aims at assessing personality, the level of maturity, and mental health.

Age: 3–10.

Time: 20–45 min.

Scores/norms: Several scoring systems have been proposed [see overview in 74].

Publication date: 1949.

References: [75].

3.2.3. Tell-Me-A-Story Test (TEMAS)

Description: The TEMAS (the Spanish word for themes) is a multicultural narrative test based on 23 colored picture test cards presenting social situations. Eleven of the cards are gender specific. The minority cards show predominantly Hispanic and Black individuals, while the nonminority cards depict mostly nonminority people. The child is presented the set of cards and asked to create a narrative of the situation depicted.

Aim: The test aims at screening both minority and nonminority children for emotional and behavior problems.

Age: 5–18.

Time: Not specified.

Scores/norms: The test scores 9 personality aspects: interpersonal relations, aggression, anxiety and depression, achievement and motivation, delay of gratification, self-concept, sexual identity, moral judgment, reality testing, and functions not pulled; 7 affects: Happy, sad, angry, fearful, neutral, ambivalent, inappropriate affect; and 18 cognitive functions including reaction time, total time, inquiries, fluency, omissions, sequencing, imagination, relationships, transformations, and conflicts.

Normative tables for white, black, Puerto Rican, and other Hispanic children and adolescents are available. Data are based on 600 children (aged 5–13 years).

Publication date: 1982.

References: [76, 77].

3.2.4. Fairy Tale Test (FTT)

Description: The test material contains 21 cards in 7 sets of 3 cards each. The child is presented the 3 cards of the set and asked questions specified in the manual.

The 7 sets of cards show Little Red Riding Hood (2 sets), Snow White and the Seven Dwarfs, and characters of witches, dwarfs, wolves, and giants.

Aim: The FTT can be used to assess the child's personality dynamics, including personality traits, and their interrelations. "The FTT can be effectively employed for: (1) personality assessment for research purposes (developmental, cross cultural and longitudinal studies), (2) diagnostic evaluation of clinical studies (severe psychopathology or disturbance as an outcome of ephemeral traumatic or stressful events, and (3) evaluation of psychotherapeutic treatment [78]."

Age: 6–12.

Time: about 45 min.

Scores/norms: Quantitative interpretation of 30 variables in six categories: impulses (9 items), desires (3), needs (5), ego functions (8), emotional states (3), and object relations (2). These comprehend: adaptation of content, unusual measures, relation to the mother, relation to the father, fear of aggressions, fears, desire for superiority, dominant aggression, oral needs, oral aggression, sense of property, desire of material wealth, desire for affection, aggression type A (exploiting, nonemotional, nonaroused), defensive aggression, envious aggression, retaliative aggression, sense of belonging, altruism, ambivalence, depression, self-esteem, moral, need for protection, sexuality, and repetitions.

Qualitative interpretation evaluates defense mechanisms, family dynamics, anxiety, and Ego functioning with synthetic-integrative functioning, regulation and control of impulses, mastery, and judgment and the quality of thought process.

Standardization is available for the FTT from data of 760 children aged 7–12 in a first study, and 873 children aged 6–7 in a second study.

Publication date: 1995.

References: [79].

3.2.5. Rorschach inkblot technique

Description: The proband is presented 10 inkblot tables in a standardized order. At the first sight, all tables seem to be symmetrical. Some of the tables are colored, some are depicted in grayscale. The proband is asked to describe what is seen on the plates. There is no limit in the answers with regard to number, or time.

Aim: Originally, Rorschach envisioned the use of plates as a diagnostic tool for schizophrenia. Later, the Rorschach inkblot technique aimed at describing and classifying personality traits of the proband.

Age: 5+.

Time: Not specified.

Scores/norms: There are several scoring systems available, which are all based on the same categories, including location (whole responses, detail responses with tiny details, edge details, interior details, and rare details, and space responses), determinants (responses relying to form, movement, color, shading, achromatic color, texture, chiaroscuro [=distribution of light and shade], "X-ray," variations of shading, reflection, pair) and content (human, animal, anatomy, human, and animal objects, "objects," "pathognomonic," and disturbing, popular and original) [36, p. 24–51, 80, 81]. One of the most elaborated scoring systems is the "Exner system" aka "Comprehensive System [82–84]."

Publication date: 1921.

References: [13, 85].

3.2.6. *Holtzman inkblot test/technique (HIT)*

Description: The proband is presented 45 plates containing inkblots after 2 trial blots, and asked to produce a single response per blot. There are two independent forms (A, B) available.

Aim: The HIT aims at describing and classifying the personality of the proband.

Age: 5+.

Time: Not specified.

Scores/norms: The scoring system is based on 22 variables in 6 clusters (or "dimensions), including "movement, integration, human, barrier, popular, color, shading, form definiteness (reversed), pathognomonic verbalization, anxiety, hostility, movement, form appropriateness, location, reaction time, rejection, animal (reversed), penetration, anatomy, and sex [86]." Norms are available from 1400 individuals without psychopathology, schizophrenia, depression, and mental retardation.

Publication date: 1961.

References: [87].

3.2.7. *Rotter incomplete sentences blank (RISB)*

Description: The proband is presented a list of 40 incomplete short sentences, consisting of 1–2 word sentences. The proband is asked to complete the respective sentence.

Aim: The RISB is described as a screening instrument for adolescents and adults and aims at measuring adjustment.

Age: There are three different forms available, one for school children, one for college students, and one for adults.

Time: 20–40 min.

Scores/norms: A scoring system has been developed on a scale from 0 to 6 for each answer according to empirically derived answers for males and females. Norms have been provided for college students [88].

Publication date: 1950 (revised 1992).

References: [89, 90].

3.2.8. Hand test

Description: The proband is shown 10 picture cards showing line drawings of a hand in various positions. The cards are administered one after another and the proband is asked to explain what each hand is doing.

Aim: measure action tendencies, especially acting-out and aggressive behavior in children and adults.

Age: 5+.

Time: 10 min.

Scores/norms: Means, cut-off scores, and typical score ranges for normal and various diagnostic groups are provided. Quantitative scores comprise aggression, exhibition, communication, dependence, acquisition, tension, and withdrawal, whereas qualitative scores aim at discovering underlying feelings and motivations. Six summary scores, including an index of overall pathology and an acting-out ratio, are provided. The latter is used to predict aggressive behavior.

Publication date: 1962.

References: [91, 92].

3.2.9. Family Relations Test (FRT)

Description: The test material consists of 20 stereotypic figure shapes made out of paper/cardboard. These figures represent persons of different age and function, e.g. child, parent(s), grandparent(s), and most importantly, the "Nobody" figure. There is a small container attached to the figures, in which the child can place tokens, or the small question cards.

The child is first asked to pick the relevant figures of his/her family, and is then asked questions about family members, for example, questions like "This person in the family is very nice to me." Then the child is asked to place the card with the question into the box attached to the figure shape.

Aim: The FRT has been used in questions of child welfare, child protection, and family placement.

Age: 3–7, 7–15 (2 versions).

Time: 30 min.

Scores/norms: For scoring, the number(s) of each card is noted with regard to the respective figure chosen. The interpretation is based on "incoming" (*from* the person) and "outgoing" (*towards* the person) attitudes, or feelings.

Normalization is available for British [93] and German children, aged 4.0–5.11 [94] and 6.0–11.11 [95].

Publication date: 1957.

References: [96, 97].

3.2.10. Patte Noire (PN) test [Schweinchen-Schwarzfuß-Test (SFT)]

Description: The test material consists of 16 pictures of a piglet, named "Patte Noire" (French for black foot), which serves as identification figure. Members of the pig family (mother, father, and siblings), other animals, and humans are shown.

The child is shown all picture cards, asked to pick some, or all, pictures, and to create a story out of these pictures. Preferred and rejected pictures are noted.

Special care should be taken with regard to cultural and religious attributions to pigs. For example, using this test with Moslem or Jewish children may not give valid results.

Aim: The test aims at detecting drive tendencies and defense mechanisms in a psychoanalytical interpretation.

Age: 7–13.

Time: 60–90 min.

Scores/norms: Psychoanalytic themes can be identified due to developmental stages, typical conflicts such as sibling rivalry.

Publication date: 1969.

References: [20, 98].

Note: Deliberate care should be taken applying this test to children with Islamic or Jewish background, where pigs are regarded as impure.

3.2.11. Madeleine Thomas completion stories test

Description: The proband is presented with 15 story stems, and is asked to complete the story.

Aim: The test aims at describing the child's attitude towards the presented fields, for example such as family and living conditions, school and learning situation, interaction with peers, and the fantasy life of an identification figure (presented as a boy or girl of the same age and sex as the proband).

Age: 3+.

Time: Not specified.

Scores/norms: Not available.

Publication date: 1937.

References: [24, 99].

3.2.12. Düss fable method (Despert fables)

Description: The proband is presented 10 story stems, some with animal characters (thus the test is called fable method). The proband is asked to complete the story.

Later the stories have been expanded to 20.

Aim: The method aims at presenting a psychoanalytic access to the child's main themes. The interpretation may give information about structure, conflicts, and relations.

In the later version, a categorization of themes including "dependency, hostility, identification, sibling rivalry, Oedipal issues, and fears" [45, p. 84] has been added.

Age: Not specified.

Time: Not specified.

Scores/norms: Not available.

Publication date: 1940 [French], 1946 [English].

References: [25, 100, 101].

3.2.13. Rosenzweig Picture Frustration test (PFT)

Description: The PFT consists of 24 sketches of a situation, in which one person tells another person a frustrating sentence in a speech bubble. The other speech bubble is empty, and the proband is instructed to fill out a suitable answer.

Aim: The PFT aims at describing a person's frustration tolerance.

Age: 6–14 (child version), 14–85 (adult version).

Time: 15–20 min.

Scores/norms: A frustrations profile can be depicted, containing aggressive reactions, self-incrimination, resignation, evasive manoeuvres, and personal initiative.

There are norms available from 320 probands containing quartiles and median values.

Publication date: 1957.

References: [27].

3.2.14. MacArthur Story Stem Battery (MSSB)

Description: The material in the MSSB consists of human miniature figures, for example, bendable dolls, or Playmobil® figures. The figures should include "mother, father, grandmother, older and younger siblings [...], additional children [...], and a family dog. It is important that the figures can stand up and that they match the child's racial background if human figures are used [26]." Additional material can be provided, such as furniture, dishes, etc.

Then the child is presented the beginning of one of 14 "story stems," all dealing with moral and relationship dilemmas. The child is asked to "show and tell what happens next." The answers are videotaped and rated later on.

Aim: The story stem techniques aims at creating a narrative of specific interpersonal situations. It has been used in attachment studies as well as in mood disorders, or aggressive behaviour.

Age: 4–8 (but other ages may also be included).

Time: Not specified.

Scores/norms: Several approaches for rating scales have been developed with regard to "(1) story content or themes, (2) theme organization or coherence, (3) emotional expression, and (4) interaction with the interviewer," [26] for example the MacArthur Research Network on Early Childhood Transitions (1983–1992, www.macfound.org), published the MacArthur Narrative Coding System (MNCS) [102].

Publication date: 1992.

References: [103, 104].

3.3. Playing arts

3.3.1. Lowenfeld Mosaic Test (LMT)

Description: The test contains of five colored wooden shapes: square, isosceles triangle, equilateral triangle, scalene triangle, and rhomboid. Each shape is available in red, blue, yellow, black, green, and white and arranged in a box in this order. Then the box is presented to the child together with a tray containing white paper. Recently, templates have been provided with different patterns, which may be useful for younger children, or for standardization purposes.

Aim: The LMT has been used to assess mental ability and developmental state, school readiness, mental disorders like schizophrenia and traumatic brain injury. It can be applied for assessing the functional capability of patients or clients, or as a tool for the expression of an inner world. The LMT has been used for diagnostics and psychotherapy. Moreover, it has been used in anthropological studies, as a means on nonverbal communication.

Age: Not specified.

Time: Not specified.

Scores/norms: The picture can be seen under the aspects of the individuality of the answer [105]. The child is asked to describe the picture, for example, it representation, or abstract pattern, with regard to its meaning. Additionally, the way of choosing the material and composing the picture is of interest.

Publication date: 1950.

References: [28, 106, 107].

3.3.2. Structured doll play test (SDP)

Description: The test consists of pictures of backgrounds and furniture and cardboard figures of a doll family. The child is presented with 18 structured situations and asked to make behavioral choices.

Aim: The test aims at finding mature and immature behavioral responses as well as at identifying.

Age: 3–11.

Time: Not specified.

Scores/norms: Not available.

Publication date: 1959.

References: [30, 108].

3.3.3. Sceno test

Description: The Sceno test consists of 16 doll-like figurines of different sex and age (8 adults and 8 children), animals (chicken, crocodile, and a big cow), wooden bricks, small dishes, a train, a deck chair, a lavatory and several others.

The child is instructed to build "a scene, as on stage, or for a movie" on the tray provided.

Aim: The Sceno aims at depicting relations and conflicts of the child's inner and outer world. It can be used to assess mental ability, psychodynamics of relations, conflicts, and structure.

Age: 3+.

Time: Not specified.

Scores/norms: The Sceno Test can be evaluated with regard to the playing behavior (attitude, presentation, verbal accompaniment, attention and "flow," handling of the material), final scene (formal aspects like number of figures used, order of the tray, relation of the figures) and the following exploration of the child (reality, desire, and fears).

Data on several hundreds of patients are available [summarized in 109], mainly children with behavioral disorders, organic brain disease, or "neurotic" and psychosomatic disturbances [110]. There are data available on reliability, validity and objectivity of the test.

Publication date: 1951 [1938].

References: [109, 111–113].

3.3.4. Children's World test [Kinder-Welt-Test] (KWT)

Description: The Children's World test consists of nine themes (family, school, fairy tales, science fiction, warriors, wildlife animals, domestic animals, water world, and rescue and help). The material is mostly from Playmobil® (figures and animals), supplemented with wooden blocks and fence posts. (The manual describes 31 blocks, but this is not apodictic: 19 larger blocks, 8 blocks with holes, and 4 fencing posts.)

The theoretical basis of this test is the gestalt therapy, and systemic approaches.

Aim: The tests aims at describing the formal storyline, the choice of the theme in the context of actual and biographical data, formal aspects of the gestalt therapy with regard to a polarity profile [114].

Age: 4–13.

Time: max. 30 min.

Scores/norms: Not available.

Publication date: 2006.

References: [115].

3.3.5. World technique/sandplay therapy/expressive sandwork

Description: In the 1920s, Margaret Lowenfeld developed a method later called the World technique, which uses sand trays, miniature figures, models, and toys to express feelings and thoughts without words.

In the 1950s, Dora M. Kalff transferred some aspects of the World technique into the Sandplay therapy. Now, the sand tray is standardized ($72 \times 57 \times 7$ cm^3), but the material used in the sand is not specified. Mostly, each therapist collects material on his / her own. Miniaturied figures of human and super-human beings, animals, plants and woods, inanimate nature like rocks and stones, fossils, or shells, can be found. The theoretical background is laid on the work of C. G. Jung.

In the 1990s, the term expressive sandwork was created.

Aim: The aim of these techniques is to create and activate an imaginal realm in which the unconscious can be expressed symbolically. In a nonverbal, nondirective approach, a sand image is created, containing archetypal, symbolic, and interpersonal elements of the inner and outer world.

Age: Not specified, but 3+ recommended.

Time: Not specified.

Scores/norms: Not applicable.

Publication date: 1929 (World Technique), 1980 (Sandplay Therapy); 2002 (Expressive Sandwork).

References: [31, 32, 116].

3.3.6. Miniature figure play with the PlaymoCase (Plämokasten)

Description: The PlaymoCase [Plämokasten] is composed of plastic figures from Playmobil® sets. The figures are sorted thematically in three levels in a metal case.

Level 1 contains humans, subdivided in men, women, adolescents, children, a royal family, knights, pirates, American Indians, fantasy figures like ghosts, a mummy, a fairy, goblins, and unicorns. Then there are wildlife and zoo animals, like deer, elephants, apes, giraffes, a camel, fish, a shark, lions and tigers, a crocodile, and farm and domestic animals like horses, cows, pigs, sheep, chicken, rabbits, hedgehogs, squirrels, dogs, and cats.

Level 2 contains boxes and baskets, trees, fences, material for a construction site, a garden, furniture from a living room, and objects from a household, like knives, spoons, forks, and dishes. Then there is a treasure, weapons, carpets, flowers, and alimentary goods. Next, furniture from a kitchen and a bedroom is provided. Next a classroom and a room in a pediatric hospital.

Level 3 contains larger components like plastic bases for a fortress, the jungle, and the construction site.

In a nondirective play therapy approach, the child is free to choose any material required from the case.

Aim: The case can be used for diagnostic and therapeutic purposes. The technique aims at providing a projective space for the child to create a scene or sequence of its unconscious. Moreover, an interaction with the therapist is possible, enabling interpretation and dialogue.

Age: 3+.

Time: Not specified or restricted. An individual session can last the whole hour of therapy.

Scores/norms: Not available. Currently, an empirical clinical study is being initiated to address this question.

Publication date: 2013.

References: [19, 117].

4. Projective approaches in play therapy

In the previous section, we have seen the use of projective techniques for diagnostic purposes. Additionally, projection is an important means of therapy. Hence, specific therapeutic approaches have been developed making use of the mechanisms of projection. These approaches include psychoanalysis, imaginary therapies, and play therapy. Whereas play therapy is seldomly used in the counseling of adult patients, it seems to be a standard procedure in child therapy, often even implicitly, meaning that sometimes the therapist is not aware of the projective (and counter-projective) elements in the therapy. In the definition of the Association for Play Therapy (APT, www.a4pt.org), play therapy is "the systematic use of a theoretical model to establish an interpersonal process wherein trained play therapists use the therapeutic powers of play to help clients prevent or resolve psychosocial difficulties and achieve optimal growth and development [118]." In the following section, we will concentrate on play therapy and describe several projective techniques in play therapy.

4.1. Typical forms of children's play

Child's play has been grouped in to different subtypes [46] such as (i) toy and object-based play, for example using balls, dolls, or puppets, (ii) narrative plays, such as story-telling and reading / book-based approaches, (iii) role-playing, including costumes and masks, (iv) creative arts, which comprehends drawing, painting, sculpting, for example with clay, wood, or stone, dancing, or playing music instruments, (v) fantasy approaches using figurines and miniature world material, and (vi) game play techniques such as strategy and cooperative games, squiggles, or chance games involving boards and cards.

In our view, there is a certain overlap in play therapy approaches, since the before mentioned definition is based on objects or material, not methods. Despite the respective approaches chosen, projection can occur with all of these.

4.2. Projection in child play

In the early twentieth century, play therapy was developed by psychoanalysts in the context of psychoanalysis for children, since it has become obvious that a "talking cure" based on a highly developed system of speech to express-free associations was not suitable for the therapy of children.

In a main assumption of the psychodynamic theory, intrapsychic elements are projected onto outer objects such as play material, especially figurines [119]. This, for example, opens the way for identification and, thus, projective identification. Of note, there is a clear difference between identification processes and the interpretation of the therapist [120]. Even "obvious" scenes occurring during play may have a totally different origin and background. Therefore, it is wise for the therapist not to provide interpretation of the patient's creation, but to reveal its meaning for and with the patient. For example, the therapist's interpretation based on (counter-) projection and projective identification, in a technique making use of externalization in cases of domestic violence or sexual abuse, and anorexia nervosa, may trivialize and minimize the problem, and may lead to misinterpretation [121].

Children make use of figurines for example to describe the dynamics in their relationships to their parents, siblings, friends and classmates, teachers, and other people of their world. Moreover, figurines give the child the possibility to externalize different inner self-objects and attribute their properties to different characters.

Play is not only an ethological component of child development, but also a therapeutic tool. A number of therapeutic factors of play have been identified and described as the "Therapeutic Powers of Play [122]." These include play as a form of self-expression and nonverbal communication, a possibility of gaining access to the unconscious, a direct and indirect form of teaching, a possibility for stress inoculation, a method for counter-conditioning of negative effects, abreaction and catharsis, chance of the creation of positive effects, the enhancement of attachment and amelioration of relationships, the development of moral judgment, empathy, and sublimation, the exertion of power and control, mastery, the increase of competence and self-control, a growing sense of self, developmental acceleration, encouraging creative problem solving, fantasy compensation, reality testing, behavioral rehearsal, and rapport building [122, 123].

4.3. Special forms of play therapy using projective mechanisms

In general, two main approaches in play therapy can be distinguished. Directive play therapy describes interventions in which the therapist initiates and structures the patients play activities, whereas nondirective play therapy approaches leaves the responsibility and direction of the play during each session to the patient [124]. Both approaches enable projection as a mechanism to address intrapsychic issues, but in general nondirective approaches makes the occurrence of projective mechanisms much easier. Moreover, in psychodynamic therapies, projection is necessary for the technique applied. A not exhaustive overview over current forms of play therapies is presented in **Table 2**.

In the following sections, two approaches are described in more detail, sandplay therapy, and a form of psychodynamic play therapy.

1. Psychodynamic Therapies
Psychoanalytic Play Therapy (A. Freud, M. Klein, D. W. Winnicott)
Adlerian Play Therapy (A. Adler)
Jungian Play Therapy (C. G. Jung)
Sandplay Therapy (D. Kalff)
2. Person-Centered (nondirective) Play Therapy
Child-Centered Play Therapy (V. Axline)
Relationship Play Therapy (C. Moustakas)
Experiential Play Therapy (B. Norton, C. Norton)
3. Other Forms
Gestalt Play Therapy (F. Perls, V. Oaklander)
Art Therapy
Ecosystemic Play Therapy (K. O'Connor)
Ericksonian Play Therapy (M. Erickson)
Solution-Focused Play Therapy (M. Selekman)
Animal-Assisted Play Therapy (AAPT)
4. Behavioral Play Therapy
Cognitive-Behavioral Play Therapy (CBPT) (S. M. Knell)
Parent-child Interaction Therapy (PCIT) (T. L. Hembree-Kigin, C. B. Mcneil)
5. Systemic (Family) Play Therapy
Dynamic Family Play Therapy (S. Harvey)
Strategic Family Play Therapy (S. Ariel)
Family Play Therapy for young children (T. G. Hardaway, L. Carey, E. F. Wachtel)
6. Preschool Children Play Therapy
Filial Therapy (FT) (B. Gurney, L. Gurney)
Developmental Play Therapy (DPT) (V. A. Brody)
Theraplay (A. M. Jernberg, P. B. Booth)

Table 2. Forms of play therapy (compiled from [10, 124, 125]).

4.3.1. World technique/sandplay therapy/expressive sandwork

Description: In the 1920s, Margaret Lowenfeld developed a method later called the World Technique, which uses sand trays, miniature figures, models, and toys to express feelings and thoughts without words.

In the 1950s, Dora M. Kalff transferred some aspects of the World Technique into the Sandplay Therapy. Now, the sand tray is standardized ($72 \times 57 \times 7$ cm^3), but the material used in the sand is not specified. Mostly, each therapist collects material on his/her own. Miniaturized figures of human and super-human beings, animals, plants and woods, inanimate nature like rocks and stones, fossils, or shells, can be found. The theoretical background is laid on the work of C. G. Jung.

In the 1990s, the term expressive sandwork was created. It is based on the assumption that any sand tray creation is an expression of the client's inner world.

Aim: The aim of these techniques is to create and activate an imaginal realm in which the unconscious can be expressed symbolically. In a nonverbal, nondirective approach, a sand image is created, containing archetypal, symbolic, and interpersonal elements of the inner and outer world.

Age: Not specified, but 3+ recommended.

Time: Not specified.

Scores/norms: Not applicable.

Publication date: 1929 (World Technique), 1980 (Sandplay Therapy); 2002 (Expressive Sandwork).

References: [31, 32, 116].

4.3.2. Psychodynamic play therapy with miniature figures using the PlaymoCase (Plämokasten)

Description: The PlaymoCase [Plämokasten] is composed of plastic figures from Playmobil® sets. The figures are sorted thematically in three levels in a metal case.

Level 1 contains humans, subdivided in men, women, adolescents, children, a royal family, knights, pirates, American Indians, fantasy figures like ghosts, a mummy, a fairy, goblins, unicorns. Then there are wildlife and zoo animals, like deer, elephants, apes, giraffes, a camel, fish, a shark, lions and tigers, a crocodile, and farm and domestic animals like horses, cows, pigs, sheep, chicken, rabbits, hedgehogs, squirrels, dogs, and cats.

Level 2 contains boxes and baskets, trees, fences, material for a construction site, a garden, furniture from a living room, and objects from a household, like knives, spoons, forks, and dishes. Then there is a treasure, weapons, carpets, flowers, and alimentary goods. Next, furniture from a kitchen and a bedroom is provided. Next a classroom and a room in a pediatric hospital.

Level 3 contains larger components like plastic bases for a fortress, the jungle, and the construction site.

In a nondirective play therapy approach, the child is free to choose any material required from the case.

Aim: The case can be used for diagnostic and therapeutic purposes. The technique aims at providing a projective space for the child to create a scene or sequence of its unconscious. Moreover, an interaction with the therapist is possible, enabling interpretation and dialogue.

Age: 3+.

Time: Not specified or restricted. An individual session can last the whole hour of therapy.

Scores/norms: Not available. Currently, an empirical clinical study is being initiated to address this question.

Publication date: 2013.

References: [19, 117].

5. Discussion and conclusions

Projective methods are widely used tools in the assessment of child and adolescent mental health. Whereas in adult assessment, projective techniques lost their predominant position over the last decades [126–129], they are in second position in child and adolescent outpatient clinics after intelligence testing [130]. Moreover, the discussion about the psychometric properties of projective tests is unsolved. With regard to the literature, one must carefully address each test: there are tests with excellent validation parameters, large study samples, normalization data, and standardized evaluation, whereas others remain obscure in technique and interpretation and provide unsound results.

The classification of projective tests has been stable since more than 50 years, but there is a certain shift and extension towards the use of computers from the paper-and-pencil–based approaches. Surprisingly, the stimulus material did not change over the years, sometimes there is revised material (for example, modern plastic figurines instead of dolls, or updated pictorial material in thematic apperceptive tests), but in general, the basic principles associated with the material remains constant.

The theoretical background of projective methods has been enlarged by both the expansion of the psychoanalytic theories and neurobiological findings, such as mirror neurons as morphological basis of the mechanisms of mentalization [131]. Moreover, the field of affective neuroscience provided evidence for the neuroanatomical location of drives through emotional circuits, corresponding to Freud's concept of the dynamic unconscious [132].

With regard to therapy, projection is the main mechanism in play therapy approaches. Having introduced the concepts of play therapy, two forms of play therapy approaches are described in detail. In this sense, projection is also the main constitute of a therapeutic agent.

In conclusion, projective methods provide useful methods for the assessment of psychological questions when appropriately used. Novel standardization of psychodynamic processes can help to reevaluate the benefit of projective methods.

Author details

Martin H. Maurer

Address all correspondence to: martin.maurer@alumni.uni-heidelberg.de

University of Heidelberg, Heidelberg, Germany

References

[1] Freud S. On the grounds for detaching a particular syndrome from neurasthenia as "anxiety-neurosis". Internationale Zeitschrift für Ärztliche Psychoanalyse. 1913 (1895);1 (4):359–62.

[2] Murstein BI, Pryer RS. The Concept of Projection: A Review. Psychol Bull. 1959;56 (5):353–74.

[3] Freud S. Totem and Taboo. Leipzig, Wien: Hugo Heller; 1913.

[4] Horney K. New Ways in Psychoanalysis. New York, NY: Norton; 1939.

[5] Lilienfeld SO, Wood JM, Garb HN. The scientific status of projective techniques. Psychol Sci Public Interest. 2000 Nov;1(2):27–66.

[6] Hibbard S. A critique of Lilienfeld et al.'s (2000) "The scientific status of projective techniques". J Pers Assess. 2003 Jun;80(3):260–71.

[7] Freud S. Selbstdarstellung. In: Grote LR, ed. *Die Medizin der Gegenwart in Selbstdarstellungen*. Leipzig: Felix Meiner; 1925.

[8] Freud S. Zur Psychopathologie des Alltagslebens. Über Vergessen, Versprechen, Vergreifen, Aberglaube und Irrtum. Berlin: S. Karger; 1904.

[9] Stross L, Shevrin H. Hypnosis as a method for investigating unconscious thought processes. A review of research. J Am Psychoanal Assoc. 1969 Jan;17(1):100–35.

[10] von Gontard A, Lehmkuhl G. Play therapy—psychotherapy with play as the medium: I. General introduction, psychoanalytic and client-centered approaches. Praxis der Kinderpsychologie und Kinderpsychiatrie. 2003;52(1):35–48.

[11] The OPD Task Force, Resch F, Romer G, Schmeck K, Seiffge-Krenke I, eds. OPD-CA-2 operationalized psychodynamic diagnosis in childhood and adolescence. Theoretical Basis and User Manual. Boston, MA: Hogrefe; 2016.

[12] American Psychiatric Association, ed. Diagnostic and Statistical Manual of Mental Disorders (DSM-5). Arlington, VA: American Psychiatric Association Publishing; 2013.

[13] Schafer R. Psychoanalytic interpretation in Rorschach testing: theory and application. New York: Grune & Stratton; 1954.

[14] Schafer R. Some applications of contemporary psychoanalytic theory to projective testing. J Proj Tech. 1954 Dec;18(4):441–7.

[15] Lindzey G. Projective Techniques and Cross-Cultural Research. New York: Appleton-Century-Crofts; 1961.

[16] Kernberg OF. Object-Relations Theory and Clinical Psychoanalysis. New York: Jason Aronson; 1976.

[17] Kohut H. The Analysis of the Self. New York, NY: International University Press; 1971.

[18] St. Claire M. Object Relations and Self Psychology: An Introduction. 2nd ed. Pacific Grove, CA: Brooks/Cole; 1996.

[19] Wienand F, ed. Projektive Diagnostik bei Kindern, Jugendlichen und Familien: Grundlagen und Praxis-ein Handbuch. Stuttgart: Kohlhammer; 2015.

[20] Corman L. Der Schwarzfuss-Test: Grundlagen, Durchführung, Deutung und Auswertung. München: Reinhardt; 1977.

[21] Lindzey G. On the classification of projective techniques. Psychol Bull. 1959 Mar;56 (2):158–68.

[22] Jung CG. Die Assoziationsmethode. Vorlesung aufgrund der Einladung der Psychologischen Abteilung der Clark University, Worcester, Massachusetts im September 1909. *Gesammelte Werke 2 "Experimentelle Untersuchungen"*. Olten: Walter; 1910:461–87 §§ 939–98.

[23] Loevinger J. Technical Foundations for Measuring Ego Development: The Washington University Sentence Completion Test. Mahwah, NJ: Erlbaum; 1998.

[24] Thomas M. Méthode des histoires à compléter (pour le dépistage des complexes enfantins). Arch Psychol. 1937;26:209–84.

[25] Düss L. The method of fables in psychoanalysis. Arch Psychol. 1940;28:1–51.

[26] Bretherton I, Oppenheim D. The MacArthur Story Stem Battery: Development, Administration, Reliability, Validity, and Reflections about Meaning. In: Emde RN, Wolf DP, Oppenheim D, eds. *Revealing the Inner Worlds of Young Children: The MacArthur Story Stem Battery and Parent–Child Narratives*. New York, NY: Oxford University Press; 2003:55–80.

[27] Rosenzweig S. The picture-association method and its application in a study of reactions to frustration. J Pers. 1945 Sep;14:3–23.

[28] Lowenfeld M. The Lowenfeld Mosaic Test. London: Newman Neame; 1954.

[29] Wells HG. Floor Games. London: J. M. Dent and Sons; 1911.

[30] Lynn DB. Structured Doll Play Test (SDP): A Projective Test for Use with Children. Denver, CO: Test Developments; 1959.

[31] Kalff DM. Sandplay. Boston, MA: Beacon; 1980.

[32] Pattis Zoja E. Sandplay Therapy in Vulnerable Communities: A Jungian Approach. Abingdon: Routledge; 2011.

[33] Ammann R. Healing and Transformation in Sandplay: Creative Processes Become Visible. LaSalle, IL: Open Court; 1991.

[34] Frank LK. Projective methods for the study of personality. J Psychol: Interdisc Appl. 1939;8:389–413.

[35] Frank LK. Projective Methods. Springfield, IL: Charles C. Thomas; 1948.

[36] Semeonoff B. Projective Techniques. London; New York: Wiley; 1976.

[37] Murray HA. Thematic Apperception Test. Cambridge, MA: Harvard University Press; 1943.

[38] Schmalt H-D, Sokolowski K. The current status of motive measurement. Diagnostica. 2000;46:115–23.

[39] Müller L, Petzold HG. Projektive und semiprojektive Verfahren für die Diagnostik von Störungen, Netzwerken und Komorbidität in der Integrativen Therapie von Kindern und Jugendlichen. Integrative Therapie. 1998;3–4:396–438.

[40] Jadad AR, Moore RA, Carroll D, Jenkinson C, Reynolds DJ, Gavaghan DJ, et al. Assessing the quality of reports of randomized clinical trials: is blinding necessary? Control Clin Trials. 1996 Feb;17(1):1–12.

[41] Hayes RB, Sackett DL, Guyatt GH, Tugwell P. Clinical Epidemiology. Philadelphia, PA: Lippincott Williams & Wilkins; 2005.

[42] Machover K. Personality projection: in the drawing of a human figure. Springfield, IL: Charles C. Thomas 1949.

[43] Murstein BI. Theory and Research in Projective Techniques (Emphasizing the TAT). New York, NY: Wiley; 1963.

[44] Rabin AI. Projective Techniques in Personality Assessment: A Modern Introduction. New York: Springer Pub. Co.; 1968.

[45] Reynolds CR, Kamphaus RW, eds. Handbook of Psychological and Educational Assessment of Children: Personality, Behavior, and Context. New York, NY: Guilford Press; 2003.

[46] Schaefer CE, Cangelosi DM. Essential Play Therapy Techniques: Time-Tested Approaches. New York, NY: Guilford Press; 2016.

[47] Hersen M. Comprehensive Handbook of Psychological Assessment. Hoboken, NJ: John Wiley & Sons; 2004.

[48] Vass Z. A Psychological Interpretation of Drawings and Paintings. The SSCA Method: A Systems Analysis Approach. Pecs: Alexandra Publishing; 2012.

[49] Goodenough F. Measurement of Intelligence by Drawings. New York, NY: World Book Co.; 1926.

[50] Ziler H. Der Mann-Zeichentest (MZT/det) in detail-statistischer Auswertung. Münster/Westfalen: Aschendorff; 1958.

[51] Brosat H, Tötemeyer N. Der Mann-Zeichen-Test nach Hermann Ziler. 11 ed: Aschendorff; 2007.

[52] Williams SD, Wiener J, MacMillan H. Build-a-Person Technique: an examination of the validity of human-figure features as evidence of childhood sexual abuse. Child Abuse Negl. 2005 Jun;29(6):701–13.

[53] ter Laak J, de Goede M, Aleva A, van Rijswijk P. The Draw-A-Person Test: an indicator of children's cognitive and socioemotional adaptation? J Genet Psychol. 2005 Mar;166 (1):77–93.

[54] Harris DB. Children's Drawings as Measures of Intellectual Maturity. New York, NY: Harcourt, Brace & World, Inc.; 1963.

[55] Buck JN, Warren WL. The House-Tree-Person Projective Drawing Technique: Manual and Interpretive Guide. Revised edition. Los Angeles: Western Psychological Services; 1970.

[56] Burns RC, Kaufman SH. Kinetic Family Drawings (K-F-D): An Introduction to Understanding Children Through Kinetic Drawings. New York, NY: Brunner/Mazel; 1987.

[57] Avé-Lallemant U. Der Sterne-Wellen-Test. 3rd ed. München: Reinhardt; 2006 [1994].

[58] Biermann G, Kos M, Haub G. The graphic test "the enchanted family" and its application in educational counselling and paediatric clinics (author's transl). Padiatr Padol. 1975;10(1):19–31.

[59] Biermann G, Kos M. Die verzauberte Familie: ein tiefenpsychologischer Zeichentest. München: Reinhardt; 1973.

[60] Biermann G, Kos-Robes M. The Drawing Test Battery Tree-Person-Enchanted Family. Prax Kinderpsychol Kinderpsychiat. 1986;35:214–22.

[61] Koch K. Der Baumtest. Der Baumzeichenversuch als psychodiagnostisches Hilfsmittel. 11 ed. Bern: Huber; 2003 [1952].

[62] Avé-Lallemant U. Baumtests. Mit einer Einführung in die symbolische und graphologische Interpretation. Ölten-Freiburg/Br.: Walter; 1976.

[63] Wartegg E. Gestaltung und Charakter. Ausdrucksdeutung zeichnerischer Gestaltung und Entwurf einer charakterologischen Typologie. Leipzig: Barth; 1939.

[64] Avé-Lallemant U. Der Wartegg-Zeichentest in der Lebensberatung. 4 ed. München: Reinhardt; 2010.

[65] Roivainen E. A brief history of the Wartegg Drawing Test. Gestalt Theory. 2009;31(1):55–71.

[66] Tamminen S, Lindeman M. Wartegg: a valid personality test or magical thinking? Psykologia. 2000;35(4):325–31.

[67] Soilevuo Gronnerod J, Gronnerod C. The Wartegg Zeichen Test: a literature overview and a meta-analysis of reliability and validity. Psychol Assess. 2012 Jun;24(2):476–89.

[68] Winnicott DW. Therapeutic Consultation in Child Psychiatry. London: Hogarth Press; 1971.

[69] Günter M. Playing the Unconscious: Psychoanalytic Interviews with Children Using Winnicott's Squiggle Technique. London: Karnac; 2007.

[70] Cramer P. The Development of Defense Mechanisms: Theory, Research, and Assessment. New York, NY: Springer; 1991.

[71] Westen D. Clinical assessment of object relations using the TAT. J Pers Assess. 1991 Feb;56(1):56–74.

[72] Westen D. Social cognition and object relations. Psychol Bull. 1991;109:429–55.

[73] Westen D. Revision of Social Cognition and Objects Relations Scale: Q-Sort for projective stories (SCORS-Q). Unpublished manuscript. Cambridge, MA: Department of Psychiatry, Cambridge Hospital and Harvard Medical School; 1995.

[74] Lis A, Mazzeschi C, Salcuni S, Zennaro A. The children's apperception test evaluation form: initial data. Psychol Rep. 2005 Jun;96(3 Pt 1):755–68.

[75] Bellak L, Bellak SS. Children's Apperception Test (C.A.T.). Gracie Station, NY: Consulting Psychologists Press; 1949.

[76] Costantino G, Malgady R, Rogler L. TEMAS (Tell-Me-A-Story) Manual. Los Angeles, CA: Western Psychological Services; 1988.

[77] Cambias R, Killian G, Faust J. Tell-Me-A-Story Test (TEMAS). In: Keyser D, Sweetland R, eds. *Test Critiques, Vol IX*. Kansas City, MO: Test Corporation of America 1991:545–60.

[78] Coulacoglou C. FTT Application. 2016 [cited 2016 Jun 14]; Available from: http://www.fairytaletest.com/index.php?dispatch=pages.view&page_id=3

[79] Coulacoglou C, Kline P. The Fairy Tale Test: A novel approach in projective assessment. Brit J Proj Psychol. 1995;40(2):10–32.

[80] Burstein AG, Loucks S. Rorschach's Test: Scoring and Interpretation; Abingdon-on-Thames: Routledge, 1989.

[81] Burstein AG, Loucks S. A Comprehensive Scoring Manual for Rorschach's Test. Br J Proj Psych Personality Study 1985;30(2):3–16.

[82] Exner JE. The Rorschach. A Comprehensive System. Volume 1: Basic Foundations. 4th ed. New York, NY: Wiley; 2002.

[83] Exner JE, Erdberg P. The Rorschach: A Comprehensive System. Volume 2: Advanced Interpretation. 3rd ed. New York, NY: Wiley; 2005.

[84] Exner JE, Weiner IB. The Rorschach: A Comprehensive System. Volume 3: Assessment of Children and Adolescents. 2nd ed. New York, NY: Wiley; 1994.

[85] Rorschach H. Psychodiagnostik. Methodik und Ergebnisse eines wahrnehmungsdiagnostischen Experiments (Deutenlassen von Zufallsformen). Bern: E. Bircher; 1921.

[86] Cohen RJ, Swerdlik ME, Sturman ED. Psychological Testing and Assessment: An Introduction to Tests and Measurement. 8th ed. Columbus, OH: McGraw Hill Higher Education; 2012.

[87] Holtzman WH, Thorpe JS, Swartz JD, Herron EW. Inkblot Perception and Personality. The Holtzman Inkblot Technique. Austin, TX: Hogg Foundation for Mental Health, University of Texas Press; 1961.

[88] Lah MI, Rotter JB. Changing college student norms on the Rotter Incomplete Sentences Blank. J Consult Clin Psychol. 1981 Dec;49(6):985.

[89] Rotter JB, Rafferty JE. The Rotter Incomplete Sentences Blank. Manual, College Form. New York, NY: The Psychological Corporation; 1950.

[90] Rotter JB, Lah MI, Rafferty JE. Rotter Incomplete Sentences Blank, Second Edition (RISB-2) San Antonio, TX: Pearson; 1992.

[91] Wagner EE. The Hand Test, Revised. Manual. Los Angeles: Western Psychological Services; 1983.

[92] Young GR, Wagner EE. The Hand Test: Advances in Application and Research. Malabar, FL: Krieger Pub. Co.; 1999.

[93] Bene E, Anthony EJ. Manual for the Children's Version of the Family Relations Test. Windsor: NFER Publishing Company; 1978.

[94] Beelmann W, Schmidt-Denter U. Standardization of the German version of the Family Relations Test (FRT) for children, ages 4–5 years. Prax Kinderpsychol Kinderpsychiatr. 1999 Jul-Aug;48(6):399–410.

[95] Flämig J, Wörner U. Standardization of a German version of the Family Relations Test (FRT) for children between 6 and 11 years of age. Prax Kinderpsychol Kinderpsychiatr. 1977 Jan;26(1):5–11.

[96] Anthony EJ, Bene E. A technique for the objective assessment of the child's family relationships. J Ment Sci. 1957 Jul;103(432):541–55.

[97] Bene E, Anthony EJ. Familiy Relations Test (FRT). Children's version. Göttingen: Hogrefe; 1985.

[98] Schröfl S. [The use of the Patte Noire Tests in children]. Prax Kinderpsychol Kinderpsychiatr. 1977 Jul;26(5):184–93.

[99] Mills ES. The Madeleine Thomas completion stories test. J Consult Psychol. 1953 Apr;17 (2):139–41.

[100] Despert JL. Psychosomatic study of fifty stuttering children; social, physical and psychiatric findings. Am J Orthopsychiatry. 1946 Jan;16:100–13.

[101] Fine R. Use of the Despert fables in diagnostic work with children. Rorschach Res Exch J Proj Tech. 1948;12(2):106–18.

[102] Robinson J, Mantz-Simmons L. The MacArthur Narrative Coding System: One approach to highlighting affective meaning making in the MacArthur Story Stem Battery. In: Emde RN, Wolf DP, Oppenheim D, eds. *Revealing the Inner Worlds of Young Children: The MacArthur Story Stem Battery and Parent–Child-Narratives.* New York, NY: Oxford University Press; 2003:81–105.

[103] Emde RN, Wolf DP, Oppenheim D, eds. Revealing the Inner Worlds of Young Children: The MacArthur Story Stem Battery and Parent–Child Narratives. New York, NY: Oxford University Press; 2003.

[104] Robinson JL. Story stem narratives with young children: moving to clinical research and practice. Attach Hum Dev. 2007 Sep;9(3):179–85.

[105] Woodcock TM-Y. Expressing the Shape and Colour of Personality: Using Lowenfeld Mosaics in Psychotherapy and Cross-Cultural Research. Eastbourne: Sussex Academic Press; 2006.

[106] Woodcock T. The use of the Lowenfeld mosaic test in child psychotherapy. Proj Psychol. 1984 December ;29(2): 11–18.

[107] Ames LB. The Lowenfeld Mosaic Test: a review of its use. J Pers Assess. 1986;50(3):428–35.

[108] Lynn DB, Lynn R. The structured doll play test as a projective technique for use with children. J Proj Tech. 1959 Sep;23:335–44.

[109] Ermert C. Scenotest-Handbuch. Bern: Hans Huber; 1997.

[110] Biermann G, Galm D, Kassian A, Klüwer K, Schmeer G, Six M. Die Tätigkeit der Psychosomatischen Beratungsstelle für Kinder bei der Universitäts-Kinderpoliklinik München. Prax Kinderpsychol Kinderpsychiat. 1963;12:193 u. 246.

[111] von Staabs G. Der Scenotest. Beitrag zur Erfassung unbewußter Problematik und charakterologischer Struktur. Stuttgart: Huber; 1964.

[112] Biermann G, Biermann R. The sceno game in the course of time. Prax Kinderpsychol Kinderpsychiat. 1998;47(3):186–202.

[113] Fliegner J. "Sceno-R": Eine Materialrevision des Scenotests. Prax Kinderpsychol Kinderpsychiat. 1995;44(6):215–21.

[114] Yontef GM. Awareness, Dialogue and Process: Essays on Gestalt Therapy. Highland, NY: Gestalt Journal Press; 1993.

[115] Baulig I, Baulig V. Kinderwelttest. Weinheim: Beltz; 2006.

[116] Lowenfeld M. The World Technique. London; Boston, MA: Allen & Unwin: Institute of Child Psychology; 1979.

[117] Reiffen-Züger B, Lehmhaus D. Begleitheft Plämokasten. München: Ärztliche Akademie für Psychotherapie von Kindern und Jugendlichen e.V.; 2015.

[118] Association for Play Therapy. A definition of play therapy. Association for Play Therapy Newsletter. 1997;16(1):7.

[119] Winnicott DW. Playing and Reality. New York, NY: Basic Books; 1971.

[120] O'Connor KJ. The value and use of interpretation in play therapy. Prof Psychol Res Pr. 2002;33(6):523–8.

[121] Freeman J, Epston D, Lobovits D. Playful Approaches to Serious Problems: Narrative Therapy with Children and Their Families. New York, NY: Norton; 1997.

[122] Schaefer CE, Drewes AA. The Therapeutic Powers of Play and Play Therapy. In: Drewes AA, Schaefer CE, eds. *School-Based Play Therapy.* New York, NY: Wiley; 2016:3–15.

[123] Kaduson HG. Release Play Therapy for Children with Posttraumatic Stress Disorder. In: Kaduson HG, Schaefer CE, eds. *Short-Term Play Therapy for Children.* New York, NY: Guilford Publications; 2016:3–21.

[124] Schaefer CE, Peabody MA. Glossary of Play Therapy Terms (2016). Int J Play Therapy. 2016;25(3):23–4.

[125] von Gontard A, Lehmkuhl G. Playtherapies — Psychotherapies with the medium of play: II. New developments. Prax Kinderpsychol Kinderpsychiatr. 2003;52(2):88–97.

[126] Gleser GC. Projective methodologies. Annu Rev Psychol. 1963;14:391–422.

[127] Molish HB. Projective methodologies. Annu Rev Psychol. 1972;23:577–614.

[128] Klopfer WG, Taulbee ES. Projective tests. Annu Rev Psychol. 1976;27:543–67.

[129] Fisher S. Projective methodologies. Annu Rev Psychol. 1967;18:165–90.

[130] Bölte S, Adam-Schwebe S, Englert E, Schmeck K, Poustka F. Test-usage in German child and adolescent psychiatry: report on a survey. Z Kinder-Jugendpsychiatr. 2000;28 (3):151–61.

[131] Solms M, Turnbull O. The Brain and the Inner World: An Introduction to the Neuroscience of Subjective Experience. New York, NY: Other Press; 2002.

[132] Panksepp J. Affective Neuroscience: The Foundations of Human and Animal Emotions. Oxford: Oxford University Press; 2004.

6

Parenting Adolescents in India: A Cultural Perspective

Roshni Sondhi

Abstract

Contemporary parenting has witnessed a multitude of adaptations over the past decade across various cultural settings. Adolescent attachment patterns with parents have been explored in varying cultural contexts. These attachment patterns have been extensively studied in the light of adolescence as a turbulent phase of development. This chapter offers a systematic review of the cultural factors influencing parenting, with a theoretical analysis specific to adolescents within the Indian context. Based on the exploration of these cultural influences on parenting, the chapter further explores the relevance of mindfulness-based approaches within the Indian culture, with an applicability of a model of mindful parenting specifically with adolescents in India. The conceptualization of mindfulness-based approaches stems from both Eastern and Western cultures, which have significant influences on parenting of adolescents. The components of mindful parenting have shown applicability within the dynamic context of parental-adolescent attachment patterns, especially considering the culture-specific concept of interdependence in a collectivistic culture like India. Such findings have potential implications for the formulation of parenting strategies toward the future of adolescent mental health in the country.

Keywords: India, parenting, mindfulness, adolescent mental health, cultural factors

1. Introduction

Ever since the conceptualization of parenting has evolved, it has been universally identified as one of the most crucial roles. Extensive research has further propelled its significance by highlighting its far-reaching consequences for the offspring, parents, siblings, and significant others. With growing awareness, parenting is increasingly being considered as a skill that needs to be honed through experience and training. As a result, many parents find themselves struggling to become a 'perfect' mother or father. Without a clearly defined thumb-rule to perfect parenting, this is undoubtedly a challenge, more so during the growing years of adolescence.

In an attempt to gain a comprehensive understanding of parenting, it becomes important to recognize the multiple factors within the family as well as the dynamics of the family with the larger community [1]. Extensive research has vouched for the influence of cultural contexts on parent-child relationship, for example, see Refs. [2–4]. Therefore, the impact of these factors on the development of child-rearing practices within a particular culture assumes greater implications. The past few decades have witnessed significant adaptations in parenting approaches globally, for example, see Refs. [5–7]. With changing times, it is not only the practices of parenting that are evolving but also the attachment patterns and perceptions encompassed, especially within a parent-adolescent relationship. This chapter attempts to highlight such cultural influences interplaying within the parenting of adolescents, while also exploring mindfulness-based parenting strategies, with specific applicability to the evolving contemporary Indian cultural settings.

2. Evolving approaches to parenting: From then to now

Parenting has often been metaphorically described as an exciting and rewarding journey, providing a sense of fulfillment that is said to be incomparable to most other significant milestones of life. However, the same journey has also been regarded as a potential source of tremendous stressors and challenges, both for the parents and for the significant others involved. These very sentiments about parenting adolescents have been aptly expressed as being a source of "excitement and of anxiety; of happiness and of troubles; of discovery and of bewilderment; and of breaks with the past and yet of links with the future" [8]. With the evolving advancements and progress in our society over the past few decades, parenting practices as well as perceptions about parenting have undoubtedly witnessed adaptations in accordance with the changing times.

2.1. Theoretical background

Parenting as a variable has been extensively explored in the course of human development studies [9]. The theoretical background of parenting has emerged from the groundbreaking work by Baumrind, with the conceptualization of three specific parenting styles, namely authoritarian, permissive and authoritative, along with the identification of parental responsiveness and parental demand as the two fundamental elements of parenting [10, 11]. According to this traditional classification, parents with an authoritarian style tend to be strict, directive, and emotionally detached; parents with a permissive style tend to set less restrictions or limits; while parents with an authoritative style tend to give clear and firm direction, with moderate discipline, warmth, and flexibility [12].

A parenting style is a representation of the standard strategies used by parents to raise their offspring(s) [12], and therefore, as a psychological construct is dependent on the behavior and attitude of the parents. In fact, a parenting style need not always fit into specific theoretical paradigms and instead could also be a creation by the parents themselves; it could be derived from a combination of multiple variables, further evolving over time as their wards begin to develop their own individual personalities and experience transitions across varying stages of life [13].

2.2. Traditional parenting

Endeavors to trace the journey of how parenting would have begun with new parents who did not have any support from researchers and theorists, and efforts to identify a single original 'tradition' of parenting, would unfortunately, be in vain. This is so because parenting patterns tend to exhibit variations based on a variety of factors, including culture, personality, parental background, educational level, socioeconomic status, family size, religion, etc. [14]. From a traditional point of view, most parenting styles tend to emanate from the way the parents themselves had been parented. However, this need not involve a repetition of similar parenting practices but could in contradiction involve discarding or avoiding such a repetition. This could simply be because these are the only practices of parenting that they have any knowledge about, or with the intention of learning from one's own parents' mistakes, or unconsciously relying on a vicarious learning of the same. In fact, even contemporary parents believe that their parenting styles are largely influenced by the way they were raised by their own parents, thereby serving as the departure point for beginning one's own journey as a parent [15, 16].

As it has been established that parenting styles are largely based on the cultural value systems that have been internalized within the family, it would seem appropriate and befitting to this chapter to gain an understanding of the traditional parenting practices within an Indian context. At the same time, it is important to keep in mind the paucity of research studies exploring such factors in contemporary India [17]. Based on the documented evidence about the collectivistic nature of the Indian society, it does not come as a surprise that traditional Indian parenting would also be pivoted around the promotion of social cohesion and interdependence [18]. The value of such parental goals helps Indian families provide for nurturance, emotional bonding, and social support [17]. Given the strong hierarchical kinship structure within traditional Indian families, an emphasis on obedience to authority can be clearly expected. Finally, as a culture which tends to give higher value to affiliation and contact, traditional Indian parenting does emphasize greater physical proximity between the parent and the child, including closeness to the body, frequent massaging, and co-sleeping, especially as an infant [19, 20].

2.3. Changes in contemporary parenting approaches

Parenting practices are bound to have evolved with changing demands over a period of time. With a constancy in the main objective of parenting, the methods and strategies used to attain such an objective have undergone significant adaptations. Over the decades, historical changes have been noted, including greater autonomy being provided by the parents, in terms of both private self-expression by the offspring and expressions of defiance toward parents [21]. There has also been a decrease in autonomy being provided by the parents for freedom of movement and a delayed acceptance of meaningful responsibilities [21]. The traditionally authoritarian style of parenting, involving an unquestioned obedience is now almost obsolete, instead being substituted by a preference for a sense of parental control [22]. Such transitions have been witnessed through a qualitative analysis of parental advice columns, with findings suggesting that parents, at the beginning of the previous century, lacked awareness regarding the offspring's whereabouts, and emphasized completion of chores and obedience as a parental goal; but changing times have led to a reversal in the degree of importance attached to these same goals, with more emphasis on the freedom of expression within the home, greater restrictions on their independence outside the home, and emphasis on chores being replaced by value being given to academics [21].

Consequently, evolutions in the parenting styles, especially among urban educated parents, have led to an orientation toward a sense of connectedness, autonomy as well as control, with parenting practices becoming more permissive, child-centered, and responsive; and therefore seeming to fit in more with Baumrind's authoritative parenting style, as compared to a traditional authoritarian approach [10, 22, 23]. In fact, there is evidence to suggest a dialectical synthesis of both material independence and psychological interdependence as a characteristic of contemporary models of parenting within urban settings of India [22]. With the advent of technological invasion, especially the increasing role of the social media, a definite change in the nature of communication patterns in families can be witnessed [24]. In addition, there have been changes within the family size and structures [17], for example, increase in dual-income families (with working parents), or increase in number of single parents, among others, are also underlying significant changes in parenting trends. Such familial adaptations have been associated with a new form of parental indulgence, as parents are spending more time, energy, and resources on their children's educational and career options, ironically assuming a more demanding role in terms of parental expectations of achievement and success [22].

At the same time, contemporary parents seem to be receptive toward reviewing their parenting approach in an effort toward building a better relationship with their child or adolescent [16]. With the dawn of globalization, better education and increased exposure to the Western cultures, both parents and adolescents have come to recognize the importance of independence and self-reliance in the contemporary world [25]. In tandem with such exposure, this growing awareness is also enabling a greater parental sensitivity, which in itself could lead to potential implications toward a 'kid-glove handling' approach to parenting in the future. Such an interface thus leads to an amalgamation of traditional parenting wisdom being integrated with the recent ideas and advancements in the field of childcare and parenting [20].

3. Parenting an adolescent

Adolescence as a phase is characterized by rapid developments including, both physical and psychological changes. It is a crucial stage of development, not only for the adolescent but also for the parents, bringing with it a set of apprehensions and worries. It is not uncommon to hear parental concerns regarding the approaching teenage years, being associated with changing expectations and relationships. In fact, a majority of parents have been found to consider adolescence as being the most difficult stage for childrearing [13, 26]. This section examines the attachment patterns of adolescents in relation to their developmental needs, along with exploring the influence of various cultural variables within this interplay.

3.1. Parent-adolescent attachment patterns

While there has been abundant research on attachment patterns arising from the seminal work by Bowlby and Ainsworth, for example, see Ref. [27]; most of the emphasis has been on the transmission of attachment patterns in infancy and childhood [28]. Ever since the work of these pioneers, it has been agreed upon, that an attachment with the parent (or caregiver) typically begins from infancy. However, as a child approaches the developmental stage of adolescence, it is not uncommon to note a shift in such attachments, seemingly to be directed more toward peers [29]. The function of attachment with parents has been found to change from the phase of childhood to adolescence [30]. While parental attachment with an adolescent does not necessitate the same degree of physical proximity as compared to childhood years, there is, however, a greater need for parental sensitivity during these teenage years [31].

It is also common for parents to feel isolated while parenting adolescents, which could possibly be attributed to this shift in attachment patterns. However, it is vital for them to recognize the significance of their role as a parent and to persist in their efforts toward increased awareness of the adolescent's subjective world, while being available to provide guidance, direction, and support, especially in the contemporary world [13].

3.2. Need for autonomy

As adolescence serves as a transitional period between childhood and adulthood, achieving a sense of autonomy has been identified as one of the salient characteristics of this phase of development. It has also been recognized as a period of transition from dependence on adult direction and protection to self-direction and self-determination [13]. Adolescents tend to adopt an exploratory approach, with the major objective of attaining independence. As Erikson described in his developmental theory, the primary psychosocial task of adolescence is the formation of an identity [32]. Therefore, it is during this phase that adolescents are likely to demonstrate a shift in their focus from the parents and the family, instead, striving toward greater interactions with the systems outside the family [33]. Recognition of such a shift reinforces the fact that the attachment of an adolescent with a parent cannot be viewed as similar to that of a child-parent relationship.

Moreover, it is also important to note that the desire for achieving autonomy does not necessarily imply a decrease in the attachment between an adolescent and his/her parents. However, normal adolescent development has been characterized by such a gradual shift from the importance of familial relationships toward interpersonal relationships with peers, with the objectives of socialization, self-definition, friendship, and support systems [13]. An adolescent would simply aim at reducing dependence on parents and, consequently, would tend to form attachments with peers, neighbors, and other members of the community. Moreover, there could also be instances when adolescents feel lost or overwhelmed with their independence, and this is the time when they could rely on their parents serving as a secure base for them [27]. In addition, a positive relationship between adolescents and their parents can often serve as a predictor for the adolescent's ability to develop a sense of autonomy [34].

It is also necessary to mention the role of cultural factors interplaying with such a developmental need, though these factors shall be discussed in more detail in the next sections. Commonly, a large extent of conflicting interests between parents and adolescents is attributed to this need for autonomy. Such a conflict could often be exaggerated within the Indian context, with parental emphasis on interdependence as an inherent part of the collectivistic culture of India. This discrepancy is often attributed to be a manifestation of adolescent rebellion or parental conservativeness. However, the role of cross-cultural variables needs to be reiterated here, as in individualistic cultures, parenting goals tend to value independence, while on the other hand Indian parenting goals are more likely to value obedience and good manners [28]. In addition, it has also been demonstrated that the parenting practices of Asian American parents who adhere to traditional Asian values may be incongruent with their children's level of acculturation, which could also breed further conflicts [35].

Simultaneously, there is growing contradictory evidence from the universalistic perspective, which demonstrates the importance of fulfilling the need for autonomy across both individualistic and relatively more collectivistic societies [36]. However, such apparent contradictions stem from the varying definitions of autonomy by both warring perspectives [37, 38]. Finally, it is necessary to note that there exists a gap in the extant research on this aspect of parenting, which has mainly been based on Western populations and thereby does not take into consideration the cross cultural differences in developmental pathways [28].

3.3. Role of cultural factors

Despite the progressing advancements, the traditional cultural value systems and beliefs still play a significant role in influencing parenting, parental attachments, and perceptions of parenting practices [21, 39–41]. Such influences can not only be attributed to the psychosocial and cultural factors influencing the immediate environment but also extending to the experience of these parents during their own upbringing. The role of a culture-parenting nexus has been recognized, both in constructing and in maintaining a pattern of parenting [2]. Recent evidence highlights the influence of both the parents' and the children's temperaments on the parenting style adopted by the parents, also being largely influenced by their own parenting and culture [13]. Therefore, it seems apt to devote the next subsections in exploring such cultural variations influencing the adolescent attachments and perceptions across cultural settings.

3.3.1. Cultural differences in parental-adolescent attachment

An analysis of the earlier research seems to suggest that most attachment theorists have focused on universals, with their measures being based on Western values like individuation and exploration; consequently, the role of cultural differences seems to have been neglected [42]. Cultural variations within the development of attachment could include differences in the subjective meaning of parental sensitivity, perceptions of parental acceptance or control, and in the meanings attached to various parenting practices [28, 43].

Research has identified that changes in parental attachments differ cross-culturally due to differences in the developmental pathways, which are characterized by culture-specific concepts of independence or interdependence. This suggests that individualistic cultures tend to have a greater emphasis on the developmental pathway of independence, as compared to the construct of interdependence prevailing in collectivistic cultures [43, 44]. Culturally significant differences in the parental-adolescent relations have also been evidenced, for instance, a symbiotic harmony characterizes their relationship in Asian cultures like Japan, maintaining a stable relationship with both parents and peers; on the other hand, in Western cultures like in the USA, the parental-adolescent relationship is characterized by a generative tension, with a transferring of close relationships from parents to peers, consequently leading to a challenging of parental values, and conflicts between the adolescents and their parents [43]. Elaborating on the culture-specific functional role of attachment, it can be understood that such a symbiotic and interdependent relationship fulfills a need for assurance and further serves as an agency to provide for the universally underlying need for competence in such cultures; this is opposed to the striving for independence and separateness leading to competence within a Western culture [45]. Therefore, a parental-adolescent attachment could be viewed as being dependent on the cultural perceptions and interpretations of their needs, including competence, autonomy, and relatedness, which are considered to be three basic psychological needs of an individual [37, 46].

3.3.2. Cultural perceptions of parental control vs. parental sensitivity

Cross-cultural factors have also been found to influence the perceptions of parental practices. For instance, the degree of parental control as perceived by individuals across cultures cannot be generalized, more so because the research findings related to parental control tend to focus more on culturally heterogeneous samples [47].

Especially from a culturally relativistic perspective, family climates with more emphasis on dependence are likely to demonstrate a greater degree of parental control, as compared to family climates emphasizing achievement [38]. According to a research study, parental control could have two specific expressions: a dependency-oriented control, involving the use of pressure to ensure greater physical and emotional proximity to the parent; and an achievement-oriented control, involving the use of pressure to strive toward excellence in performance-based situations [48]. In alignment with the same, the role of culturally significant differences in these expressions of parental control has also been evidenced [38].

Depending on their cultural orientation, adolescents' interpretation of parental control, sensitivity, and the affective connotation attached with it is likely to differ [38]. An individualistic culture is likely to have adolescent perceptions of parental control as being intrusive and hostile, as a constraint, contradictory to a relatively benign and appropriate perception in the form of a supportive and more sensitive approach, in collectivistic cultures [49, 50].

Greater parental control could be correlated with detrimental effects on the adolescents, specifically in terms of stifled independence, along with an encouraged dependency. However, such negative effects of parental control would be relevant only to cultural contexts where independence is highly valued, being inconsistent with the prevailing cultural values [38]. Based on such differences in cultural orientations, parental control in Asian countries is likely to be perceived as an expression of parental involvement and care, being in alignment with their traditional cultural values [51]. Therefore, positive meanings of sensitivity could be attached to the parental control in families wherein loyalty, parental involvement, and cooperation are valued [38]. However, it is important here to highlight the role of increasing westernization, growing exposure through education and media, and a greater cultural awareness, which could in turn lead to evolving cultural values influencing an adolescent's perceptions of the parental control.

3.3.3. *Individualistic vs. collectivistic cultures*

An exploration of the cultural variables influencing Indian parenting would be incomplete without an understanding of the nature of collectivism characterizing Indian culture. As discussed above, adolescence is earmarked by the development of autonomy and relatedness as a universal task. However, there is research evidence that supports cultural factors influencing the degree of importance given to each of these two tasks; for example, individualistic cultures emphasize autonomy relatively more than collectivistic cultures, which emphasize parental control and family obligations [28, 44]. Research on parenting within Indian families is suggestive of greater emphasis on interdependence [52]. This difference could be attributed to variations in the family size and structure across cultures, with smaller family units' parenting goals focussing on raising autonomous and independent individuals, and dependence being discouraged as being psychologically unhealthy [41].

Interdependence is a culture-specific construct highlighting the role of family relationships and obligations, which is emphasized in a collectivistic culture like in India [28]. This can be evidenced by the strength of the kinship networks and extended families that have been prevailing in India [53]. Therefore, such a cultural backdrop tends to emphasize loyalty toward family values; consequently, seeking an independence from parents could actually be disapproved of in such a cultural setting.

Upon examining cultural differences in parenting styles, Asian parents have been found to exhibit an authoritarian style of parenting [54]. Specifically, Indian fathers have traditionally been the patriarchal figures dominating their households [55]. Internalizing the values of collectivistic cultures within the process of parenting, the expression of an individual's own needs is typically inhibited in deference to valuing the needs of others; subsequently, it is common to note more authoritarian and restraining parenting, with a greater expectation of obedience dependence and sociability; on the contrary, parents from individualistic cultures tend to value self-reliance, self-interest, and autonomy within the socialization process, thereby having greater parental expectations of exploration and independence with an authoritative style of parenting [56]. At the same time, it is vital to note that the restrictive and normative parenting in collectivistic cultures is not necessarily associated with parents being rejecting or lacking in warmth [57–60].

Finally, it is also essential to mention that although Asian countries are often depicted as being uniformly collectivistic in nature, such a static characterization of cultures in general could be overly simplistic [61]. Simultaneously, it is interesting to observe multiple instances of Indians persisting to value familial unity and filial piety, despite the impact of increased exposure being considered responsible for the waning of traditional values over decades [62].

And therefore, the prevailing cultural factors within a family need to be explored as independent entities with significantly potential implications toward the relationship between parents and adolescents.

4. Mindfulness-based approach to parenting

According to the teachings of Buddha, mindfulness, being ubiquitous in nature, can be useful everywhere [63]. As a fundamental parenting practice, mindfulness in the context of parenting and parent training has been suggested as a significant force toward improving the effectiveness of parenting interventions [64]. Such an approach not only could improve the quality of the parental-adolescent relationship but can also influence parental self-efficacy.Given the pressure felt by most parents to "get parenting right," along with the parents' concern about their level of confidence in their parenting [16], adopting a mindfulness-based approach could be extremely beneficial. With the growing popularity of the concept of mindfulness, and increasing evidence indicating its benefits within the field of mental health and applied research, incorporating such an approach within our parenting practices undoubtedly can unfold its potential toward improving the experience of parenting for both the parent and the adolescent.

4.1. Historical underpinnings of mindfulness

The roots of mindfulness as a practice have been borrowed from the Eastern meditative and Western Christian contemplative traditions, specifically from the teachings and practices associated with Buddhist traditions [65]. The term "mindfulness" is an English translation of the Pali word *sati*, in the language of Buddhist psychology 2500 years ago, connoting awareness, attention, and remembering [66]. While this is not the first instance of borrowing components of Buddhist practice and other Eastern meditative practices, many such integrations between Buddhism and Western psychology have been developed in the past few decades, ranging from such inclusions within the original psychoanalytical traditions to more recent integrations within the cognitive-behavioral traditions [67, 68]. The construct of mindfulness has now carved a niche for itself as an established component of several contemporary psychotherapies, including Mindfulness-Based Stress Reduction, Mindfulness-Based Cognitive Therapy and its derivatives, Dialectical Behavior Therapy, Acceptance and Commitment Therapy, Compassion-Focused Therapy, and Mindfulness-Based Relationship Enhancement [67, 69].

According to Marsha Linehan, who developed the model of Dialectical Behavior Therapy, core mindfulness is one of the fundamental modules of the skills training program, aiming at improving an individual's control of attention and the mind, which has also been found as a promising intervention for adolescents [70, 71]. The practice of mindfulness has been defined as "the awareness that emerges through paying attention, on purpose, in the present moment, and nonjudgmentally to the unfolding of experience moment by moment" [72]. More Western psychological perspectives are also in alignment, describing mindfulness as "a receptive attention to and awareness of present events and experience" [73].

4.2. Model of mindful parenting

Mindful parenting was first proposed as a concept by Myla and Jon Kabat-Jinn in 1997, identifying sovereignty, acceptance, and empathy as the salient features of parenting [74]. According to them, sovereignty is described as the process of recognizing the child's "wholeness" by "seeing beneath behavior"; and acceptance refers to "an attempt to come to terms with the nature of things", within the parent, the child, or a particular situation [74]. The parental attitudes of compassion, acceptance and kindness, along with them being fully present during their interactions with their offspring, are key characteristics of mindful parenting [75, 76].

While there is not much empirical evidence as yet to explore the application of mindfulness within parenting, there is sufficient evidence supporting its role within a preventive paradigm toward mental health [77]. A model of mindful parenting could be considered as a framework in which parents intentionally bring moment-to-moment awareness to the parent-child relationship, through an integration of various components of core mindfulness; these could include attending behavior, emotional awareness, self-regulation, and nonjudgmental acceptance as integral parts of the parenting practice [78]. Further elaborating on this model, a recent research operationalized mindful parenting consisting of six dimensions, which involved (i) listening with full attention, (ii) having compassion for the child, (iii) a nonjudgmental acceptance of parental functioning, (iv) an emotional nonreactivity in parenting, (v) an emotional awareness of the child, and (vi) an emotional awareness of the self [79]. A combination of these dimensions enables parents to be mindful, maintaining a consistency with their parenting goals and values, within the realm of the parent-child relationship [78].

Integrating a mindfulness-based approach within parenting practices enables a shift in parental awareness toward the present-moment parenting experience, thereby becoming one of the most significant aspects of the parental relationship [78]. In fact, an application of such an approach to parenting creates a demarcation between the parenting goals being predominated by parent-oriented or child-oriented motivations [80]. The model of mindful parenting reiterates such a distinction, encouraging parents' mindful awareness and acceptance of the child's needs, thereby improving their relationship with the child [78].

5. Applicability for adolescents within an Indian context

Drawing from the implications suggested above, with an integration of the various cultural factors influencing parenting, it seems interesting to explore the applicability of such a mindfulness-based model of parenting in India. Such an approach could be advocated especially for the parenting of an adolescent population, considering the characteristic challenges associated with this phase of development. Undoubtedly, the role of parenting does not come without its challenges, it being easier to find faults in retrospect. In fact, with increasing stressors, it is indeed becoming difficult to parent effectively in the contemporary world [7]. In light of research supporting the benefits of mindfulness within daily living, such a model can also have potential implications not just toward the parental-adolescent relationship but also toward reducing parental stresses and enhancing their own well-being [73].

5.1. Incorporating mindfulness within communication patterns

As the value of interdependence within the Indian culture has previously been established, the application of one of the most significant components of the model of mindful parenting can potentiate significant implications. Parents' mindful listening, i.e., with full attention and awareness being given to the present moment experiences, can have significant implications toward the relationship between the parent and the offspring. As the parental attachment undergoes a shift during adolescence, such mindful listening can enhance the quality of attachment and security. Furthermore, this can be appreciated by adolescents who are commonly heard complaining of 'not being understood' by their parents.

This model can also play a significant role in shaping the perceptions of the parental sensitivity toward the adolescent. This is expected to be reflected in their accurate and increased awareness of the adolescent's verbal as well as behavioral cues, along with a simultaneous reduction in parental expression of expectations from the adolescent. This assumes a greater significance considering the lack of parental awareness of the adolescent's whereabouts in the outer world [81].

Finally, recent preliminary evidence suggests that self-reported mindful parenting can be associated with the interactions between the parents and the youth [82]. Further, such mindful attention and awareness is likely to improve the accuracy of parental perceptions of adolescents' thoughts and feelings, thereby leading to a significant decrease in the amount of conflicts or disagreements, and deceptiveness by the adolescents, which are considered characteristic of this phase [81, 83].

5.2. Adopting a nonjudgmental stance

Given the magnitude of conflicts between adolescents and parents, a mindfulness-based model of parenting advocates a nonjudgmental acceptance of both the self and the adolescent [78]. In combination with an enhanced and mindful understanding of the adolescent's thoughts and feelings, such a stance enables the parents to be accepting of the presence of struggles within the parental-adolescent relationship. Such an acceptance brings with it a more realistic set of expectations, along with an enhanced sense of parenting self-efficacy.

Mindfulness within parenting approaches has been hypothesized to reduce parental preoccupation and/or negative bias [77]. It also enables parents to identify their interactions with the adolescent, which could contribute to a relational disconnect [84]. Therefore, the parental goal shifts from evading such conflicts toward gaining a more complete and nonjudgmental understanding of the present moment (based on mindful attention). Such a perspective can serve as a foundation for a preventive approach toward parenting conflicts, and in turn improving the parental-adolescent relationship.

6. Implications: Way forward

Mindfulness-based parenting can serve as a foundation for enhancing crucial parent-adolescent relationships. As has been suggested by Duncan [78, 82], the implementation of a mindfulness-based model of parenting can help in the creation of family contexts that are more conducive for a satisfying parental relationship with the child. Such a model has immense potential toward a preventive approach to adolescents' parenting. Adolescents' perceptions and attitudes toward their parents can largely be impacted by this model, consequently improving the quality of the parent-adolescent attachments.

Incorporating a mindfulness-based approach within our parenting styles can be instrumental in altering the nature of responsiveness toward the adolescent's emotions. It is also likely to reduce the expression of negative affect within the parent-adolescent relationship. In addition, mindful parents tend to develop more adaptive coping mechanisms, thereby equipping them to deal with their parental stresses as well. Therefore, this model brings with it a two-fold benefit for adolescents' as well as parents' well-being.

Finally, the success of such a mindfulness-based approach is expected to have a greater receptivity, given the nature of spirituality rooted within the Indian culture. In spite of the research supporting mindful parenting as a preventive model, there is a need for empirical investigations of the efficacy of such mindfulness-based parenting, as a means to foster positive outcomes for the adolescent [77, 85]. It is imperative that future research exploring the efficacy of such a model can extend this discourse, as well as formulate more culturally sensitive parenting practices within the societal realm of India.

Author details

Roshni Sondhi

Address all correspondence to: roshnisondhi@yahoo.com

Department of Mental Health and Behavioral Sciences, Fortis Healthcare, New Delhi, India

References

[1] Deater-Deckard K. Parenting Stress. USA: Byword Books; 2011. 220 p.

[2] Bornstein M. H. Cultural approaches to parenting. Parenting: Science and Practice. 2012;**12**(2–3):212–221. DOI: 10.1080/15295192.2012.683359

[3] Spicer P. Cultural influences on parenting. Zero to Three. 2010;**30**(4):28–32.

[4] Chang M. Cultural differences in parenting styles and their effects on teens' self-esteem, perceived parental relationship satisfaction, and self-satisfaction [thesis]. CMU; 2007. 47 p. Available from: http://repository.cmu.edu/cgi/viewcontent.cgi?article=1084&context=hsshonors

[5] Lee D. L. Overview of societal change factors affecting parenting practices. In: Nicolas G., Bejarano A., Lee D. L., editors. Contemporary Parenting: A Global Perspective. New York: Taylor and Francis; 2016. pp. 60–67.

[6] Collishaw S., Gardner F., Maughan B., Scott J., Pickles A. Do historical changes in parent-child relationships explain increases in youth conduct problems? Journal of Abnormal Child Psychology. 2012;**40**(1):119-132. DOI: 10.1007/s10802-011-9543-1

[7] Long N. The changing nature of parenting in America. Pediatric Dentistry. 2004;**26**(2): 121–124.

[8] Lerner R. M., Noh E. R., Wilson C. The parenting of adolescents and adolescents as parents: A developmental contextual perspective [Internet]. 1998. Available from: http://parenthood.library.wisc.edu/Lerner/Lerner.html [Accessed: 3rd August 2016].

[9] Baldwin D. R., McIntyre A., Hardaway E. Perceived parenting styles on college students' optimism. College Student Journal. 2007;**41**(3):550.

[10] Baumrind D. Current patterns of parental authority. Developmental Psychology Monographs. 1971;**4**:1–103.

[11] Maccoby E., Martin J. Parent-child relationships. In: Mussen P., Hetherington E. M., editors. Handbook of Child Psychology—Socialization, Personality and Social Development. New York: Wiley; 1983. pp. 1–1043.

[12] Kordi A., Baharudin R. Parenting attitude and style and its effect on children's school achievements. International Journal of Psychological Studies. 2010;**2**(2):217–222.

[13] Laxmi A. H. M. V., Kadapatti M. Analysis of parenting styles and interpersonal relationship among adolescents. International Journal of Scientific and Research Publications. 2012;**2**(8):1–5.

[14] Amos P. M. Parenting and culture – Evidence from some African communities. In: Seidl-de-Moura M. L., editor. Parenting in South American and African Contexts. Croatia: In-Tech; 2013. pp. 65-77. DOI: 10.5772/56967

[15] Belkin L. It's not your mom and dad's parenting [Internet]. 2009. Available from: http://parenting.blogs.nytimes.com/2009/08/17/changes-in-parenting-over-generations/?_r=0 [Accessed: 28th August 2016].

[16] Tucci J., Mitchell J., Goddard C. The Changing Face of Parenting – Exploring the Attitudes of Parents in Contemporary Australia. Australia: Australian Childhood Foundation; 2005. 29 p.

[17] Sonawat R. Understanding families in India: A reflection of societal changes (Translated from—Compreendendo as Famílias na Índia: Uma Imagem das Mudanças na Sociedade). Psicologia: Teoria e Pesquisa. 2001;**17**(2):177–186.

[18] Chadda R. K., Deb K. S. Indian family systems, collectivistic society and psychotherapy. Indian Journal of Psychiatry. 2013;**55**(2):S299–S309. DOI: 10.4103/0019-5545.105555

[19] Liu S., Volcic Z., Gallois C. Introducing Intercultural Communication: Global Cultures and Contexts. London: Sage; 2011. 328 p.

[20] Tuli M. Beliefs on parenting and childhood in India. Journal of Comparative Family Studies. 2012;**43**(1):81–91.

[21] Rutherford M. B. Children's autonomy and responsibility: An analysis of childrearing advice. Qualitative Sociology. 2009;**32**(4):337–353. DOI: 10.1007/s11133-009-9136-2

[22] Sharma V., Sandhu G. K. A community study of association between parenting dimensions and externalizing behaviours. Journal of Indian Association for Child and Adolescent Mental Health. 2006;**2**(2):48–58.

[23] Saraswathi T. S., Ganapathy H. Indian parents ethno theories as a reflection of Hindu scheme of child and human development. In: Keller H., Poortinga Y. H., Scholmerich A., editors. Between Culture and Biology: Perspectives on Ontogenetic Development. Cambridge: Cambridge University Press; 2002. pp. 79–88.

[24] Bala K. Social media and changing communication patterns. Global Media Journal—Indian Edition. 2014;**5**(1):1–6.

[25] Casalina A. Education builds self-reliance in a changing world [Internet]. 2014. Available from: http://www.huffingtonpost.in/entry/education-builds-selfreli_b_4892967 [Accessed: 2nd August 2016].

[26] Dobson J. Preparing for Adolescence—How to Survive the Coming Years of Change. Washington, DC: Revell; 2005. 162 p.

[27] Bretherton I. The origins of attachment theory: John Bowlby and Mary Ainsworth. Developmental Psychology. 1992;**28**:759–775.

[28] Albert I., Trommsdorff G., Mishra R. Parenting and adolescent attachment in India and Germany. In: Zheng G., Leung K., Adair J. G., editors. Perspectives and Progress in Contemporary Cross-Cultural Psychology. USA: International Association for Cross-Cultural Psychology, Inc.; 2008. pp. 97–108.

[29] Allen J., Land D. Attachment in adolescence. In: Cassidy J., Shaver P., editors. Handbook of Attachment. New York: Guilford; 1999. pp. 319–335.

[30] Trinke S. J., Bartholomew K. Hierarchies of attachment relationships in young adulthood. Journal of Social and Personal Relationships. 1997;**14**:603–625.

[31] Moretti M. M., Peled M. Adolescent-parent attachment: Bonds that support healthy development. Pediatric Child Health. 2004;**9**(8):551–555.

[32] Erikson E. H. Identity and the Life Cycle; Selected Papers, with a Historical Introduction by David Rapaport. New York: International University Press; 1959.

[33] Sokol J. T. Identity development throughout the lifetime: An examination of Eriksonian theory. Graduate Journal of Counseling Psychology. 2009;**1**(2):139-148.

[34] Weiss R. S. Attachment in adult life. In: Parkes C. M., Stevenson-Hinde J., editors. The Place of Attachment in Human Behaviour. New York: Basic; 1982. pp. 171–184.

[35] Park Y. S., Kim B. S. K., Chiang J., Ju C. M. Acculturation, enculturation, parental adherence to Asian cultural values, parenting styles, and family conflict among Asian American college students. Asian American Journal of Psychology. 2010;**1**(1):67–79.

[36] Vansteenkiste M., Lens W., Soenens B., Luyckx K. Autonomy and relatedness among Chinese Sojourners and Applicants: Conflictual or independent predictors of well-being and adjustment? Motivation and Emotion. 2006;**30**:273–282.

[37] Deci E. L., Ryan R. M. The "What" and "Why" of goal pursuits: Human needs and the self determination of behavior. Psychological Inquiry. 2000;**11**:227–268.

[38] Soenens B., Park S.-Y., Vansteenkiste M., Mouratidis A. Perceived parental psychological control and adolescent depressive experiences: A cross-cultural study with Belgian and South-Korean adolescents. Journal of Adolescence. 2012;**35**:261–272. DOI: 10.1016/j.adolescence.2011.05.001

[39] Mishra R., Mayer B., Trommsdorff G., Albert I., Schwarz B. The value of children in urban and rural India: Cultural background and empirical results. In: Trommsdorff G., Nauck B., editors. The Value of Children in Cross-Cultural Perspective—Case Studies from Eight Societies. Lengerich: Pabst Science; 2005. pp. 143–170.

[40] Saraswathi T. S., Pai S. Socialization in the Indian context. In: Kao H. S. R., Sinha D., editors. Asian Perspectives on Psychology. US: Sage Publications; 1997. pp. 79–88.

[41] Zervides S., Knowles A. Generational changes in parenting styles and the effect of culture. E-Journal of Applied Psychology. 2007;**3**(1):65–75.

[42] Rothbaum F., Weisz J., Pott M., Miyake K., Morelli G. Attachment and culture: Security in the United States and Japan. American Psychologist. 2001;**55**(10):827–829. DOI: 10.1037//0O03-066X.56.10.827

[43] Rothbaum F., Pott M., Azuma H., Miyake K., Weisz J. The development of close relationships in Japan and the United States—Paths of symbiotic harmony and generative tension. Child Development. 2000;**71**(5):1121–1142.

[44] Greenfield P. M., Keller H., Fuligni A., Maynard A. Cultural pathways through universal development. Annual Review of Psychology. 2003;**54**(1):461–490.

[45] Rothbaum F., Trommsdorff G. Do roots and wings oppose or complement one another? The socialization of autonomy and elatedness in cultural context. In: Grusec J. E., Hastings P. D., editors. The Handbook of Socialization: Theory and Research. New York: Guilford Press; 2007. pp. 461–489.

[46] Chen X., Rubin K. H., editors. Socioemotional Development in Cultural Context. New York: Guilford Press; 2011. 342 p.

[47] Pomerantz E. M., Wang Q. The role of parental control in children's development in Western and East Asian countries. Current Directions in Psychological Science. 2009;**18**:285–289.

[48] Soenens B., Vansteenkiste M., Luyten P. Toward a domain-specific approach to the study of parental psychological control: Distinguishing between dependency-oriented and achievement-oriented psychological control. Journal of Personality. 2010;**78**:217–256.

[49] Chao R. K. Beyond parental control and authoritarian parenting style: Understanding Chinese parenting through the cultural notion of training. Child Development. 1994;**65**:1111–1119.

[50] Trommsdorff G. Parent-adolescent relations in changing societies: A cross-cultural study. In: Noack P., Hofer M., Youniss J., editors. Psychological Responses to Social Change: Human Development in Changing Environments. Berlin: Walter de Gruyter; 1995. pp. 189–218.

[51] Chao R. K., Aque C. Interpretations of parental control by Asian immigrant and European American youth. Journal of Family Psychology. 2009;**23**:342–354.

[52] Seymour S. Women, Family and Child Care in India: A World in Transition. New York: Cambridge University Press; 1999. 344 p.

[53] Roopnarine J. L., Hossain Z. Parent-Child Socialization in Diverse Cultures. Norwood: Ablex; 1992.

[54] Pong S.-L., Hao L., Gardner E. The roles of parenting styles and social capital in the school performance of immigrant Asian and Hispanic adolescents. Social Science Quarterly. 2005;**86**(4):928–950. DOI: 10.1111/j.0038-4941.2005.00364.x

[55] Ranganath V. M., Ranganath V. K. Asian Indian children. In: Johnson-Powell G., Yamamoto J., editors. Transcultural Child Development: Psychological Assessment and Treatment. New York: Wiley; 1997. pp. 103–125.

[56] Yaman A., Mesman J., van IJzendoorn M. H., Bakermans-Kranenburg M. J., Linting M. Parenting in an individualistic culture with a collectivistic background: The case of Turkish immigrant families with toddlers in the Netherlands. Journal of Child and Family Studies. 2010;**19**(5):617–628. DOI: 10.1007/s10826-009-9346-y

[57] Deković M., Pels T., Model S., editors. Child Rearing in Six Ethnic Families: The Multi-Cultural Dutch Experience. New York: Edwin Mellen Press; 2006. 306 p.

[58] Rudy D., Grusec J. E. Correlates of authoritarian parenting in individualist and collectivist cultures and implications for understanding the transmission of values. Journal of Cross-Cultural Psychology. 2001;**32**:202–212. DOI: 10.1177/0022022101032003007

[59] Rudy D., Grusec J. E. Authoritarian parenting in individualist and collectivist groups: Associations with maternal emotion and cognition and children's self-esteem. Journal of Family Psychology. 2006;**20**(1):68–78.

[60] Güngör D., Bornstein M. H. Gender, development, values, adaptation, and discrimination in acculturating adolescents: The case of Turk heritage youth born and living in Belgium. Sex Roles: A Journal of Research. 2008;**60**:537–548. DOI: 10.1007/s11199-008-9531-2.

[61] Tamis-LeMonda C. S., Way N., Hughes D., Yoshikawa H., Kalman R. K., Niwa E. Y. Parents' goal for their children: The dynamic coexistence of individualism and collectivism in cultures and individuals. Social Development. 2008;**17**:182–209.

[62] Lieber E., Nihira K., Mink I. T. Filial piety, modernization, and the challenges of raising children for Chinese Immigrants: Quantitative and qualitative evidence. Ethos. 2004;**32**(3):324–347.

[63] Sujato B. A History of Mindfulness—How Insight Worsted Tranquillity in the Satipatthana Sutta. India: Santipada; 2012. 260 p.

[64] Dumas J. E. Mindfulness-based parent training: Strategies to lessen the grip of automaticity in families with disruptive children. Journal of Clinical Child and Adolescent Psychology. 2005;**34**(4):779–791.

[65] Holt R. W., Cottone R. R. Mindfulness: An overview for human services professionals. Journal of Human Services. 2014;**34**(1):52–69.

[66] Germer C. K., Siegel R. D., Fulton P. R., editors. Mindfulness and Psychotherapy. New York: Guilford; 2005. 333 p.

[67] Paulson J. The Psycheyana: Historical roots of contemporary mindfulness practices and future implications for social work education. International Research in Higher Education. 2016;**1**(2):149–154. DOI: 10.5430/irhe.v1n2p149

[68] Tirch D., Silberstein L. R., Kolts R. L. Buddhist Psychology and Cognitive-Behavioural Therapy: A Clinician's Guide. New York: Guilford Press; 2015. 266 p.

[69] Carson J. W., Carson K. M., Gil K. M., Baucom D. H. Mindfulness-based relationship enhancement. Behaviour Therapy. 2004;**35**:471–494. DOI: 10.1016/S0005-7894(04)80028-5

[70] Linehan M. Dialectical behaviour therapy (DBT) for borderline personality disorder [Internet]. 2003. Available from: http://www.dbtselfhelp.com/html/linehan_dbt.html [Accessed: 27th July 2016].

[71] Fleischhaker C., Bohme R., Sixt B., Bruck C., Schneider C., Schulz E. Dialectical behavioural therapy for adolescents (DBT-A): A clinical trial for patients with suicidal and self-injurious behaviour and borderline symptoms with a one-year follow-up. Child and Adolescent Psychiatry and Mental Health. 2011;**5**(3):1–10.

[72] Kabat-Zinn J. Mindfulness-based interventions in context: Past, present and future. Clinical Psychology. 2003;**10**:144–156. DOI: 10.1093/clipsy/bpg016

[73] Brown K. W., Ryan R. M. The benefits of being present: Mindfulness and its role in psychological well-being. Journal of Personality and Social Psychology. 2003;**84**(4):822–848.

[74] Kabat-Zinn M., Kabat-Zinn J. Everyday Blessings: The Inner Work of Mindful Parenting. New York: Hyperion; 1998. 416 p.

[75] Bogels S., Restifo K.. Mindful Parenting: A Guide for Mental Health Practitioners. New York: Springer; 2013. 328 p. DOI: 10.1007/978-1-4614-7406-7

[76] Coatsworth J. D., Duncan L. G., Greenberg M. T., Nix R. L. Changing parents' mindfulness, child management skills and relationship quality with their youth: Results from a

randomized pilot intervention trial. Journal of Child and Family Studies. 2010;**19**:203–217. DOI: 10.1007/s10826-0099304-8

[77] Bogels S. M., Lehtonen A., Restifo K. Mindful parenting in mental health care. Mindfulness. 2010;**1**:107–120. DOI: 10.1007/s12671-010-0014-5

[78] Duncan L. G., Coatsworth J. D., Greenberg M. T. A model of mindful parenting: Implications for parent-child relationships and prevention research. Clinical Child and Family Psychology Review. 2009;**12**:255–270. DOI: 10.1007/s10567-009-0046-3

[79] Geurtzen N., Scholte R. H. J., Engels R. C. M. E., Tak Y. R., van Zundert R. M. P. Association between mindful parenting and adolescents' internalizing problems: Non-judgmental acceptance of parenting as core element. Journal of Child and Family Studies. 2015;**24**:1117–1128. DOI: 10.1007/s10826-014-9920-9

[80] Dix T., Branca S. Parenting as a goal-regulation process. In: Kuczynski L., editor. Handbook of Dynamics in Parent-Child Relations. CA: Sage; 2003. pp. 167–188.

[81] Smetana J. G., Metzger A., Gettman D. C., Campione-Barr N. Disclosure and secrecy in adolescent-parent relationships. Child Development. 2006;**77**:201–217.

[82] Duncan L. G., Coatsworth J. D., Jochebed G. G., Geier M. H., Greenberg M. T. Can mindful parenting be observed? Relations between observational ratings of mother-youth interactions and mothers' self-report mindful parenting. Journal of Family Psychology. 2015;**29**(2):276–282. DOI: 10.1037/a0038857

[83] Hastings P. D., Grusec J. E. Parenting goals as organizers of responses to parent-child disagreement. Developmental Psychology. 1998;**34**(3):465–479.

[84] Altmaier E., Maloney R. An initial evaluation of a mindful parenting program. Journal of Clinical Psychology. 2007;**63**:1232–1238.

[85] Cohen J. A. S., Semple R. J. Mindful parenting: A call for research. Journal of Child and Family Studies. 2010;**19**:145–151. DOI: 10.1007/s10826-009-9285-7

7

Influence of Drugs on Cognitive Functions

Claudia Juárez-Portilla, Tania Molina-Jiménez, Jean-Pascal Morin, Gabriel Roldán-Roldán and Rossana Citlali Zepeda

Abstract

Disorders related to the misuse of certain drugs represent not only a worldwide public health problem, but also an economic and social issue. Adolescents and children represent the most vulnerable population for drug consumption and addiction. At this early stage in life, a crucial phase of the neurodevelopmental process, substance abuse can induce brain plasticity mechanisms that may produce long-lasting changes in neural circuitry and ultimately behavior. One of the consequences of these changes is the impairment of cognitive functions, with academic negative impact in the acquisition of new knowledge. In this chapter, we will describe the effects of illicit substances of abuse, both stimulants and depressants as well as prescription drug misuse and its influence of on learning and memory processes. Recent evidence on the new so-called smart drugs is also discussed.

Keywords: abuse, cognition, performance, nootropic, smart, stimulants, depressant, memory, impairment, adolescent

1. Introduction

According to United Nations Office on drugs and Crime, in 2015, around a quarter of a billion people used drugs, and approximately 29.5 million showed drug use disorders, including dependence [1]. Drug abuse produces health disruption. Disorders related to the use of certain drugs are associated with an important worldwide rate of morbidity. A wide range of drug-induced neurobiological modifications have been described; some of which can affect learning and memory functions. Stimulant drugs, like nicotine and amphetamine, improve cognitive function at lower doses but impair memory performance at higher doses. Depressant drugs, like alcohol, can cause long-term effects on prefrontal cortex function, disrupting cognitive abilities.

Several studies have suggested that the influence of psychoactive drugs on learning and memory might be explained, at least in part, because of the shared neurobiological mechanisms involved in learning and memory processes and the drug-induced structural and functional changes in the brain. Anatomically, there is an important overlap between the neural substrates of learning and memory and those of addiction. Some of the areas that show overlap include the cerebral cortex, hippocampus, amygdala and striatum [2]; all of them are components of the mesolimbic dopaminergic system.

Adolescence is a sensitive period in brain development characterized by a decrease in gray matter and an increase in white matter. The diminution of gray matter is thought to be due, at least in part, to the process of synaptic pruning, which is the developmental refinement of brain circuits by removal of superfluous synapses [3]. Early drug exposure is associated with frontal lobe damage, low cognitive performance and emotional learning, as well as other behaviors. Moreover, it has been demonstrated that adolescent exposure to both prescription and social drugs impairs cognition, as well as other behaviors, in the adulthood [4].

There is a clear bidirectional relationship between abuse of drugs and poor academic achievement. It has been suggested that cognitive deficits could make adolescents more vulnerable to substance abuse than others; conversely, other proposals argue that substance abuse is the source of cognitive impairments [5–7]. Of course the two possibilities are not mutually exclusive; teenagers with poor academic performance may be more prone to abusing illicit drugs, which may impair their results at school even further. While the several social science theories have been proposed to try to explain each of these phenomena [6], in the following text, we will focus on the cognitive consequences of adolescent substance abuse on the functioning of the nervous system that may have a deleterious impact on cognitive abilities, academic achievement and long-term satisfaction with life in general.

2. Stimulant drugs

Memory is the natural counterpart of learning; both are necessary for behavioral change that precedes survival of species. Substance abuse has been demonstrated to exert detrimental impact upon learning and memory. According to the United Nations Office on Drugs and Crime through World Drug Report 2017, 29.5 million people globally suffer from drug use disorders [8]. Cognitive impairment is a well-established consequence of long-term substance abuse, with stimulants as nicotine, methamphetamine (MA) and cocaine leading deficits in the area of executive function. Stimulants are a class of illicit drugs that can have negative impact on individuals who use them, although this impact might be masked by the believed benefits (**Table 1**) [9].

2.1. Nicotine

Nicotine is the main psychoactive component of tobacco and the responsible agent of tobacco dependency. According to the World Health Organization, despite its severe health consequences, about one billion people smoke worldwide.

Drug	Cognitive process	Effect	Model	Reference
Stimulant drugs	Attention Vigilance Memory	*Acute*: Improving selective visuospatial attention, spatial working memory and associative memory	Monkey Rat Mice Zebrafish Human	[10, 11]
		Chronic: Tolerance Withdrawal syndrome Mild deficits in memory and inhibition response Disruption in prospective and visual memory, verbal ability, reasoning and decision making	Human Rat	[13, 25–27, 29]
Depressant drugs	Attention Memory	*Acute/low doses*: Facilitation in working memory, verbal fluency and executive functions Impaired working memory, verbal fluency and executive functions	Human	[37, 38, 41, 55–57]
		Chronic/high doses: Disruption in working and episodic memory, consolidation memory, attention and memory Also, presence of blackouts	Human	[39, 61–67]

Table 1. Effects of the stimulants and depressant drugs in cognitive functions.

When nicotine is administered acutely, it produces positive effects improving cognitive functions, including sustained attention, vigilance, visuospatial selective attention, spatial working memory and associative memory, both in animal models [10] and in humans [11]. Conversely, a vast amount of literature has showed that chronic nicotine use leads to tolerance, and 1 h after cessation of nicotine exposure, nicotine withdrawal syndrome emerges and it is characterized by mild cognitive deficits. In other words, nicotine tends to improve cognitive function at lower doses and impair performance at higher doses [12]. Furthermore, heavy smokers under acute abstinence from smoking experience decreased neurocognitive functions, including impairments in sustained attention, working memory and response inhibition [13]. Strong activation of memory-related brain regions that include the dorsolateral prefrontal cortex and hippocampus has been correlated with smoking-related cues in adult heavy smokers [14]. These areas are involved in emotional learning and reward-related learning.

Some reports have shown that nicotine and nicotinic agonists, as mecamylamine, evoked cognitive enhancement by potentiating the release of dopamine [12, 15]. Working memory is critically reliant on dopaminergic neurotransmission. In addition, rodent studies have revealed a direct relationship between dopamine release in the prefrontal cortex and on memory task accuracy [16]. Moreover, cholinergic systems and nicotinic receptors are essential for cognitive processes and have been implicated in diseases associated with cognitive impairment [17].

2.2. Methamphetamine (MA)

MA abuse represents a serious public health issue associated with a high likelihood of relapse. By 2008, nearly 25 million people worldwide were estimated to have used MA, with abuse being among younger age groups [18]. MA used is mainly for recreational purposes and it is known to induce a variety of desirable effects, including increased energy levels, positive mood, euphoria, reduced appetite, weight loss, enhanced mental acuity and social and sexual disinhibition [19]. In addition, MA-dependent individuals often claimed enhancement of cognitive function and ability to focus following drug administration. However, this drug induces long-term changes in the brain structure and function, changes in synaptic plasticity, cell death via apoptosis and neurotoxicity, and consequently, it causes dependence and withdrawal syndrome [20].

Anatomically, MA has a preferential neurotoxic effect on the frontostriatal systems that contributes to both emotion dysregulation and neurocognitive impairment [21]. For instance, MA addicts showed impaired performance on tests of cognitive flexibility, which measures the ability to modify behavior when presented with new information or changing outcomes. These deficits may impair MA addicts from altering their habitual drug abuse behavior, leading to an inability to initiate abstinence or resist relapse [22]. Cellular mechanism of this MA impairment has been associated with long-term downregulation of dopamine transporters, suggesting that there are structural changes in some of the dopamine nerve terminals [23]. Other findings suggest that MA use causes changes in the metabolism of the insula and striatum [24]. In a study in humans, MA-dependent participants had significantly lower results than control participants on memory tasks, including prospective memory and visual memory [25]. Accordingly, studies in young adult MA abusers have shown impaired verbal ability, deficits in psychomotor processing [26], reasoning deficits reflecting problematic decision-making abilities as well as retrospective memory task impairment [27].

The evidences pointed that acute administration of MA improves cognitive functions, while chronic consumption of MA deteriorates them.

2.3. Cocaine

Cocaine has long been one of the most common recreational stimulants, especially for adolescents. A recent estimate indicates that half a million of United States habitants use this drug weekly; in this sense, cocaine addiction represents a substantial burden for societies worldwide, linked to adverse outcomes such as violence, suicide and disability, as well as high rates of chronic relapse [28]. In the brain, crack cocaine use has been shown to cause toxic effects, particularly in the prefrontal cortex. These abnormalities are associated with neuropsychological impairments.

Abundant evidence has shown that cocaine withdrawal induces memory decline after its chronic use. It has been reported that chronic cocaine users showed significant harm on verbal memory and fluency as well as deficits in cognitive flexibility, but not in spatial memory, after acute withdrawal. Further, Briand and colleagues observed that object recognition was disturbed after withdrawal from chronic exposure to cocaine by an object recognition task in 2-week abstinent rats [29]. Several reports have shown that the insular and prefrontal cortices, involved in cognitive control, show reduced activity on selective attention and inhibitory control tasks in cocaine addicts [30]. These brain areas may be involved in the maintenance and relapse of drug use [31]. Individuals with cocaine abuse and dependence show higher insula, frontal and/or striatum activation in response to cocaine-related cues, reflecting heightened attention in response to this drug [32, 33]. Furthermore, imaging data have revealed that gray matter volume loss over time is twice as fast among cocaine addicts as in healthy individuals. Given that gray matter volume in prefrontal cortex has been related to working memory performance, these findings are in keeping with the idea that long-term cocaine use may cause sustained deleterious effect on working memory.

3. Depressant drugs

Adolescence is the critical period for initiation of alcoholic beverage consumption. Epidemiologic studies reveal that alcohol use is remarkably common among teenagers, with increasing rates of alcohol abuse in the US including heavy episodic drinking [33]. After alcohol and tobacco, marijuana is the social drug most frequently consumed by this cohort. Additionally, a high percentage of alcohol abusers also consume marijuana [34]. Several studies have shown that both alcohol and marijuana tend to alter the structure and function of the brain and are associated with impaired decision-making, memory and impulsivity in young adults and adolescents (**Table 1**).

3.1. Ethanol

Evidence shows a direct correlation between early onset of alcohol intake and alcohol-related problems in adulthood, suggesting that adolescent exposure to the reinforcing properties of this drug increases the probability of its abuse later [35]. However, as for other addictive substances, the effect of exposure to alcohol depends to a great extent on how much and for how long it is consumed.

Acute alcohol intake has a biphasic effect on brain activity, causing excitation and euphoria at low blood concentration and depression as it increases [36]. However, regarding cognitive functions, experimental data have been inconsistent using a variety of cognitive tests. Thus, low or moderate doses of alcohol, relative to placebo, produced facilitation [37, 38], deficits [39] or no change [40] in memory performance at subtoxic amounts (<65 mg/dl). Moreover, it apparently does not produce adverse effects and may even slightly improve working memory in nonproblem drinkers, regardless of sex [41]. However, as the dose of alcohol increases, confusion, loss of awareness and selective attention begin to occur, significantly diminishing the execution of working memory and its long-term consolidation. The effect of alcohol on long-term memory formation is much greater than its impact on the capacity to remember previously consolidated memories or to retrieve short-term memory. It is well known that if subjects are asked to repeat newly acquired information following short delays (seconds) after its presentation while intoxicated, they often do fine [42]. Likewise, they are able to retrieve information acquired before acute intoxication. On the contrary, subjects perform very poorly using delays longer than 20 min, particularly if they are distracted between the stimulus presentation and testing [43].

As studies indicate that the extent of alcohol-induced memory deficits increases with the dose but maintains the same pattern (i.e., greater difficulty at forming new long-term memories than recalling the existing ones), it appears that this drug mostly affects memory consolidation.

Unfortunately, during adolescent life, repeated intoxication with high doses of alcohol becomes more frequent and memory impairments are more profound, commonly resulting in blackouts, that is, a complete incapability to remember all or part of a drinking event [44]. Heavy alcohol drinking associated with blackouts [45] does not necessarily involve loss of consciousness, but rather a failure to transfer information from short- to long-term memory [46]. Individuals with a history of blackouts show episodic memory impairments while intoxicated [47], particularly at retrieving the spatiotemporal context of events [48]. Moreover, long-term (3 years) heavy alcohol intake in adolescents between 15 and 19 years of age induced memory deficits [49] as well as volume reduction in subcortical and temporal regions [50].

The mechanisms underlying alcohol-induced memory disruption are still elusive. Throughout several decades, it was supposed that alcohol produces a nonspecific general depression of brain activity. Later, research led to assumption that alcohol depressed the activity of neurons by altering the fluidity of the neuronal membrane and consequently the activity of proteins, including ion channels that might, in turn, produce synaptic dysfunctions [51].

It was not until recently that new pharmacological information regarding the effects of alcohol on neural cells revealed that this drug has actually very selective effects on various neurotransmitter systems, both excitatory, e.g., glutamatergic and cholinergic, and inhibitory, such as GABAergic, glycinergic and serotonergic among others. Alcohol could alter the activity of specific receptor subtypes as well [52]. All these neurotransmission mechanisms have a deep impact on cognitive functions. Paradoxically, repeated alcohol exposure might promote the formation of a particular drug-reward–associated implicit memory that could underlay its addiction [53].

The main risk of alcohol ingestion early in life is that the adolescent brain is still in a maturation period and drug intoxication greatly affects its development and the individual's future life.

3.2. Cannabis

Recently, endocannabinoids, endogenous ligands that bind to and activate the same receptors as 9-delta-tetrahydrocannabinol (THC), the psychoactive component of cannabis, were found to play an important role in the diminution of gray matter [3]. Cannabis is the third most prevalent drug of abuse among teenagers, behind alcohol and tobacco [54]. Many studies in humans have shown that chronic cannabis consumption, especially when initiated early in life, correlates with a range of cognitive impairments in adulthood, including learning and memory deficits. Meanwhile, the evidence remained equivocal, partly due to the myriad of confounding factors, characteristic of human studies, as well as different methodology employed by the distinct studies, some unveiling clear effects, while others finding marginal or no effects [55]. However, in recent years, a clearer picture is emerging, which seems to suggest that teenage cannabis consumption may indeed have long-term detrimental effects on cognitive processes, including memory. The present section surveys the evidence linking adolescent cannabis consumption and prevailing memory deficits. We will further discuss the present state of knowledge on such questions as how is it that cannabis consumption can affect memory? Is memory homogenously affected or are there certain types of memory more impaired? Also, if cannabis intake during adolescence affects brain function in the long-term, are such sequelae reversible?

First, as for the acute effects of marijuana consumption, impaired working memory during the acute phase of cannabis intoxication has been observed in several studies [55, 56]. For instance, randomized clinical trials with dronabinol, a synthetic derivate of THC, revealed impaired verbal fluency, working memory and executive functions in healthy subjects during and in the hours following intoxication [57]. On the other hand, other works on healthy subjects found that performance on verbal working memory was left unaffected but that the tasks elicited a higher activation of parahippocampal areas, which may indicate either "neurophysiological inefficiency" or alternate/compensatory neural mechanisms in these subjects [58]. This is consistent with another fMRI study that was conducted on otherwise healthy adults that were current marijuana users and that showed hyperactivation during a verbal working memory challenge, which the authors suggest may be related to suboptimal efficiency during cognitive challenge in this group [59]. Finally, another study by the same group showed that the frequency of cannabis use is positively correlated to blood oxygenation level–dependent signal in the left parahippocampal gyrus during a visual associative memory task, regardless of the age of onset (early vs. late adolescence) [60].

But beyond the acute intoxication phase, one obvious question is whether cannabis consumption produces long-term sequelae on cognition. Working memory performance appears to be especially sensitive to cannabis consumption in the early teenage years (before the age of 16–17). Testing 122 long-term heavy cannabis users on a corroborated 28-day abstinence period and 87 control subjects, Pope and collaborators showed that although adult-onset cannabis users hardly differed from controls, those that started before the age of 17 were impaired in a series of cognitive tests, most especially in verbal memory [61]. Further research has shown that the observed cannabis-induced deficits may prevail even after 6 weeks of discontinuation; although after 3 months of complete discontinuation, no difference was observed between previous heavy users and controls [62]. However, a more recent study in adolescents 18–20 years old with a history of chronic, heavy cannabis use, while performance in a verbal memory test was comparable to that of age-matched controls, a significant bilateral atrophy was observed, even after 6 months of supervised drug abstinence [63]. The putative detrimental effects of cannabis use appear to be dose-dependent. For example, performance in the Rey Auditory Verbal Learning Test correlated negatively with the number of years of cannabis misuse [64].

However, these results did not allow to determine whether cannabis had long-term detrimental effects on the cognitive abilities and brain functioning of these youths once they reached adulthood or whether a preexisting set of slight cognitive deficiencies such as lower verbal memory somewhat predisposed these youths to maladaptive behaviors including early-onset cannabis consumption. More to the point, as the authors pointed out, even if the toxic effects of cannabis were the culprit, it was impossible to determine in the light of these results, whether the observed differences were due to long-term effects of cannabis on these subjects or more short-term effects during adolescence that made them perform poorly at school and therefore made them less prone to develop these cognitive skills through adulthood.

In this regard, a recent widely reaching analysis from the Cannabis Cohorts Research Consortium using data from three distinct longitudinal studies started to shed light on this issue [57]. The study found that young adults that were cannabis users as teenagers were more likely to experience adverse outcomes as diverse as cannabis addiction, suicide attempt and high-school dropout. Importantly, the authors report that controlling for the potential confounding factors present, both before and during adolescence and spanning individual, parental and peer factors, failed to abolish most of the associations observed. Along with the fact that they also observed a dose-response relation, heavy users having the poorest outcomes as adults, the findings support the hypothesis that teenage marijuana consumption has long-term detrimental effects on cognition, memory and general well-being. Finally, preclinical research brought further support for a causal relationship between teenage cannabis consumption and adult cognitive impairments; chronic consumption of cannabis in rats during adolescence, but not adulthood, impaired spatial working memory when tested as adults [65, 66].

4. Prescription drugs

According to the Anxiety and Depression Association of America, mental disorders are common among children in the United States. Anxiety and major depression disorders are usually diagnosed in children between 8 and 15 years of age (National Health and Nutrition Examination Survey). The treatment of metal disorders in children and adolescents depends on the impairment degree. However, these treatments usually include drugs that affect cognitive functions. On the other hand, during childhood and adolescence, sports activities, especially at college levels, are frequently a cause of painful injuries that requires acute or chronic treatment of anti-inflammatory and/or analgesic drugs. All these treatments that are administered to school students could have an impact on cognitive functions and therefore on academic achievement. In this section, we will discuss the effects of nonsteroidal anti-inflammatory, anxiolytic and antidepressant drugs (**Table 2**).

4.1. Nonsteroidal anti-inflammatory drugs (NSAIDs)

NSAIDs are therapeutic agents commonly used in clinical practice for their analgesic, anti-inflammatory and antipyretic activity [67]. Although these chemical compounds are structurally different, they all inhibit both isoforms of the cyclooxygenase enzyme, COX-1 and COX-2, an enzyme responsible for inflammation and pain, which is necessary for prostaglandins and prostanoid synthesis [68]. Normally, COX-2 is expressed in dendritic spines of hippocampal and cortex neurons and has been implicated in synaptic modification, because its expression increases during long-term potentiation [69]. Moreover, astrocytes express prostaglandin E2 receptors (EP) and prostaglandin E2 (PGE2), which regulate membrane excitability, synaptic transmission and synaptic plasticity implicated in learning and memory processes [70]. Also, the administration of misoprostol, an agonist of PGE2 receptors, ameliorates the long-term deficits observed in Huntington disease R6/1 mice by increasing the branching in hippocampal neurons and stimulating the synthesis of brain-derived neurotrophic factor (BDNF) [71].

Drug	Cognitive process	Effect	Model	Reference
Prescription drugs	Spatial memory impairment	Acute administration: Neuroprotection Subchronic administration: improving cognitive functions Chronic administration: improve spatial memory impairment	Rat Mouse	[70–75]
	Cognitive and emotional alterations	Reestablishment of the deterioration in memory and spatial learning Diminish despair and memory impairment Chronic administration: increase cell proliferation in hippocampus Increase of BDNF levels	Human Rat	[78, 81–86]
	Memory and learning impairment	Restore cognitive impairment Improve executive function Increase spatial memory	Mouse	[88–90]
Cognition-enhancing drugs	Formation of memories and performing tasks	Enhancing cognitive performance in Alzheimer's disease patients Improve cognitive functions as: verbal memory, attention memory, information processing, executive function and memory mood	Human	[95, 96]
	Alertness and enhance cognition	Improves attention, memory and executive function in sleep-deprived individuals Limited effects in nonsleep deprived Mental performance of subjects with low baseline performance	Human	[101–105]
	Attention deficit/ hyperactivity disorder	Improve cognition processes as: working memory, speed of processing, verbal learning and memory and attention	Human Rat	[107–109, 111]

Table 2. Effects of the prescription and cognition-enhancing drugs in cognitive functions.

Furthermore, subchronic administration of acetylsalicylic and ascorbic acids increases expression of receptors related with cognitive function such as learning and memory, while chronic treatment of acetylsalicylic acid lessens the spatial memory impairment observed in an experimental model of Alzheimer's disease [72]. Several reports indicate that celecoxib, a selective COX-2 inhibitor, reduces oxidative stress in a model of hypoxia reoxygenation, reducing the activation of microglia and astrocytes in the neonatal rat brain and improving cognitive function, suggesting that celecoxib may have neuroprotective actions [73]. In addition, multiple exposures to sevoflurane, a model that mimics the neurotoxicity induced by anesthesia, produces an increase in proinflammatory cytokines and deterioration in cognitive function in young mice, effects that were attenuated by the administration of ketorolac [74]. Another study showed that meloxicam ameliorated the depressive-like behavior, cognitive impairment and neuroinflammation in hippocampus caused by chronic unpredictable mild stress [75]. Then, NSAIDs indirectly could disrupt cognitive functions.

4.2. Antidepressant drugs

Major depression is a common mental disorder affecting adolescents in the United States. According to the National Institute of Mental Health, in 2015, an estimated of 3 million adolescents aged 12–17 in the United States had, at least, one major depressive episode. Major depressive disorder is a long-term disabling condition occurring with relapse and recurrences, which could become a chronic condition [76]. Among all the symptoms presented in this psychopathology, memory and attention deficits are considered an important clinical manifestation of major depressive disorder [77]. Furthermore, cognitive and emotional alterations observed in depressive patients have been associated with changes in neuronal activity of prefrontal cortex, cingulate cortex and hippocampus. In major depressive disorder, orbitofrontal, ventromedial and prefrontal cortices are hypoactive, and postmortem evidence indicates histopathological changes in orbitofrontal and prefrontal cortex [78]. Additionally, significant hyperactivity in anterior cingulated cortex, inferior frontal gyrus and occipitoparietal regions has been observed in adolescents with major depressive disorder [79]. Also, a reduction in the volume of the hippocampus was reported, which is related to the severity and the duration of the major depressive disorder [80]. All these alterations were shown to contribute to changes in cognitive and emotional processing in depressive patients. Nevertheless, antidepressant treatment contributed to reestablish mood and cognitive functions. For instance, the chronic administration of deprenyl, a monoamine-oxidase-B inhibitor, reestablished the deterioration in memory and spatial learning and also diminished the lipid peroxidation and the neuronal loss in prefrontal cortex, striatum and hippocampus [81]. Moreover, treatment with desipramine, a norepinephrine reuptake inhibitor, caused reestablished long-term potentiation and diminished despair and memory impairment, through activation of CREB in the hippocampus [82]. Similar effects were observed with fluoxetine (serotonin reuptake inhibitor); rats receiving a chronic treatment of fluoxetine increased cell proliferation and BDNF in hippocampus associated to a memory and learning improvement [83]. These studies suggest that antidepressants revert memory and learning deterioration observed in animal models of depression.

Regarding clinical studies, patients with major depressive disorder showed lower levels of BDNF in plasma, which correlates with memory function deficits; hence, BDNF levels increased after the antidepressant treatment [84]. Nevertheless, the impairment in psychomotor and memory processes observed in depressed treated patients has no significance for clinical purposes [85]. Moreover, some evidence has shown that conventional antidepressant treatment selectively diminishes cognitive dysfunction [86].

The involvement of antidepressant drugs in cognitive functions is not clear; however, animal model studies have shown that synaptic plasticity is increased in neuronal regions involved in mood and memory processing [81–84].

4.3. Anxiolytics

Cognitive impairments have been consistently reported in anxiety disorders. Benzodiazepine, which acts in a specific site of the GABA A receptor, has been, for many years, the first-line therapy for the treatment of anxiety disorders. Although benzodiazepines are attractive for their rapid therapeutic effect, these drugs have undesirable side effects both in the short term (e.g., sedation) and in the long-term (e.g., dependence and memory impairment [87]). Some reports have indicated that GABAergic neurotransmission in the hippocampus is involved in the modulation of learning and memory functions [88]. Also, the administration of an inverse agonist of $\alpha 5$ subtype GABA A receptors (RO4938581) enhances long-term potentiation in hippocampus, restores the cognitive impairment caused by the scopolamine treatment and improves the executive function in monkeys without affecting emotional state [89]. Furthermore, a partial inverse agonist of $\alpha 5$ subtype GABA A receptors increased spatial memory [90]. These studies indicate that GABAergic neurotransmission regulates memory and learning processes, which opens the possibility of designing new selective molecules with clinical utility, not just for treating anxiety disorders, but also for improving cognitive functions.

5. Cognition-enhancing drugs

The search for drugs that improve cognitive functions to treat several diseases, including Alzheimer disease (AD), attention deficit disorder (ADD), attention deficit hyperactivity disorder (ADHD), has derived a wide number of synthetic drugs that, in turn, increase learning, executive functions, or creativity in healthy people. These drugs, also named "smart drugs" or "nootropics," have different chemical origins and mechanisms and in general have showed little or no effect in improving learning and memory tasks. There is a growth in the consumption of these drugs by adolescents [91, 92], mainly due to academic demands and competitiveness [93]. According to the Federal Substance Abuse and Mental Health Services Administration, every year around 137,000 college students in the US begin to use psychostimulants. Furthermore, consumption of stimulant drugs of abuse increases in key academic dates (**Table 2**) [94].

Nootropics have focused their targets on modulation of neurotransmission, hormones, transduction systems and neuron metabolism. However, we will focus on legal stimulants commonly used by students to improve academic performance: acetylcholinesterase inhibitors, memantine, modafinil and methylphenidate.

5.1. Antidementia drugs

5.1.1. Acetylcholinesterase inhibitors (AChEIs)

Most of the drugs that are used to enhance cognitive functions, both in patients and in healthy volunteers, work through acetylcholine (ACh) neurotransmission. ACh is a neurotransmitter closely involved in synaptic transmission and also in the formation of memories and performing tasks. Donepezil, rivastigmine or galantamine had good results enhancing cognitive performance in patients with mild to moderate AD, when compared with placebo [95]. However, diverse studies conducted in healthy volunteers have showed that AChEIs lightly improve verbal memory after semantic processing of words, attention memory, information processing, executive function and memory mood [96].

5.1.2. Memantine

Memantine is a psychostimulant used to treat moderate to severe AD. It acts on the glutamatergic system by antagonizing N-methyl-D-aspartate (NMDA) receptors. This drug has been showed to slightly improve cognitive functions as monotherapy of AD [97]. There are few studies about the cognitive-enhancing capacity of memantine on healthy volunteers. The studies published were tested with acute single dose of memantine, finding that this drug does not increase mental performance significantly [96].

5.2. Modafinil

Modafinil is a psychostimulant indicated in the treatment of narcolepsy, shift work sleep disorder and excessive daytime sleepiness [98]. Since approval by FDA, in 1998, modafinil has been widely used not only to treat wakefulness disorders, but also to increase alertness and enhance cognition. Modafinil exhibits advantages among other psychostimulants, including the lack of unwanted side effects (e.g., tolerance, abuse potential, sleep rebound and locomotor excitability) [99], and, in most countries, it is not a controlled substance; therefore, it can be easily purchased online. Modafinil exerts its actions through an unknown mechanism. Still, it is recognized that modafinil inhibits dopamine and noradrenaline uptake, elevates catecholamine's levels, therefore raises extracellular serotonin, glutamate, histamine and orexin and reduces GABA's concentration [100]. Although the effects of modafinil as a wakefulness promoter have been proven [101], its properties as cognitive enhancer are still controversial. In sleep-deprived individuals, modafinil improves attention, memory and executive function [102], while the effects of modafinil in non–sleep-deprived adolescents are limited [103]. Other reports have found that modafinil actually improves several cognitive functions [104]. Interestingly, modafinil has showed to enhance mental performance of subjects with low baseline performance or IQ on several tasks evaluated [105].

5.3. Methylphenidate (MPH)

MPH (Ritalin©) is a psychostimulant approved for the treatment of attention deficit/hyperactivity disorder (ADD/ADHD) [106]. Additionally, MPH is one of the most effective cognitive enhancers used by healthy people [107], because it acts through a mechanism analogous to that of cocaine: increases the levels of the catecholamines, dopamine, norepinephrine and serotonin, by blocking their transport [108]. This drug improves working memory, speed of processing, verbal learning and memory and attention [102]. Nevertheless, MPH effects are not restricted to spatial problems, since it also improves digit span test score [109]. Although MPH has demonstrated to be effective and safe in most of the patients when used in the short term, several side effects have been reported: decrease of appetite, insomnia, headache, irritability, weight loss, sadness, abdominal pain, nausea, somnolence, dizziness, among others.

Several studies have reported that MPH treatment during childhood produces "permanent" changes in behavioral responses to other psychostimulants [110]. Moreover, a recent study made on rats has showed that acute and long-term exposure of adolescents to MHP has important effects on reward-dependent learning and decision [111].

5.4. Considerations about use and misuse of cognition-enhancing drugs

There are some difficulties evaluating the efficacy of smart drugs, mainly due to the heterogeneity of subjects and the differences in the cognitive evaluation methods. Besides, the disparities in the design of the studies have been challenging the evaluation of smart drugs in healthy subjects. However, there are some studies that have used systematic methodology to analyze the literature published on healthy volunteers [96, 97]. According to these reviews, antidementia drugs, AChEIs and memantine enhance cognitive functions in patients with AD; nevertheless, their effects on healthy volunteers appear to be very poor [107]. Another aspect to consider is the interindividual variability of volunteers, because it could be an important reason that masks the cognitive effect of these drugs.

There are also several ethical considerations about the use of psychostimulants in healthy people. Currently, caffeine is the stimulant most commonly used to get alertness. However, the misuse of MPH and modafinil is growing among students, since these drugs are cheap and easy to obtain illegally.

6. Perspectives

Drug abuse and addiction to legal and illegal substances have become a major challenge in western developed and developing societies. Growing evidence has shown that the onset age of drug consumption is around 15 years. At this age, the central nervous system is still under maturation. Childhood and adolescence are critical stages for neural and social development. Therefore, worldwide increasing prevalence of drug abuse among teenagers will certainly have an effect on scholar performance. All the evidence described in the present review suggests that teenagers that consume drugs risk deleterious consequences in their academic growth, since the neural mechanisms targeted by these drugs may have long-term impacts on cognitive functions. Therefore, prevention initiatives and public health programs must be implemented in schools to protect children and teenagers from escalating drug use.

7. Conclusion

In summary, the evidence regarding the possible long-term detrimental effects of teenage drug consumption on learning and memory adds to the increased risk of developing mental disorders, and therefore it should be included in public health information campaigns that seek to encourage delaying and/or reducing drug consumption at this stage of life. The scientific information obtained from studies such as those described above will be of little use without adequate public policies aimed at alleviating this serious problem.

Author details

Claudia Juárez-Portilla[1], Tania Molina-Jiménez[2], Jean-Pascal Morin[3], Gabriel Roldán-Roldán[3] and Rossana Citlali Zepeda[1]*

*Address all correspondence to: rzepeda@uv.mx

1 Biomedical Research Centre, University of Veracruz, Xalapa, Veracruz, Mexico

2 Faculty of Chemical Pharmaceutical Biologist, and Faculty of Biology, University of Veracruz, Xalapa, Veracruz, Mexico

3 Department of Physiology, Faculty of Medicine, National Autonomous University of Mexico, Mexico City, Mexico

References

[1] United Nations Office on Drugs and Crime through World Drug Report 2017. Available from: https://www.unodc.org/wdr2017/field/Booklet_1_EXSUM.pdf [Accessed: 2017-08-29]

[2] Kelley AE. Memory and addiction: Shared neural circuitry and molecular mechanisms. Neuron. 2004;**44**:161-179. DOI: 10.1016/j.neuron.2004.09.016

[3] Bossong MG, Niesink RJM. Adolescent brain maturation, the endogenous cannabinoid system and the neurobiology of cannabis-induced schizophrenia. Progress in Neurobiology. 2010;**92**(3):370-385. DOI: 10.1016/j.pneurobio.2010.06.010

[4] Robbins T, Everitt B, David N, editors. The neurobiology of addiction. 1st ed. The Royal Society; 2008. Available from: https://global.oup.com/academic/product/the-neurobiology-of-addiction-9780199562152?cc=mx&lang=en Accessed 2017-09-21

[5] Henry KL. Academic achievement and adolescent drug use: An examination of reciprocal effects and correlated growth trajectories. The Journal of School Health. 2010;**80**(1):38-43. DOI: 10.1111/j.1746-1561.2009.00455.x

[6] Bryant AL, Zimmerman MA. Examining the effects of academic beliefs and behaviors on changes in substance use among urban adolescents. Journal of Education & Psychology. 2002;**94**(3):621-637. DOI: 10.1037/0022-0663.94.3.621

[7] Crosnoe R. The connection between academic failure and adolescent drinking in secondary school. Sociology of Education. 2006;**79**(1):44-60 https://www.ncbi.nlm.nih.gov/pmc/articles/PMC2834180/

[8] Jasper LE. Working Memory and Long-Term Abstinence from Substance Use. 2016. PhD Thesis, George Fox University

[9] Hall FS, Der-Avakian A, Gould TJ, Markou A, Shoaib M, Young JW. Negative affective states and cognitive impairments in nicotine dependence. Neuroscience and Biobehavioral Reviews. 2015;**58**:168-185. DOI: 10.1016/j.neubiorev.2015.06.004

[10] Grundey J, Amu R, Ambrus GG, Batsikadze G, Paulus W, Nitsche MA. Double dissociation of working memory and attentional processes in smokers and non-smokers with and without nicotine. Psychopharmacology. 2015;**232**(14):2491-2501. DOI: 10.1007/s00213-015-3880-7

[11] Jasinska AJ, Zorick T, Brody AL, Stein EA. Dual role of nicotine in addiction and cognition: A review of neuroimaging studies in humans. Neuropharmacology. 2014;**84**:111-122. DOI: 10.1016/j.neuropharm.2013.02.015

[12] Ashare RL, Falcone M, Lerman C. Cognitive function during nicotine withdrawal: implications for nicotine dependence treatment. Neuropharmacology. 2014;**76**(Pt B):581-591. DOI: 10.1016/j.neuropharm.2013.04.034

[13] Gould TJ, Leach PT. Cellular, molecular, and genetic substrates underlying the impact of nicotine on learning. Neurobiology of Learning and Memory. 2014;**107**:108-132. DOI: 10.1016/j.nlm.2013.08.004

[14] Freedman R. Agonistas del receptor α7-nicotínico de la acetilcolina para la mejora cognitiva en la esquizofrenia. Revisión Anual de la Medicina. 2014;**65**:245-261. DOI: 10.1146/annurev-med-092112-142937

[15] Robbins TW, Arnsten AF. The neuropsychopharmacology of fronto-executive function: Monoaminergic modulation. Annual Review of Neuroscience. 2009;**32**:267-287. DOI: 10.1146/annurev.neuro.051508.135535

[16] Dineley KT, Pandya AA, Yakel JL. Nicotinic ACh receptors as therapeutic targets in CNS disorders. Trends in Pharmacological Sciences. 2015;**36**(2):96-108. DOI: 10.1016/j.tips.2014.12.002

[17] Harlé KM, Zhang S, Schiff M, Mackey S, Paulus MP, Yu AJ. Altered statistical learning and decision-making in methamphetamine dependence: Evidence from a two-armed bandit task. Frontiers in Psychology. 2015;**6**:1-14. DOI: 10.3389/fpsyg.2015.01910

[18] Dwoskin LP, Glaser PE, Bardo MT. Methamphetamine. In: Addiction Medicine. New York: Springer; 2010. pp. 1049-1061. DOI: 10.1007/978-1-4419-0338-9_52

[19] Bigdeli I, Nikfarjam-Haft Asia M, Miladi-Gorji H, Fadaei A. The spatial learningand memory performance in methamphetamine-sensitized and withdrawn rats. Iranian Journal of Basic Medical Sciences. 2015;**18**:234-239. Available from: https://www.ncbi.nlm.nih.gov/pubmed/25945235 [Accessed: 29-08-2017]

[20] Casaletto KB, Obermeit L, Morgan EE, Weber E, Franklin DR, Grant I, Woods SP. Depression and executive dysfunction contribute to a metamemory deficit among individuals with methamphetamine use disorders. Addictive Behaviors. 2015;**0**:45-50. DOI: 10.1016/j.addbeh.2014.08.007

[21] Cox BM, Cope ZA, Parsegian A, Floresco SB, Aston-Jones G, See RE. Chronic methamphetamine self-administration alters cognitive flexibility in male rats. Psychopharmacology. 2016;**233**(12):2319-2327. DOI: 10.1007/s00213-016-4283-0

[22] Thanos PK, Kim R, Delis F, Rocco MJ, Cho J, Volkow ND. Effects of chronic methamphetamine on psychomotor and cognitive functions and dopamine signaling in the brain. Behavioural Brain Research. 2017;**320**:282-290. DOI: 10.1016/j.bbr.2016.12.010

[23] Stewart JL, Connolly CG, May AC, Tapert SF, Wittmann M, Paulus MP. Striatum and insula dysfunction during reinforcement learning differentiates abstinent and relapsed methamphetamine-dependent individuals. Addiction. 2014;**109**(3):460-471. DOI: 10.1111/add.12403

[24] Morgan EE, Woods SP, Poquette AJ, Vigil O, Heaton RK, Grant I. Visual memory in methamphetamine-dependent individuals: Deficient strategic control of encoding and retrieval. The Australian and New Zealand Journal of Psychiatry. 2012;**46**(2):141-152. DOI: 10.1177/0004867411433212

[25] Latvala A, Castaneda AE, Peräla J, Saarni SI, Aalto-Setäla T, Lönnqvist J, Kaprio J, Suvisaari J, Tuulio-Henriksson A. Cognitive functioning in substance abuse and dependence: A population-based study of young adultsadd. Addiction. 2009;**104**:1558-1568. DOI: 10.1111/j.1360-0443.2009.02656.x

[26] Rendell PG, Mazur M, Henry JD. Prospective memory impairment in former users of methamphetamine. Psychopharmacology. 2009;**203**:609-616. DOI: 10.1007/s00213-008-1408-0

[27] Degenhardt L, Hall W. Extent of illicit drug use and dependence, and their contribution to the global burden of disease. Lancet. 2012;**379**:55-70. DOI: http://dx.doi.org/10.1016/S0140-6736(11)61138-0

[28] Amin B, Andalib S, Vaseghi G, Mesripour A. Learning and memory performance after withdrawal of agent abuse: A review. Iranian Journal of Psychiatry and Behavioral Sciences. 2016;**10**(2):e1822. DOI: 10.17795/ijpbs-1822

[29] Naqvi NH, Bechara A. The insula and drug addiction: An interoceptive view of pleasure, urges, and decision-making. Brain Structure & Function. 2010;**214**:435-450. DOI: 10.1016/j.pbb.2009.08.005

[30] Goldstein RZ, Craig AD, Bechara A, Garavan H, Childress AR, Paulus MP, Volkow ND. The neurocircuitry of impaired insight in drug addiction. Trends in Cognitive Sciences. 2009;**13**(9):372-380. DOI: 10.1016/j.tics.2009.06.004

[31] Prisciandaro JJ, Myrick H, Henderson S, McRae-Clark AL, Brady KT. Prospective associations between brain activation to cocaine and no-go cues and cocaine relapse. Drug and Alcohol Dependence. 2013;**131**:44-49. DOI: 10.1016/j.drugalcdep.2013.04.008

[32] Prisciandaro JJ, McRae-Clark AL, Myrick H, Henderson S, Brady KT. Brain activation to cocaine cues and motivation/treatment status. Addiction Biology. 2014;**19**(2):240-249. DOI: 10.1111/j.1369-1600.2012.00446.x

[33] Stewart JL, Connolly CG, May AC, Tapert SF, Wittmann M, Paulus MP. Cocaine dependent individuals with attenuated striatal activation during reinforcement learning are

more susceptible to relapse. Psychiatry Research. 2014;**223**(2):129-139. DOI: 10.1016/j.pscychresns.2014.04.014

[34] Martin CS, Kaczynski NA, Maisto SA, Tarter RE. Polydrug use in adolescent drinkers with and without DSM-IV alcohol abuse and dependence. Alcoholism, Clinical and Experimental Research. 1996;**20**:1099-1108. DOI: 10.1111/j.1530-0277.1996.tb01953.x

[35] Vitali M, Napolitano C, Berman MO, Minuto SF, Battagliese G, Attilia ML, Braverman ER, Romeo M, Blum K, Ceccanti M. Neurophysiological measures and alcohol use disorder (AUD): Hypothesizing links between clinical severity index and molecular neurobiological patterns. Journal of Addiction Research & Therapy. 2016;**5**(2):1-17. DOI: 10.4172/2155-6105.1000181

[36] Harrison NL, Skelly MJ, Grosserode EK, Lowes DC, Zeric T, Phister S, Salling MC. Effects of acute alcohol on excitability in the CNS. Neuropharmacology. 2017;**122**:36-45. DOI: 10.1016/j.neuropharm.2017.04.007

[37] Gilbertson R, Ceballos NA, Prather R, Nixon SJ. Effects of acute alcohol consumption in older and younger adults: perceived impairment versus psychomotor performance. Journal of Studies on Alcohol and Drugs. 2009;**70**(2):242-252. Available from: https://www.ncbi.nlm.nih.gov/pmc/articles/PMC2653610/pdf/jsad242.pdf Accessed: 2017-08-29

[38] Sklar AL, Gilbertson R, Boissoneault J, Prather R, Nixon SJ. Differential effects of moderate alcohol consumption on performance among older and younger adults. Alcoholism, Clinical and Experimental Research. 2012;**36**(12):2150-2156. DOI: 10.1111/j.1530-0277.2012.01833.x

[39] Friedman TW, Robinson SR, Yelland GW. Impaired perceptual judgment at low blood alcohol concentrations. Alcohol. 2011;**45**:711-718. DOI: 10.1016/j.alcohol.2010.10.007

[40] Dry MJ, Burns NR, Nettelbeck T, Farquharson AL, White JM. Dose-related effects of alcohol on cognitive functioning. PLoS One. 2012;**7**(11):e50977. DOI: 10.1371/journal.pone.0050977

[41] Hoffman L, Nixon SJ. Alcohol doesn't always compromise cognitive function: Exploring moderate. Doses in young adults. Journal of Studies on Alcohol and Drugs. 2015;**76**(6):952-956. DOI: 10.15288/jsad.2015.76.952

[42] Ryback RS. The continuum and specificity of the effects of alcohol on memory. A review. Quarterly Journal of Studies on Alcohol. 1971;**32**(4):995-1016

[43] Acheson SK, Stein RM, Swartzwelder HS. Impairment of semantic and figural memory by acute ethanol: Age-dependent effects. Alcoholism, Clinical and Experimental Research. 1998;**22**(7):1437-1442. DOI: 10.1111/j.1530-0277.1998.tb03932.x

[44] White AM, Jamieson-Drake DW, Swartzwelder HS. Prevalence and correlates of alcohol-induced blackouts among college students: Results of an e-mail survey. Journal of American College Health. 2002;**51**(3):117-119 (122-131). DOI: http://dx.doi.org/10.1080/07448480209596339

[45] Wetherill RR, Fromme K. Alcohol-induced blackouts: A review of recent clinical research with practical implications and recommendations for future studies. Alcoholism, Clinical and Experimental Research. 2016;**40**(5):922-935. DOI: 10.1111/acer.13051

[46] White AM. What happened? Alcohol, memory blackouts, and the brain. Alcohol Research & Health. 2003;**27**(2):186-196. Available from: https://pubs.niaaa.nih.gov/publications/arh27-2/186-196.pdf [Accessed: 29-08-2017]

[47] Wetherill RR, Fromme K. Acute alcohol effects on narrative recall and contextual memory: An examination of fragmentary blackouts. Addictive Behaviors. 2011;**36**(8):886-889. DOI: 10.1016/j.addbeh.2011.03.012

[48] Wetherill RR, Schnyer DM, Fromme K. Acute alcohol effects on contextual memory BOLD response: Differences based on fragmentary blackout history. Alcoholism, Clinical and Experimental Research. 2012;**36**(6):1108-1115. DOI: 10.1111/j.1530-0277.2011.01702.x

[49] Squeglia LM, Pulido C, Wetherill RR, Jacobus J, Brown GG, Tapert SF. Brain response to working memory over three years of adolescence: Influence of initiating heavy drinking. Journal of Studies on Alcohol and Drugs. 2012;**73**(5):749-760. DOI: https://doi.org/10.15288/jsad.2012.73.749

[50] Squeglia LM, Rinker DA, Bartsch H, Castro N, Chung Y, Dale AM, Jernigan TL, Tapert SF. Brain volume reductions in adolescent heavy drinkers. Developmental Cognitive Neuroscience. 2014 Jul;**9**:117-125. DOI: 10.1016/j.dcn.2014.02.005

[51] Chin JH, Goldstein DB. Effects of low concentrations of ethanol on the fluidity of spin-labeled erythrocyte and brain membranes. Molecular Pharmacology. 1977;**13**(3):435-441. Available from: http://molpharm.aspetjournals.org/content/13/3/435.long [Accessed: 30-08-2017]

[52] Criswell HE, Simson PE, Duncan GE, McCown TJ, Herbert JS, Morrow AL, Breese GR. Molecular basis for regionally specific action of ethanol on gamma-aminobutyric acid A receptors: Generalization to other ligand-gated ion channels. The Journal of Pharmacology and Experimental Therapeutics. 1993;**267**(1):522-537. Available from: http://jpet.aspetjournals.org/content/267/1/522.long [Accessed: 29-08-2017]

[53] Bernier BE, Whitaker LR, Morikawa H. Previous ethanol experience enhances synaptic plasticity of NMDA receptors in the ventral tegmental area. Journal of Neuroscience. 2011;**31**(14):5205-5212. DOI: 10.1523/JNEUROSCI.5282-10.2011

[54] Degenhardt L, Chiu WT, Sampson N, Kessler RC, Anthony JC, Angermeyer M, Bruffaerts R, de Girolamo G, Gureje O, Huang Y, Karam A, Kostyuchenko, Lepine JP, Medina Mora ME, Neumark Y, Ormel JH, Pinto Meza A, Posada-Villa J, Stein DJ, Takeshima T, Wells JE. Toward a global view of alcohol, tobacco, cannabis, and cocaine use: Findings from the WHO world mental health surveys. PLoS Medicine. 2008;**5**(7):1053-1067. DOI: https://doi.org/10.1371/journal.pmed.0050141

[55] Schoeler T, Bhattacharyya S. The effect of cannabis use on memory function: An update. Substance Abuse and Rehabilitation. 2013;**4**(January):11-27. DOI: https://doi.org/10.2147/SAR.S25869

[56] Crean RD, Crane NA, Mason BJ. An evidence based review of acute and long-term effects of cannabis use on executive cognitive functions. Journal of Addiction Medicine. 2011;**5**(1):1-8. DOI: https://doi.org/10.1097/ADM.0b013e31820c23fa.An

[57] Silins E, Horwood LJ, Patton GC, Fergusson DM, Olsson CA, Hutchinson DM, Spry E, Toumbourou JW, Degenhardt L, Swift W, Coffey C, Tait RJ, Letcher P, Copeland J, Mattick RP. Young adult sequelae of adolescent cannabis use: An integrative analysis. The Lancet Psychiatry. 2014;**1**(4):286-293. DOI: https://doi.org/10.1016/S2215-0366(14)70307-4

[58] Bossong MG, Jager G, Bhattacharyya S, Allen P. Acute and non-acute effects of cannabis on human memory function: A critical review of neuroimaging studies. Current Pharmaceutical Design. 2014;**20**(13):2114-2125. DOI: https://doi.org/10.2174/1381612811 3199990436

[59] Becker B, Wagner D, Gouzoulis-Mayfrank E, Spuentrup E, Daumann J. The impact of early-onset cannabis use on functional brain correlates of working memory. Progress in Neuro-Psychopharmacology & Biological Psychiatry. 2010b;**34**(6):83745. DOI: https:// doi.org/10.1016/j.pnpbp.2010.03.032

[60] Becker B, Wagner D, Gouzoulis-Mayfrank E, Spuentrup E, Daumann J. Altered parahippocampal functioning in cannabis users is related to the frequency of use. Psychopharmacology. 2010a;**209**(4):361-374. DOI: https://doi.org/10.1007/s00213-010-1805-z

[61] Pope HG, Gruber AJ, Hudson JI, Cohane G, Huestis MA, Yurgelun-Todd D. Early-onset cannabis use and cognitive deficits: What is the nature of the association? Drug and Alcohol Dependence. 2003;**69**(3):303-310. DOI: https://doi.org/10.1016/S0376-8716 (02)00334-4

[62] Schweinsburg AD, Brown SA, Tapert SF. The influence of marijuana use on neurocognitive functioning in adolescents. Current Drug Abuse Reviews. 2008;**1**(1):99-111. Available from: http://www.ncbi.nlm.nih.gov/pubmed/19630709 [Accessed: 29-08-2017]

[63] Ashtari M, Avants B, Cyckowski L, Cervellione KL, Roofeh D, Cook P, Gee J, Sevy S, Kumra S. Medial temporal structures and memory functions in adolescents with heavy cannabis use. Journal of Psychiatric Research. 2011;**45**(8):1055-1066. DOI: https://doi.org/10.1016/j.jpsychires.2011.01.004

[64] Auer R, Vittinghoff E, Yaffe K, Künzi A, Kertesz SG, Levine DA, Albanese E, Whitmer RA, Jacobs DR Jr, Sidney S, Glymour MM, Pletcher MJ. Association between lifetime marijuana use and cognitive function in middle age. JAMA Internal Medicine. 2016;**176**(3):352-361. DOI: https://doi.org/10.1001/jamainternmed.2015.7841

[65] Renard J, Krebs MO, Jay TM, Le Pen G. Long-term cognitive impairments induced by chronic cannabinoid exposure during adolescence in rats: A strain comparison. Psychopharmacology. 2013;**225**(4):781-790. DOI: https://doi.org/10.1007/s00213-012-2865-z

[66] Renard J, Rushlow WJ, Laviolette SR. What can rats tell us about adolescent cannabis exposure? Insights from preclinical research. Canadian Journal of Psychiatry. 2016;**61**(6): 328-334. DOI: https://doi.org/10.1177/0706743716645288

[67] Abdulla A, Adams N, Bone M, Elliott AM, Gaffin J, Jones D, Knaggs R, Martin D, Sampson L, Schofield P. British geriatric society. Guidance on the management of pain in older people. Age and Ageing. 2013;**42**:1-57. DOI: 10.1093/ageing/afs200

[68] Atkinson TJ, Fudin J, Jahn HL, Kubotera N, Rennick AL, Rhorer M. What's new in NSAID pharmacotherapy: Oral agents to injectables. Pain Medicine. 2013;**14**:S11-S17. DOI: 10.1111/pme.12278

[69] Yang H, Chen C. Cyclooxygenase-2 in synaptic signaling. Current Pharmaceutical Design. 2008;**14**:1443-1451. DOI: 10.2174/138161208784480144

[70] Furuyashiki T, Narumiya S. Stress responses: The contribution of prostaglandin E(2) and its receptors. Nature Reviews. Endocrinology. 2011;**7**:163-175. DOI: 10.1038/nrendo.2010.194

[71] Anglada-Huguet M, Vidal-Sancho L, Giralt A, García-Díaz Barriga G, Xifró X, Alberch J. Prostaglandin E2 EP2 activation reduces memory decline in R6/1 mouse model of Huntington's disease by the induction of BDNF-dependent synaptic plasticity. Neurobiology of Disease. 2016;**95**:22-34. DOI: 10.1016/j.nbd.2015.09.001

[72] DoostMohammadpour J, Hosseinmardi N, Janahmadi M, Fathollahi Y, Motamedi F, Rohampour K. Non-selective NSAIDs improve the amyloid-β-mediated suppression of memory and synaptic plasticity. Pharmacology, Biochemistry, and Behavior. 2015;**132**:33-41. DOI: 10.1016/j.pbb.2015.02.012

[73] Fan LW, Kaizaki A, Tien LT, Pang Y, Tanaka S, Numazawa S, Bhatt AJ, Cai Z. Celecoxib attenuates systemic lipopolysaccharide-induced brain inflammation and white matter injury in the neonatal rats. Neuroscience. 2013;**240**:27-38. DOI: 10.1016/j.neuroscience.2013.02.041

[74] Shen X, Dong Y, Xu Z, Wang H, Miao C, Soriano SG, Sun D, Baxter MG, Zhang Y, Xie Z. Selective anesthesia-induced neuroinflammation in developing mouse brain and cognitive impairment. Anesthesiology. 2013;**118**:502-515. DOI: 10.1097/ALN.0b013e3182834d77

[75] Luo Y, Kuang S, Li H, Ran D, Yang J. cAMP/PKA-CREB-BDNF signaling pathway in hippocampus mediates cyclooxygenase 2-induced learning/memory deficits of rats subjected to chronic unpredictable mild stress. Oncotarget. 2017;**8**:35558-35572. DOI: 10.18632/oncotarget.16009

[76] Kessler RC, Bromet EJ. The epidemiology of depression across cultures. Annual Review of Public Health. 2013;**34**:119-138. DOI: 10.1146/annurev-publhealth-031912-114409

[77] Rock PL, Roiser JP, Riedel WJ, Blackwell AD. Cognitive impairment in depression: A systematic review and meta-analysis. Psychological Medicine. 2013;**44**:1-12. DOI: https://doi.org/ 10.1017/S0033291713002535

[78] Klauser P, Fornito A, Lorenzetti V, Davey CG, Dwyer DB, Allen NB, Yücel M. Cortico-limbic network abnormalities in individuals with current and past major depressive disorder. Journal of Affective Disorders. 2015;**173**:45-52. DOI: 10.1016/j.jad.2014.10.041

[79] Colich NL, Ho TC, Foland-Ross LC, Eggleston C, Ordaz SJ, Singh MK, Gotlib IH. Hyperactivation in cognitive control and visual attention brain regions during emotional interference in adolescent depression. Biological Psychiatry: Cognitive Neuroscience and Neuroimaging. 2017;**2**:388-395. DOI: 10.1016/j.bpsc.2016.09.001

[80] Zhao K, Liu H, Yan R, Hua L, Chen Y, Shi J, Lu Q, Yao Z. Cortical thickness and subcortical structure volume abnormalities in patients with major depression with and without anxious symptoms. Brain and Behavior: A Cognitive Neuroscience Perspective. 2017;**7**:e00754. DOI: 10.1002/brb3.754

[81] Kiray M, Bagriyanik HA, Pekcetin C, Ergur BU, Uysal N, Ozyurt D, Buldan Z. Deprenyl and the relationship between its effects on spatial memory, oxidant stress and hippocampal neurons in aged male rats. Physiological Research. 2006;**55**:205-212. Available from: http://www.biomed.cas.cz/physiolres/pdf/55/55_205.pdf [Accessed: 21-09-2017]

[82] Wang DD, Li J, LP Y, MN W, Sun LN, Qi JS. Desipramine improves depression-like behavior and working memory by up-regulating p-CREB in Alzheimer's disease associated mice. Journal of Integrative Neuroscience. 2016;**15**:247-260. DOI: 10.1142/S02196352165 0014X

[83] Welbat JU, Sangrich P, Sirichoat A, Chaisawang P, Chaijaroonkhanarak W, Prachaney P, Pannangrong W, Wigmore P. Fluoxetine prevents the memory deficits and reduction in hippocampal cell proliferation caused by valproic acid. Journal of Chemical Neuroanatomy. 2016;**78**:112-118. DOI: 10.1016/j.jchemneu.2016.09.003

[84] Molendijk ML, Bus BA, Spinhoven P, Penninx BW, Kenis G, Prickaerts J, Voshaar RC, Elzinga BM. Serum levels of brain-derived neurotrophic factor in major depressive disorder: State-trait issues, clinical features and pharmacological treatment. Molecular Psychiatry. 2011;**16**:1088-1095. DOI: 10.1038/mp.2010.98

[85] Gorenstein C, de Carvalho SC, Artes R, Moreno RA, Marcourakis T. Cognitive performance in depressed patients after chronic use of antidepressants. Psychopharmacology. 2006;**185**:84-92. DOI: 10.1007/s00213-005-0274-2

[86] Bortolato B, Miskowiak KW, Köhler CA, Maes M, Fernandes BS, Berk M, Carvalho AF. Cognitive remission: A novel objective for the treatment of major depression? BMC Medicine. 2016;**14**:9. DOI: 10.1186/s12916-016-0560-3

[87] Rudolph U, Möhler H. GABAA receptor subtypes: Therapeutic potential in Down syndrome, affective disorders, schizophrenia, and autism. Annual Review of Pharmacology and Toxicology. 2014;**54**:483-507. DOI: 10.1146/annurev-pharmtox-011613-135947

[88] Prut L, Prenosil G, Willadt S, Vogt K, Fritschy JM, Crestani F. A reduction in hippocampal GABAA receptor $\alpha 5$ subunits disrupts the memory for location of objects in mice. Genes, Brain, and Behavior. 2010;**9**:478-488. DOI: 10.1111/j.1601-183X.2010.00575.x

[89] Ballard TM, Knoflach F, Prinssen E, Borroni E, Vivian JA, Basile J, Gasser R, Moreau JL, Wettstein JG, Buettelmann B, Knust H, Thomas AW, Trube G, Hernandez MC. RO4938581, a novel cognitive enhancer acting at GABAA alpha5 subunit-containing receptors. Psychopharmacology. 2009;**202**:207-223. DOI: 10.1007/s00213-008-1357-7

[90] Navarro JF, Buron E, Martin-Lopez M. Anxiogenic-like activity of L-655,708, a selective ligand for the benzodiazepine site of GABAA receptors which contain the alpha-5 subunit, in the elevated plus-maze test. Progress in Neuro-Psychopharmacology & Biological Psychiatry. 2002;**26**:1389-1392. DOI: https://doi.org/10.1016/S0278-5846(02)00305-6

[91] Ott R, Biller-Andorno N. Neuroenhancement among swiss students—A comparison of users and non-users. Pharmacopsychiatry. 2014;**47**:22-28. DOI: 10.1055/s-0033-1358682

[92] Schulenberg JE, Johnston LD, O'Malley PM, Bachman JG, Miech RA, Patrick ME. Monitoring the Future National Survey Results on Drug Use, 1975-2016: Volume II, College Students and Adults Ages 19-55. Ann Arbor: Institute for Social Research, The University of Michigan, The University of Michigan; 2017. 445 pp. Available from: http://monitoringthefuture.org/pubs.html#monographs [Accessed: 2017-08-29]

[93] Garasic MD, Lavazza A. Moral and social reasons to acknowledge the use of cognitive enhancers in competitive-selective contexts. BMC Medical Ethics. 2016;**17**:18. DOI: 10.1186/s12910-016-0102-8

[94] Lipari R. The CBHSQ Report: Monthly Variation in Substance Use Initiation among Full-Time College Students Rockville. Substance Abuse and Mental Health Services Administration, Center for Behavioral Health Statistics and Quality; 2015. Available from: https://www.ncbi.nlm.nih.gov/books/NBK343537 Accessed 2017-09-21

[95] Birks J. Cholinesterase inhibitors for Alzheimer's disease. The Cochrane Database of Systematic Reviews. 2006;**1**:1-3. DOI: 10.1002/14651858.CD005593

[96] Repantis D, Laisney O, Heuser I. Acetylcholinesterase inhibitors and memantine for neuroenhancement in healthy individuals: A systematic review. Pharmacological Research. 2015;**61**(6):473-481. DOI: 10.1016/j.phrs.2010.02.009

[97] Matsunaga S, Kishi T, Iwata N. Memantine Monotherapy for Alzheimer's disease: A systematic review and meta-analysis. PLoS One. 2015a;**10**(4):e0123289. DOI: 10.1371/journal.pone.0123289

[98] Kumar R. Approved and investigational uses of modafinil: An evidence-based review. Drugs. 2008;**68**(13):1803-1839. DOI: 10.2165/00003495-200868130-00003

[99] Deroche-Gamonet V, Darnaudéry M, Bruins-Slot L, Piat F, Le Moal M, Piazza PV. Study of the addictive potential of modafinil in naive and cocaine-experienced rats. Psychopharmacology (Berl). 2002;**161**:387-395. DOI: 10.1007/s00213-002-1080-8

[100] WM Q, Huang ZL, XH X, Matsumoto N, Urade Y. Dopaminergic D1 and D2 receptors are essential for the arousal effect of modafinil. The Journal of Neuroscience. 2008;**28**:8462-8469. DOI: 10.1523/JNEUROSCI.1819-08.2008

[101] Westenson NJ, Killgore WD, Balkin TJ. Performance and alertness effects of caffeine, dextroamphetamine, and modafinil during sleep deprivation. Journal of Sleep Research. 2005;**14**:255-266. DOI: 10.1111/j.1365-2869.2005.00468.x

[102] Repantis D, Schlattmann P, Laisney O, Heuser I. Modafinil and methylphenidate for neuroenhancement in healthy individuals: A systematic review. Pharmacological Research. 2010;**62**(3):187-206. DOI: 10.1016/j.phrs.2010.04.002

[103] Randall DC, Fleck NL, Shneerson JM, File SE. The cognitive-enhancing properties of modafinil are limited in non-sleep deprived middle-aged adolescents. Pharmacology Biochemistry & Behavior. 2004;**77**:547-555. DOI: 10.1016/j.pbb.2003.12.016

[104] Battleday RM, Brem AK. Modafinil for cognitive neuroenhancement in healthy non-sleep-deprived subjects: A systematic review. European Neuropsychopharmacology. 2015;**25**:1865-1881. DOI: 10.1016/j.euroneuro.2015.07.028

[105] Randall DC, Shneerson JM, File SE. Cognitive effects of modafinil in student volunteers may depend on IQ. Pharmacology Biochemistry & Behavior. 2005;**82**:133-139. DOI: 10.1016/j.pbb.2005.07.019

[106] Storebø OJ, Krogh HB, Ramstad E, Moreira-Maia C, Holmskov M, Skoog M, Holmskov M, Rosendal S, Groth C, Magnusson FL, Moreira-Maia CR, Gillies D, Buch Rasmussen K, Gauci D, Zwi M, Kirubakaran R, Forsbol B, Simonsen E, Gluud C. Methylphenidate for attention-deficit/hyperactivity disorder in children and adolescents: Cochrane systematic review with meta-analyses and trialsequential analyses of randomised clinical trials. British Medical Journal. 2015;**351**:h5203. DOI: 10.1136/bmj.h5203

[107] Advokat C, Scheithauer M. Attention-deficit hyperactivity disorder (ADHD) stimulant medications as cognitive enhancers. Frontiers in Neuroscience. 2013;**7**:82. DOI: 10.3389/fnins.2013.00082

[108] Kuczenski R, Segal DS. Effects of methylphenidate on extracellular dopamine, serotonin, and norepinephrine: Comparison with amphetamine. Journal of Neurochemistry. 1997;**68**:2032-2037. DOI: 10.1046/j.1471-4159.1997.68052032.x

[109] Agay N, Yechiam E, Carmel Z, Levkovitz Y. Non-specific effects of methylphenidate (Ritalin) on cognitive ability and decision-making of ADHD and healthy adults. Psychopharmacology (Berl). 2010;**210**:511-529. DOI: 10.1007/s00213-010-1853-4

[110] Crowley NA, Cody PA, Davis MI, Lovinger DM, Mateo Y. Chronic methylphenidate exposure during adolescence reduces striatal synaptic responses to ethanol. The European Journal of Neuroscience. 2014;**39**(4):548-556. DOI: 10.1111/ejn.12426

[111] LR A, E J-B, MS MM, JD R. Acute and long-term effects of adolescent methylphenidate on decision-making and dopamine receptor mRNA expression in the orbitofrontal cortex. Behavioural Brain Research. 2017;**324**:100-108. DOI: 10.1016/j.bbr.2017.02.019

8

Can Frames Make Change? Using Communications Science to Translate the Science of Child Mental Health

Nat Kendall-Taylor and Allison Stevens

Abstract

Mental illness in children is on the rise in the United States, but research shows that the American public does not understand the science of child mental health—what it is and what supports and disrupts it. To build public understanding of child mental health and support for the systemic solutions needed to promote it, the FrameWorks Institute developed a "core story"—a master narrative—that advocates and experts in the field can use to communicate about the issue more effectively. This research is built on interviews with experts and members of the public, cognitive analyses of frames commonly used in media stories about the issue, and surveys of frame elements such as values and metaphors. Findings show that two values—*Prosperity* and *Ingenuity*—lifted support for policies related to child mental health. The *Levelness* Explanatory Metaphor, which compares child mental health to the levelness of a table, is also effective.

Keywords: framing, communication science, health communication, mass communication theory, qualitative analysis, culture and science, interdisciplinary social science, public perception of science, child mental health

1. Introduction

Mental illness, long considered a taboo subject, is breaking into the public discourse. Lawmakers across the U.S. political spectrum, members of the American news media, and leading advocates and philanthropists in the country are increasingly paying attention to mental health issues. New laws have expanded access to mental healthcare services, and advocates are working to fulfill growing demands for treatments for a range of mental health disorders. As President Obama stated in 2016: "Mental health should be treated as part of a person's overall health, and we must ensure individuals living with mental health conditions can get the treatment they need." Nevertheless, advocates, experts, and practitioners still face significant obstacles in the way the public thinks about mental health—and particularly child mental health. We must overcome these barriers, and the cultural understandings that undergird them, if we hope to build public support for the services and supports that children and families need to promote good mental health and if we want our society to flourish in the future.

To do this, we must find new ways of talking with the public and policymakers about the science of child mental health. Mental illness in children, including conditions often diagnosed in childhood such as attention-deficit/hyperactivity disorder, behavioral disorders, and autism spectrum disorder, are on the rise [1]. And many children do not get the treatment they need when they need it. The average time between the onset of mental illness symptoms and intervention is 8–10 years, according to the National Alliance on Mental Illness (NAMI). Children with mental illness have lower educational achievement and greater involvement with the criminal justice system [2]—negative outcomes that affect individuals, families, and communities. Data clearly show that the inability of our systems to support positive child mental health is affecting our entire society.

To be sure, the national conversation does occasionally turn to child mental health, particularly in response to high-profile incidents in the news—when, say, an adolescent opens fire on his classroom peers. But these conversations do not advance the movement for better prevention strategies and much better treatment for children with mental illness. In fact, they reinforce the very patterns of public thinking that keep people from engaging productively with this issue. Part of the inability to move child mental health issues forward is due to an inhospitable communications environment—a cultural context in which messages about the science of child mental health and the importance of the systems that support it are unable to thrive and spread.

Child development scientists have made significant advances in recent decades, and the public does have more access to information about child mental health than previous generations did [3]. Yet our research, discussed below, shows that Americans do not understand the complex science behind mental health, particularly as it applies to children. They are not even sure child mental health exists—that children, and especially young ones, can in fact have "good" or "poor" mental health. Child development experts say that child mental health is a real phenomenon that requires public attention. But the public does not share this conviction; they do not appreciate the importance of this issue or the need for policies and systemic solutions.

Even when people are able to understand that children experience states of mental health, our research shows that they tend to equate good mental health with a narrow understanding of emotions and see solutions in individualistic terms rather than at the level of biology, development, or social context. According to this way of thinking, children can achieve good mental health if they have the discipline to control their emotions. Mental *illness*, on the other hand, is perceived as a genetic problem that has no cure but that can be managed to some degree by taking drugs to correct "chemical" imbalances. This way of thinking, as we discuss below, interferes with public support for potential solutions.

This lack of understanding undermines efforts to educate the public about child mental health and build public support for programs and policies that can support positive mental health and address mental health issues. When people have a better understanding of what child mental health is and when they can see what disrupts and promotes it, they are more likely to take steps to support policies and programs that promote good mental health in children and that increase access to high-quality treatment. Public support for child mental health policies, in other words, is not a matter of *opinion* but of *cognition and understanding* [4].

This chapter explores research conducted by the FrameWorks Institute, a communications think tank in Washington, D.C., to describe the "cognitive terrain" of thinking about child mental health in the United States and to provide advocates and experts with communications tools they can use to more effectively move through this terrain. It first "charts the landscape" by describing the differences between how child development experts and the American public understand child mental health and illness and then analyzes child mental health frames in use by the news media. Next, this chapter "redraws the map" by exploring the effect of communications tools and framing strategies on public understanding of the issue.

2. Charting the landscape

The Expert Story. In 2009, FrameWorks conducted extensive research on expert views of child and family mental health; public views of these issues; and of media frames. This work was undertaken in partnership with and with support from the Center on the Developing Child at Harvard University and was supplemented by initial funding from the Endowment for Health in New Hampshire. It builds on more than a decade of FrameWorks research on ways that frames—the strategic presentation of information that cues predictable responses—can build public understanding of the science of early brain and biological development. It is an important chapter in the "core story"—or master narrative—FrameWorks developed to more effectively communicate the science of early childhood.

FrameWorks undertook a two-step research process to understand the differences between how child mental health is understood by child development experts and by members of the U.S. public. First, researchers interviewed a panel of seven child development experts to distill the state of the science and refine the messages experts need to communicate with the public. This series of one-on-one hour-long interviews was supplemented by a review of relevant scholarly literature. Researchers found that—contrary to public narratives about the issue—experts emphasize that child mental health is a "real phenomenon" that has long-term implications for lifelong health and well-being [5]. They emphasized that child mental health is caused by interactions between a child's genes and the environment in which he or she lives and affects the child's ability to function in developmentally appropriate ways within the family and community. Experts often defined child mental health in negative terms—as the absence of symptoms or pathology—rather than in clear, positive ones. The science was clear, however, about the importance of early intervention and the fact that it can help prevent long-term effects for children who have symptoms of mental disorders.

The Public Story. After distillling the "expert story" about child mental health, FrameWorks researchers set out to distill the "public story" about this issue. This research is based on theories that argue that individuals use cognitive structures called cultural models to make sense of their social worlds [6]. As noted anthropologist and sociologist Evan Goffman wrote in his 1967 book:

> *Cultural models can be seen as systems of existing and consistently implied relationships, propositions, and assumptions that are implicitly applied to make sense of and organize the information and experiences that individuals are presented with. Functionally, these models are what allow us to make sense of an infinite range of incoming information and experiences expeditiously enough to interact seamlessly with the individuals and situations that we encounter [8].*

To understand the cultural models that Americans use to understand mental health, mental illness, and child mental health, FrameWorks conducted a series of in-depth open-ended interviews with 20 members of the American public in Dallas, Texas, and Cleveland, Ohio, and an additional set of "on-the-street" interviews in three other U.S. locations. The sample included 10 men and 10 women of various ages, races and ethnicities, and political identifications. While the sample was not nationally representative (nor was it intended to be), participants were selected to ensure that the cultural models identified represented shared, or cultural, patterns of thinking. Previous research shows that members of the same culture share many of the same beliefs and attitudes about social issues—even when they differ according to race, ethnicity, socioeconomic background, and other criteria [4].

2.1. Dominant cultural models

Analysis of the interviews revealed the following cultural models about mental health, mental illness, and child mental health. The FrameWorks Institute describes these models as "dominant" because of their pervasiveness throughout participants' talk. The findings are summarized in *Conflicting Models of Mind in Mind*, a report published by the FrameWorks Institute in 2009 [7].

- ***Mental* health is tantamount to *emotional* health.** Participant discussions revealed an assumption that good mental health results from experiencing positive emotions and coping with negative ones. Poor mental health, in turn, was seen to result from failing to "deal with" negative emotions. Participants also believed that individuals are responsible for controlling their emotions and, by extension, their mental health.

  Mental health, then, is seen as an individual issue, not an environmental or contextual one. This individualistic, or "mentalist," model is common in American culture. It reflects a widely shared assumption that people's outcomes are completely under their control and determined by hard work and self-discipline. When applied to issues related to child mental health, this model reduces the complex interactions between individuals and environmental and systemic factors to individual control and undermines efforts to advance systemic solutions to promote child mental health. If mental health is determined by an individual's emotional state and controlled by his or her ability to control emotions, then remediating problems is an individual's responsibility and can be accomplished through effort and discipline. Contextual supports and interventions are difficult to see as important when thinking in this way.

- **Mental *illness* is a "chemical imbalance" in the brain.** While participants saw mental health as an issue of emotions, they understood mental illness as caused by the presence or absence of certain chemicals in the brain. As such, participants saw mental health as a condition that can be controlled by the individual and mental illness as a condition over which individuals have no control. Some participants thought people might benefit from medication, but participants also assumed that the chemicals that result in mental illness are genetic and, as such, are "hard-wired" into the brain. Pharmaceuticals, they reasoned, are the only way to rebalance these chemicals.
- **Children either *do* or *do not* experience mental health.** Participants spoke in multiple and contradictory ways about child mental health and illness. Some said, for example, that children *do not* experience mental health because their brains work in different ways than adult brains do. Children, they said, cannot "really" have mental health because they "are not sufficiently aware of, do not have the ability to remember, and do not have enough understanding of their emotions to experience either good or poor mental health." Participants also said children—especially the very young—have less ability to understand and remember emotions, which they understood to determine whether children can experience meaningful mental states. Other participants, meanwhile, said children *do* experience mental health but in less complex ways than adults do. Participants compared children to "little adults" who live in "simpler worlds" with "fewer variables" (i.e., parents, the home environment, and the classroom). Reasoning from this assumption, children's narrow worlds limit their ability to experience extreme states of mental health or illness.

2.2. Implications of dominant cultural models

These dominant cultural models have significant implications for advocates and experts who are seeking to build public understanding and support for systemic solutions. Communicators who cue these models, even if inadvertently, are likely to depress public support for child mental health policies and programs. FrameWorks compares these cultural models to a swamp —a rich, wild, untamed ecosystem where advocates' messages can get "lost" in a thicket of unproductive or competing assumptions, attitudes, and beliefs about children, families, and mental health, or "eaten" by stronger, counterproductive attitudes and beliefs about these subjects. The swamp is meant to convey the complexity, depth, and multiplicity of public thinking on social and scientific issues and the fact that much of this thinking takes place at an implicit level. The swamp can help communicators see how certain ways of thinking are productive for communicating certain messages and others unproductive in creating openings to consider new information. The swamp metaphor is not meant to imply that certain ways of thinking are "right" and others "wrong." Culture is never right or wrong, but certain cultural understandings can facilitate the communication of ideas while others may block or impede the communications process.

Advocates and experts who have a map of the swamp of cultural models about child mental health will be better able to make their way through it and more successful in moving their messages and issues into the public discourse with fidelity. Their messages will not get lost in the swamp or "devoured" by other counterproductive models about child mental health—the "gators" in the swamp. The following are key implications of the swamp for those communicating about child mental health, as explained in detail in a 2009 report by the FrameWorks Institute [7].

First, if the public believes that emotional health is tantamount to mental health, and that children do not experience emotions in the same way that adults do, then people will question whether children do in fact experience mental health. This makes it difficult to effectively communicate about the importance of policies and programs that promote child mental health and for funding for such actions. This is especially true in conversations about very young children, who are perceived to have even less capacity to experience emotions.

Second, if young children cannot remember experiences, then the long-term effects of those experiences on mental health become difficult to conceptualize. This can make it difficult for people to grasp the importance of programs that promote child mental health at early ages, which experts say is deeply affected by the experiences children have in their early years.

Third, if people believe that child and adult mental health are essentially the same, then they will have difficulty understanding the need for child-specific treatments or interventions for particular developmental periods and will gravitate toward those that encourage children to take responsibility for coping with negative emotions. This is something that was frequently seen in FrameWorks research.

2.3. Recessive cultural models

Analysis of cultural models interviews revealed the following recessive cultural models about mental health, mental illness, and child mental health [9]. FrameWorks describes these models as "recessive" because they came up less often than dominant models and were pushed to the cognitive periphery when a more dominant model came into thinking.

Some participants acknowledged that a child's environment can influence whether he or she experiences good or poor mental health. Environmental factors, however, were most frequently restricted to parental behavior and home life. Participants often overlooked other factors, such as relationships with other caregivers, housing quality, neighborhood and community resources, child care and school quality, and the "built environment."

Some participants understood that stress, and specifically prolonged or repeated stress, can contribute to mental health conditions in children. As above, these participants had a narrow understanding of the source of stress; they saw it coming mainly from home and school environments. Some also talked about how children who experience strong "foundations" (i.e., nurturing and responsive interactions with caring adults during their early years) are more likely to experience good mental health and those who have poor foundations are more likely to have poor mental health.

Participants also defined the quality of a child's mental health as his or her level of functioning—the ability to participate in developmentally appropriate activities in typical ways in family and community environments. This is consonant with the views of experts, who assess a child's mental health in part by his or her functional and developmentally appropriate capabilities.

2.4. Implications of recessive cultural models

Swamps are not entirely dangerous places. In addition to giant reptiles, venomous snakes, and murky bogs, they also have things of great beauty, richness, and utility, like orchids and rare medicinal plants. The same is true for the "swamp" of cultural models of child mental health. This cultural ecology has useful thought patterns that, if activated, can help in the communications of child mental health science and increase the accessibility of key messages from the field of child development. These more recessive models represent opportunities for advocates to help members of the public better understand the science behind child mental health and build support for needed policies and programs.

For example, the fact that, with the right cues, people are able to appreciate that a child's environment can affect his or her mental health is important because it opens the door for people to access and apply scientific understandings of the influence of environmental factors such as nutrition, supportive relationships, housing quality, access to health and child care, and others, on child mental health. Even so, participants had a very limited understanding of which environmental factors *do* in fact affect mental health; they tended to focus narrowly on parents and home life and overlooked the effects of other environmental and systemic factors that shape mental health and development more generally. Also important is the fact that participants were able to understand the effects of stress—again, at certain points in their discussions—and particularly prolonged, severe stress, on children's mental health. And finally, the fact that participants could think of child mental health in terms of developmentally appropriate functioning is promising because of the consonance between this way of thinking and the science of child mental health.

2.5. Gaps in understanding

The following section summarizes the gaps between expert and public understandings of child mental health [4]. These gaps represent specific challenges for child mental health advocates to address through strategic communications and framing. Frames, as discussed in subsequent sections of this chapter, have proven effective in bridging these gaps and deepening understanding of key concepts from the field of child mental health and increasing support for a new set of solutions.

- Experts blur the line between mental health and mental illness, but the public see these as separate and distinct.
- Experts support a wide range of means to prevent and treat mental health issues and disorders, but the public has narrow understandings of effective treatments depending on whether they are thinking about mental health or mental illness. They see individuals as responsible for developing good mental health and drugs as a way to cope with—but not cure—mental illness.
- Experts believe that child mental health is a real phenomenon that requires attention, but the public frequently does not share that unequivocal conviction or the experts' sense of the salience of the issue.

- Experts have a broad understanding of the environmental factors that shape mental health, but, for members of the public, this view is limited to home and family.
- Experts believe that the genetic influence on mental health and illness is contingent on environments and experiences, while the public sees genes and the chemicals they shape as "set in stone."

2.6. The media story

Understanding cultural models about child mental health, and knowing how they differ from expert views, is a key first step in creating more effective strategies to bring science to public thinking. Understanding how the media frames the issue adds an important layer of detail about public thinking and can be a lever for shifting and expanding it. The media is a primary source of information for Americans [10] and plays a powerful role in setting and reinforcing cultural models. As explained in an earlier FrameWorks study on this subject: "Common media frames lead to common interpretations both because of their standardized content and due to the fact that repeated exposure to these frames activates and engrains a set of interpretations that become highly practiced and easy to use in 'thinking' information on an issue" [10]. Advocates and experts who understand how the media influences cultural models—specifically how they amplify some ways of thinking and suppress others—will be better able to navigate their messages through the swamp of public thinking.

To map media frames of child mental health, FrameWorks, in partnership with the Endowment for Health and the Center on the Developing Child at Harvard University, conducted a systematic analysis of articles published in major newspapers between May 2008 and May 2009. The analysis identified dominant news frames and examined how those frames affect, and are affected by, public thinking.

Overall, the findings showed that the media rarely cover children's mental *health*. Instead, the media is more likely to cover mental *illness*, but in ways that are likely to cue unproductive cultural models. For example, many articles that were included in the sample painted detailed "pictures of vivid cases" of disruptive child behavior. One story, published in the *Omaha World-Herald* in 2008, chronicles a mother's decision to leave her 11-year-old son in a U.S. hospital. The story describes how the boy tore the house apart, refused to take his medication, tortured the family pet, and physically abused his brother. The mother felt that placing her son in state care was "the only way" to help him [10]. Articles that describe children's disruptive behavior in this level of detail are likely to trigger the public's sense of hopelessness about mental illness in general and children's mental disorders in particular. When presented with such vivid accounts of severe issues, members of the public are likely to see these problems as caused by genetic factors, and "set in stone" and thus incurable [10]. Reasoning from this perspective, it is difficult to see solutions as tenable and hard to engage in the issue.

These articles also present details about the difficulties faced by families in accessing care but exclude, to a large extent, explanations about how and why children develop mental illness or about specific solutions and how they work to address issues and improve outcomes. This suppresses public thinking about programs and policies that can promote child mental health. "Without coverage that strategically frames the science of child mental health, and concretizes and specifies policies that involve all citizens, child mental health outcomes will continue to be perceived by the public as an unfortunate but unsolvable problem that affects a small subset of Americans," the study found [10].

On the other hand, researchers did find some promising aspects of media coverage of child mental health. To start, the media focus on issues of access and adopt a systemic perspective in these discussions—that is, when discussing access issues, media coverage tends to focus on the structural factors that impede or facilitate a family's ability to access treatment. This is particularly true of coverage of issues facing marginalized populations. Low-income families, or those of racial and ethnic minority groups, are frequently portrayed as facing structural factors that make it difficult for them to access the care they need for a child with a mental health issue [10]. These more systemic or "thematic" stories likely encourage readers to adopt a more structural and contextual perspective and move beyond what FrameWorks calls the *Family Bubble*—the widely shared assumption that parenting behaviors determine children's outcomes and the difficulty in seeing the wider set of factors that affect parents. Despite these more positive aspects of the media coverage, the report concludes, "The likely impact of the media's definition of the problem is to deepen the public's sense that children's mental health problems are fundamentally intractable and cannot be addressed through programs or policies that support these children and their families" [10].

3. Redrawing the map

To help advocates and experts navigate the swamp of public thinking about child mental health, FrameWorks designed and tested framing strategies for their ability to increase public understanding of child mental health issues and support for a wide range of evidence-based solutions [11]. As part of this work, FrameWorks tested the effect of six values on public thinking. Values are frame elements that orient readers to deep beliefs or principles they consider worthy and important. Four of the six values were chosen because they had performed well in prior research on early childhood development. These values were collective prosperity (we will all prosper if we promote child mental health); ingenuity (we can tackle difficult problems like child mental health with innovative solutions); future progress (we must devote resources to children because they are the key to future social progress); and responsible management (we have a responsibility to make careful decisions about how best to support child well-being). The survey also tested two values that were common in advocacy literature: vulnerable children (we must take action to support children because they are society's most vulnerable members) and health (investing in children's well-being is important because health is an important social goal). In 2010, FrameWorks followed this initial survey experiment with a subsequent one that tested two additional values: prevention (the power of prevention-focused actions in improving long-term outcomes for children and society) and interdependence (the notion that children's mental health affects the well-being of all of society) [11].

The surveys found that two values—prosperity and ingenuity—improved respondents' understanding of the importance of child mental health and elevated their support for evidence-based policies [11]. The value of prosperity was the most effective in shifting support for children's mental health policies. The value of ingenuity, meanwhile, increased efficacy by helping to counter the public's default assumption that little can be done to improve outcomes for children.

To help advocates and experts use these frames in their communications, FrameWorks developed sample iterations of these values in a report it produced in 2010 [3]. These examples follow:

> *Child well-being is important for community development and economic development. Young children with strong mental health are prepared and equipped to develop important skills and capacities that begin in early childhood. These children then become the basis of a prosperous and sustainable society—contributing to things like good school achievement, solid workforce skills, and being strong citizens. When we ensure the healthy development of the next generation, they will pay that back through productivity and responsible citizenship. Innovative states and communities have been able to design high-quality programs for children, which have solved problems in early childhood development and shown significant long-term improvements for children. As a society, we need to invent and replicate more effective policies and programs for young children.*

FrameWorks also studied the effects of "explanatory metaphors"—metaphors that enhance understanding of scientific concepts by comparing them to concrete, ordinary objects, and processes—on public thinking. This research found that comparing child mental health to the "levelness"—of a table or piece of furniture—helped members of the public understand the concept and reason about solutions in productive ways [12]. This metaphor in particular was effective in communicating that children's mental health is influenced by environmental factors and must be addressed with actions that address environments and experiences. It also tapped into people's recessive connection between child mental health and functioning. People reasoned that if a table is unstable it would not function well and that a child's mental health works in the same way. If a child is exposed to abuse, violence, or neglect, or does not have access to nourishing foods or quality health and child care, then his or her mental health may not be as "level" as it would be if he or she grew up in a more stable environment. This metaphor counters the public's assumptions that children's mental health is influenced entirely by parental behaviors.

The metaphor also takes the onus for achieving good mental health off of individual children. Tables, after all, cannot level themselves. Likewise, children cannot solve mental health problems on their own. At the same time, the metaphor conveys that interventions and treatment *can* promote stability and function. Putting a piece of cardboard under the leg of a wobbly table will increase its stability, as will moving it to more level and stable ground. Interventions work the same way; they have the potential to help children achieve better mental health. This counters the public's fatalistic attitudes, which presuppose that mental illness is genetic and therefore incurable. A sample iteration from the 2010 FrameWorks report follows [3].

> *Scientists say that children's mental health affects how they socialize, how they learn, and how well they meet their potential. One way to think about child mental health is that it's like the levelness of a piece of furniture, say, a table. The levelness of a table is what makes it usable and able to function, just like the mental health of a child is what enables him or her to function and do many things. Some children's brains develop on floors that are level. This is like saying that the children have healthy, supportive relationships and access to things like good nutrition and health care. For other children, their brains develop on more sloped or slanted floors. This means they are exposed to abuse or violence, have unreliable or unsupportive relationships, and do not have access to key programs and resources. Remember that tables cannot make themselves level—they need attention from experts who understand levelness and stability and who can work on the table, the floor, or even both. We know that it's important to work on the floors and the tables early, because little wobbles early on tend to become big wobbles later.*

These findings led to the creation of a "core story" of child mental health—a master narrative that advocates and experts can use to help the public understand what child mental health is and what needs to be done to promote it. This core story begins with an appeal to the values of prosperity and ingenuity and includes the "levelness" metaphor. Leading communication materials with messages about how our future prosperity depends on children who have good mental health and about our country's history of tackling difficult problems with innovative solutions primes the public to productively consider the policies and programs needed to promote good child mental health. Using the *Levelness* metaphor to explain the science behind and solutions to child mental health also supports productive thinking. These are the tools—the flashlights, the compasses, the protective gear—that communicators need to navigate through the "swamp" of public understanding and get their messages through to the public in productive ways. For more detail about these tools and the research that supports them are found in website visit www.frameworksinstitute.org.

Acknowledgements

This chapter draws on studies published by authors including Nat Kendall-Taylor, Lynn Davey, Moira O'Neil, Anna Mikulak, Pamela Morgan, and Adam Simon. We would like to thank them for their contributions.

Author details

Nat Kendall-Taylor and Allison Stevens*

*Address all correspondence to: astevens@frameworksinstitute.org

FrameWorks Institute, Washington, D.C., USA

References

[1] Harrison, P. Mental Illness on the Rise in America's Children. Medscape. [Internet] 2013 May [cited 2016 August 16]. Available from: http://www.medscape.com/viewarticle/804334

[2] Stagman, S., and Cooper, J. Children's Mental Health: What Every Policymaker Should Know. National Center for Children in Poverty. [Internet] 2010 April [cited 2016 August 16] Available from: http://www.nccp.org/publications/pub_929.html

[3] Davey, L. How to Talk about Child Mental Health: A FrameWorks MessageMemo. Washington, DC: FrameWorks Institute. 2010 December. Available from: http://frameworksinstitute.org/assets/files/CMH_MM.pdf

[4] Kendall-Taylor, N. Conflicting Models of Mind: Mapping the Gaps Between Expert and Public Understandings of Child Mental Health. Science Communication. 2012. 34(6): 695–726. DOI: 10.1177/1075547011429200 Available from http://scx.sagepub.com/content/early/2012/02/02/1075547011429200.abstract

[5] Kendall-Taylor, N., and Mikulak, A. Child Mental Health: A Review of the Scientific Discourse. A FrameWorks Research Report. 2009. Washington, DC: FrameWorks Institute. Available from http://www.frameworksinstitute.org/assets/files/PDF_childmentalhealth/childmentalhealthreview.pdf

[6] Quinn, N., editor. Finding Culture in Talk: A Collection of Methods (1st ed.). New York, USA: Palgrave Macmillan. 2005. 277 p.

[7] Kendall-Taylor, N. Conflicting Models of Mind in Mind: Mapping the Gaps Between the Expert and the Public Understandings of Child Mental Health as Part of Strategic Frame Analysis. Washington, DC: FrameWorks Institute. Available from http://www.frameworksinstitute.org/assets/files/PDF_childmentalhealth/childmentalhealthculturalmodels.pdf

[8] Goffman, E. Interaction Ritual: Essays in Face-to-Face Behavior. New Brunswick, New Jersey: Transaction Publishers. 1967, 280 p.

[9] Kendall-Taylor, N. Conflicting Models of Mind in Mind: Mapping the Gaps Between the Expert and the Public Understandings of Child Mental Health as Part of Strategic Frame Analysis. Washington, DC: FrameWorks Institute. 2009 July. Available from http://scx.sagepub.com/content/early/2012/02/02/1075547011429200.abstract

[10] O'Neil, M., Mikulak, A., Morgan, P., and Kendall-Taylor, N. Competing Frames of Mental Health and Mental Illness: Media Frames and the Public Understandings of Child Mental Health as Part of Strategic Frame Analysis. A FrameWorks Research Report. Washington, DC: FrameWorks Institute. 2009. Available from http://www.frameworksinstitute.org/assets/files/PDF_childmentalhealth/competingframesofmentalhealth.pdf

[11] Simon, A. Refining the Options for Advancing Support for Child Mental Health Policies: A FrameWorks Research Report. Washington, DC: FrameWorks Institute. 2010. Available from http://www.frameworksinstitute.org/assets/files/CMH_US_Values_Final.pdf

[12] Erard, M., Kendall-Taylor, N., Davey, L., and Simon, A. The Power of Levelness: Making Child Mental Health Visible and Concrete through a Simplifying Model. FrameWorks Institute: Washington, DC. 2010. Available from http://frameworksinstitute.org/assets/files/CMH_MM.pdf

9

Poverty and Mental Health Outcomes in Mexican Adolescents

Blanca Estela Barcelata-Eguiarte and
Maria Elena Márquez-Caraveo

Abstract

The purpose of this chapter is to analyze the adaptive and resilience processes in adolescents from different marginalizing communities. The theoretical and empirical foundations of the ecological-transactional perspective of adolescent development as a framework for understanding the adaptive processes and resilience in contextual adversity is reviewed, with the recognition of risk and protective factors at multiple levels and ecological settings. Under this perspective, the authors provide data supporting the predictive role of stressful life events, coping, and family functioning in adaptive and nonadaptive outcomes in adolescents living in diverse contexts of high-risk communities in Mexico City. These findings may contribute to early intervention programs based on empirical evidence with adolescents and families living in disadvantages communities in schools and in clinical settings.

Keywords: adolescents, resilience, poverty, mental health, adaptation

1. Introduction

Adolescence is a transitional and vulnerable period in the life cycle. Particularly for those living in countries where access to mental health (MH) services is low, it is necessary to promote preventive interventions based on evidence. The purpose of this chapter is to analyze the adaptive and resilience processes in adolescents from different marginalizing communities. The theoretical and empirical foundations of the ecological-transactional perspective of adolescent development as a framework for understanding the adaptive processes and resilience in contextual adversity is reviewed, with the recognition of risk and protective factors at multiple levels and ecological settings. Under this perspective, the authors provide data supporting the predictive role of stressful life events, coping, and family functioning in adaptive and nonadaptive outcomes in adolescents living diverse contexts of high-risk communities in Mexico City. These findings may contribute to early intervention programs based on empirical evidence with adolescents and families living in disadvantaged communities in schools and in clinical settings.

2. An ecological framework for understanding youth outcomes in high-risk contexts

For more than four decades, development researchers appear to be concerned with children and adolescents living in a situation of considerable adversity, including poverty or social marginalization, and thus trying to understand those mechanisms that draw them either to a path of psychopathology or to positive adaptation [1–3]. The findings provided a set of questions regarding the traditional assumption that situations of risk and stress are "inevitable" linked to psychopathology. This questioning broke down previous schemes of child development, inviting new theoretical and methodological proposals to appear. Thus, a more comprehensive and positive perspective about the human development emerged, which involves the possibility of positive adaptation together with the reconstruction, from experiences, in the face of adversity. With this, the focus extended toward the study of strengths despite significant stress and risk, also known as resilience. Its study is originated in the model of"developmental psychopathology," proposed through longitudinal investigations made by Garmezy and Rutter [4] with children living in contexts of poverty, psychosocial risk, and parents with mental disease. Likewise, the model is based on multifactorial research carried out by Werner and Smith [3], among others, with vulnerable population which, contrary to predictions, presented positive adaptation.

Developmental psychopathology represents a macroparadigm that resumes basic assumptions of both systemic [5] and bioecological approaches [6]. This perspective implies the intersection between the fields of clinical and human development and it also includes contributions from neurosciences, ethology, and psychiatry. It is focused on children and adolescents within different ecological levels that involve risk, vulnerability, adaptation, and resilience [7, 8], and it also recognizes the multidimensional nature of adaptation. For this reason, the evaluation and intervention methods are multifactorial, multilevel, and multireferential. Also known as "ecologic-transactional perspective" [9] and "organizational model" [10], this new approach assumes that adaptation is the result of an organization of different systems that interact dynamically. It also includes particular theories and approaches that frame the investigation in multiple contexts and settings, such as hospitals, schools, mental health (MH) centers, and courts and with different risks like sexual abuse [11], mental diseases in parents [12], psychosocial risk and marginalization [13], and poverty [14].

Under this perspective resilience is a multidimensional construct with two basic components: positive adaptation and the presence of significant stress, risk, and/or adversity [8]. Luthar [7] defines resilience as those behaviors within a norm and a relatively good outcome in the face of a context of risk and vulnerability. Resilience is a supraorganized construct that presents adjustment indicators both negative and positive emotional and behavioral and not always in directly observable behaviors [8]. Thus, resilience has to be inferred comparing individual's outcomes among individuals with similar experiences of adversity [12]. So the study of resilience, in terms of trajectories and outcomes, is still very useful, in order to design prevention and promotion programs aimed to strengthen the positive youth development [15, 16].

In the last years, the study of resilience has encompassed various domains, fields, and problems. Among them, an important area is the one in charge of studying positive adaptation processes in children and adolescents that live in contexts of high risk, such as poverty and low socioeconomic status (SES). In this sense, poverty is a distal multidimensional factor considered a risk factor due to its link with other adversities and sources of stress such as economic constraints [17], child maltreatment, [18], alcohol abuse [19], and negative parenting [20] which can be operating cumulatively or as a risk cascade [21]. There is evidence that economic distress may cause daily hassles and family conflicts which either directly or indirectly negatively influence the adolescent's health [22].

UNICEF [23] points out that the experience of childhood occurs each time more often in an urban environment allowing children to enjoy the advantages that urban life offers, such as education, medical services, and recreational facilities. However, a countless number of children lack basic services despite having them close. Socioeconomic inequality has an impact on adolescent health, particularly in countries with low- and middle-income, where rapid economic and urban growth leads a large number of adolescents to displacement and deprivation and finally unemployment. Therefore, this has a negative impact on mental health outcomes; for instance, an increase of suicide and also mortality related to violence [24].

It is interesting to evaluate whether this impact derives from income *per se* or also form other family conditions that coincide with an environment of poverty: monoparental families, low educational level, unemployment, and underemployment. These sociodemographic factors affect health in different moments in the life course and operate two different levels and through causal differential mechanisms [25]. It is important to identify other factors that mediate between the distal context (socioeconomic status) and adolescent results, since usually family is a mediator between the adolescent and his environment. Thus, some family factors are described as being the ones with higher prevalence in an environment of poverty. These include emotional distress (e.g., depression, irritability, emotional liability), substance abuse by parents, less solid parenting styles which are more punitive and inconsistent, mostly chaotic environments, with fewer stimulation and regular routines as well as restricted learning opportunities and reduced accessibility to parental interaction [26].

In short, multifactorial research emphasizes the importance of a balance between personal, familiar, and social protective and risk factors for resilience [18, 27, 28]. The understanding of adaptation profiles and mechanisms of adolescents, who present a relatively good outcome despite living in an environment of psychosocial risk and poverty, could be the basis for designing programs with an ecological framework based on evidence [29]. The programs should be aimed at promoting positive adaptation, teaching coping skills, and a positive parenting in both adolescents and their families in accordance with global mental health policies [30].

3. Adolescent mental health problems: risk and protective factors

The concept of risk borrowed from the medical model and then transferred to social sciences refers to those characteristics of a person, or of the environment, that limit, impede, or represent a threat for his development having as a consequence negative outcome [9, 20]. Statistically this involves a higher probability of presenting an alteration in the course of development in "critical" domains. Vulnerability entails personal and environmental factors that increase the negative effects of a risk condition [7]. Protection is a process in which individual and environmental factors participate and attenuate the impact of stress and risk. Because of their contribution to positive adaptation they are called protective and can be defined based on personal attributes such as coping, personality [31], self-efficacy, and also environmental ones like a functional family organization or family care [11]. This perspective suggests that factors of risk and protection belong to multiple levels, from individual to contextual (family, school, community) and of a diverse domain (biological, psychological, and social), and throughout life [32].

What is mental health and mental health problems (MHP)? Mental health (MH) is defined as the "successful performance of mental function that results in productive activities, fulfilling relationships with other individuals and the ability to adapt to change and cope with adversity" [33: p. 6]. Mental health problems (MHP) include signs and symptoms which are not intense or lengthy enough so as to fulfill the criteria of a certain mental disorder. The term mental or psychiatric disorder refers to the group of disorders diagnosed according to medical classification systems like DSM5 and ICD-10 [33]. These include a series of conditions characterized by thought, mood, or behavior disturbance (or a combination of them) and associated to an altered functioning or personal suffering.

Children and adolescents constitute a third of the world's population (2.2 billions) and a 90% of them live in low- and middle-income countries (LMIC) where they represent 50% of its population. Although adolescents are considered to be a healthy population group, it is during this period of their lives that they are confronted to risk processes decisive in their future health, like drugs, tobacco and alcohol consumption, unsafe sex, obesity, and lack of physical activities. Under these circumstances, mental disorders increase [34]. It is known that neuropsychiatric disorders are the main cause of global burden (accounting for 15–30% of the disability-adjusted life years, DALYs) and the world prevalence of these disorders is calculated to be among 10–20%. However, there is a gap between the need and the existing resources in these countries [35].

A recent meta-analysis of research carried out in 27 countries (regions in North America, South America, Caribbean, Europe, Africa, Asia, and Oceania) specifies a number of 13.4% of mental disorders that affect children and adolescents, just slightly below obesity (16.8%) and above asthma (8.5%) [36]. However, there is a scarcity of youth health and well-being indicators at an international level and the ones available are for high-income countries (HIC). It is therefore recommended to carry out research for those health aspects that have been ignored in adolescent health: mental health, health systems, and risk and protection factors in their immediate context.

The most prominent distal risk factor associated with mental health problems in children and adolescents is low socioeconomic status (SES). It is suggested that the study of the relationship between SES and MD includes disaggregation in its indicators in order to explain the mechanism through which poverty impacts in adolescent's results. McLauglin [37] estimated the association between SES and MD in a representative sample of U.S. students and noted that a subjective perspective of social status was one of the indicators more directly associated to mental disorder. Parents' education level is associated with a low risk of anxiety disorders and relative deprivation as a high risk for affective disorders. Another mechanism supported in research data is the inverse relationship between parents' education and the use of health services and/or treatment [38, 39]. Even in high income countries, most adolescents with a psychiatric disorder do not receive treatment and once it occurs, it is not provided by a mental health specialist [40].

In Mexico, the prevalence of mental disorders in adolescents was measured through Mexican Adolescent Mental Health Survey [38] and it revealed that 39.4% of the adolescents, from 12 to 17 years, presented a mental disorder measured by CIDI and DSM-IV criteria: 1/11 had a serious disorder; 1/5 moderate; and 1/10 mild. Anxiety disorders were the most prevalent ones in both sexes. In men, oppositional-defiant disorder and alcohol abuse appear as the second and third main ones, respectively, after specific phobia and social phobia. The most frequent disorders in women, after anxiety (phobias) were major depression and oppositional-defiant disorder. Most of them did not receive treatment. Two-thirds lived with their parents, four-fifths were students, and one-tenth had social burden. Social burdens associated to a probability of mental disorder were: being married, having a child, and working while studying. Parents' education was related to the use of treatment. The relationship between mental disorders and other indicators of well-being is not yet available in Mexico.

In comparison to other OECD [41] countries, Mexico ranked the bottom third regarding children and adolescent well-being with the next indicators: income and wealth, housing

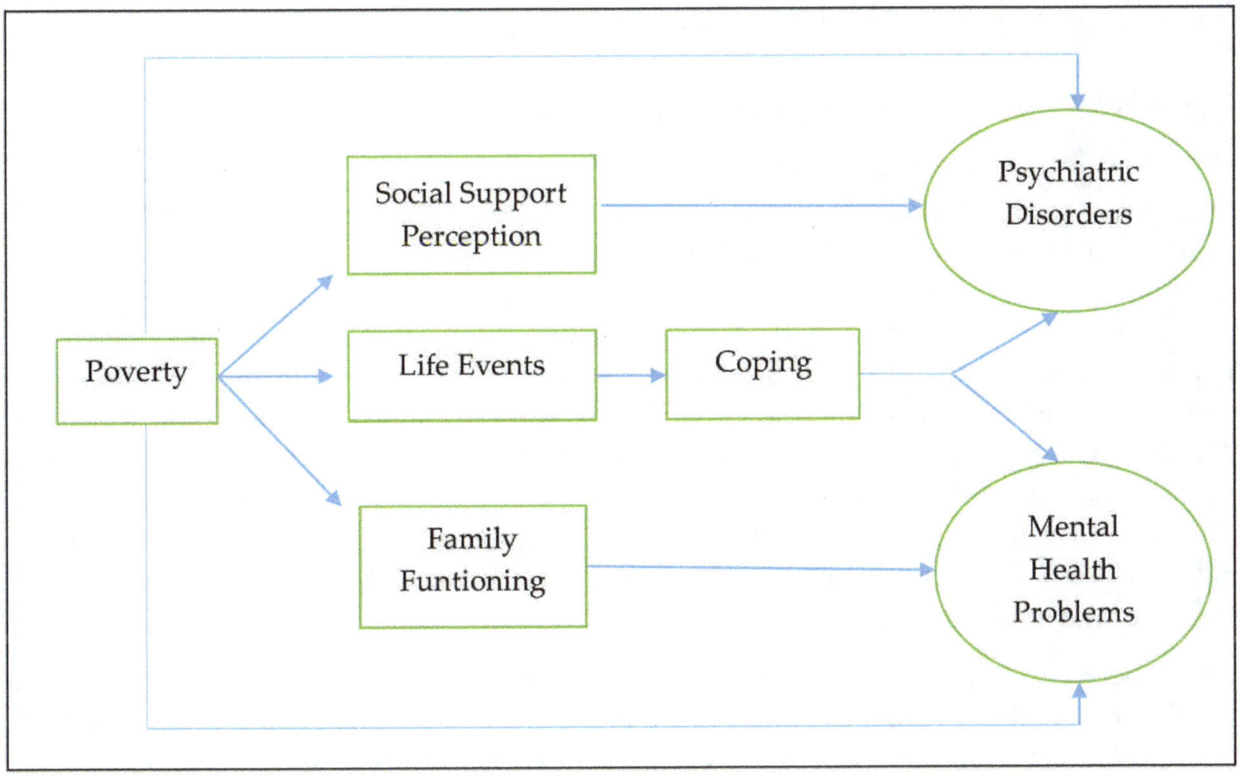

Figure 1. A research proposal-intervention for adolescents in disadvantaged communities.

condition, infant mortality, teenage birth rate, reading skills among 15 years old (PISA), and youth neither in employment nor education/training, among others. These data show the situation of Mexican adolescents and their families and at the same time represent different challenges in the ability of adapting, including the flexibility to generate new personal and familiar functioning ways. Hence, the research line proposed for adolescents living in a high risk context includes proximal and distal variables that allow, based on evidence, to identify "clue" elements for intervention and promotion of adolescent development. Literature shows how elements such as coping and familiar functioning (communication and familiar cohesion) work are protective variables in contexts of poverty that buffer the effect of psychosocial risk.

Finally, although it is proposed [35] that the risks factors are similar in HIC to those reported in LMIC, resilience research is scanty in LMIC. Hence, we propose a theoretical model aimed to understand risk/protective factors underlying adaptation and resilience in **Figure 1**. The research data that were generated is described in Section 3.

4. Adapting processes and resilience in multiple contexts

According to our previous statements, adolescents' outcomes result from a complex process involving the dynamic interaction of multiple factors at multiple levels. A salient individual factor explaining the mechanism of adaptive or maladaptive outcomes is coping. However, in the field of resilience it is needed to take into account the social context of adolescents in order to analyze the relationship between stressful life events and coping in multiple contexts, clinical and nonclinical, in disadvantaged communities.

4.1. Stress life events and coping in disadvantaged communities

Adolescent stress approaches [42–44] based in Lazarus' transactional model [45] emphasizes the importance of individual characteristics, stressors, and context. There is evidence that both, major and daily events or hassles, due to its frequency, intensity, and duration represent a high stress burden [46]. However, according to the compensatory model of resilience [8] positive events can buffer the negative effect of these stressors [46, 47]. Family stress theory [48] shows that daily stressful experiences associated to a socioeconomic disadvantage usually generate family crises and mental health problems affecting whole family system and family members [49]. The "Context Model" (e.g., risk-stress model) suggests that families in disadvantaged societies are exposed to multiple risks, most of them related to a lack of money [50]. Economic pressure represents a chronic stressor associated to mental health problems including anxiety and depression. Therefore, it supports the notion of relationship between economic hardship, family conflict, and emotional disorder [17, 22].

In a Mexican context, it is reported that around 80% has experienced an adverse event in a year and that to a higher number of adversities there was also a higher probability of psychopathology [51]. This coincides with previous data regarding stressors and internalizing an externalizing problem [22, 50, 52]. The difference between youth risk, for instance, with or without suicidal ideation [53], drug consumers or nonconsumers [54] and adolescents with or without psychopathology [55] is the number, type, and source of stressors, generally related to family, in which, even normative life events, can be perceived negatively by adolescents [46]. Regarding this, our research line[1] has been oriented to analyze adaptive processes in adolescents and families of marginalized and high-risk communities in metropolitan area of Mexico City. A cross-sectional study tested a model on resilience [56] in 538 students aged 13–18 years who were provided with the life events questionnaire [57] and the MMPI-A [58]. Findings showed an overall model (R^2 = 0.278; X^2 = 16.294; $p > 0.05$) with stressful life events as negative predictors of adaptation (β = 2.118, p = 0.000). These findings were also replicated in older adolescents confirming the contribution of stressful life events and perceived social support on resilience [59]. In concordance with previous research [17, 46, 47], data showed the negative influence of stressful life events on adaptive processes.

On the other hand, there is systemic evidence regarding coping as a relevant factor playing a mediator and/or moderator role in stressful experiences and adolescent outcomes. Resilient adolescents and families with a kind of adversity frequently present problem solving and seeking social support. The adverse effect of negative contextual experiences and parental conflict can be buffered with functional coping, being a predictor of resilience [60]. Coping reduces the negative impact of family stress which derives from economic pressure [61]. Similar data were founded in Mexican adolescents: problem solving, seeking social support, and spirituality were the strongest predictors of resilience in poor adolescents [62]. However, its protective function can be diminished due to influence of negative peers or negative models of parental and family coping [63]. On the contrary, adolescents that present an emotional problem like anxiety, depression, or aggressive behavior, basically use avoidance coping [50, 60, 64].

Recently, a cross-cultural research that compared styles and coping strategies between Mexican and Paraguayan students was carried out [65]. Participants completed the adolescent coping scale [43] and results showed that both samples used mostly productive strategies. However, problem solving and effort to achieve success was more frequent among Mexican adolescents, whereas Paraguayan reported a higher level of seeking spiritual support and slightly higher nonproductive strategies than Mexican students. Although adaptation was not assessed, results are similar to others cross-cultural studies [43, 64].

The relationship between coping and externalizing and internalizing behaviors and resilience was assessed with earlier adolescents. Results showed higher scores in productive strategies (e.g., physical recreation and seek relaxing diversions) [66] and nonproductive strategies (e.g., worry and not cope), which significantly related to both, internalizing (i) and externalizing (e) problems. When testing a model of resilience [67] active coping, perceived control, and family support predicted negatively, internalizing (R^2 = 0.364; F = 97.47; $p < 0.001$) and externalizing behaviors (R^2= 0.279; F = 63.564; $p < 0.001$). Positive qualities (e.g., prosaical behavior, positive self-concept) were predicted by positive thinking, perceived social support, and self-control (R^2 = 0.229; F = 57.597; $p < 0.001$). As hypothesized, a set of personal and familiar

[1] Current research "Adaptation and resilience in multiple contexts. Basis for the intervention in adolescence" (PAPIIT IN303714). Research granted by DGAPA, National Autonomous University of Mexico.

resources was related to all syndromes or behaviors as the literature regarding resilience has reported [13, 18, 19, 68].

In brief, coping is relevant for adolescent adaptation in adverse context, although its multidimensional character sets questions with regard to its role and the nature of its relationships with other personal, familiar, and contextual variables which also contribute to resilience.

4.2. Family functioning in clinical and nonclinical adolescent settings

Family represents the first scenario, which is at the same time the most natural and lasting one, of the individual-context interaction. Family factors are suggested to be a determinant in health during the course of life and among different cultures. Supportive parents and families are "crucial part in the improvement of global health" [24, p. 1647]. However, it is not possible to ignore the influence of macrostructural factors that shape the individual and familiar development such as the economic crisis that characterizes low- and middle-income countries (LMIC) like Mexico. The family unit is a reflection of contemporary transformation processes and there is no convergence with a unique family model as it was proposed in the sociological theories of the 1960s [69]. It is hard to build a set of understandable generalizations of how family environments relate to the developmental life course from childhood to adolescence. This may be a result of both a wide array of measurements that evaluate the same constructs and variables and the complexity of the relationships itself.

The debate about the nature and impact of the psychosocial determinants in the trajectories and outcomes of the adolescent development is still open and to a certain level mediated by genetic factors [8, 10, 21]. Still, it appears that there is a universal agreement in the understanding of human development as an interactive process between the individual and the context, particularly family context. Developmental systems theories [16] and ecological-transactional perspectives [9, 10] suggest that high social risk contexts entail a series of adversities for adolescents and their families. Risk indicators include sociodemographic characteristics and structural and psychological markers that affect family functioning and adolescents' adaptive processes. The most prominent influence in the family environment is poverty. Razavi and Razavi [70] highlight that SES influences the adolescent outcomes through parental communication, which acts as a predictor of emotional and behavioral problems. The association between low economic income, low academic level in parents, and addictions are described in the corresponding literature [9, 14, 19]. The effect of some families in the physical and mental health of their offspring has been also documented [48, 71]. The term risky families [9, 71] describes environments characterized by the presence of conflict and aggression. Family relationships in these environments are cold, neglectful, and unsupportive affecting the quality of parenting practices and contributing to adverse mental and physical outcomes in their offspring.

Schleider and Weisz [72] suggest a triadic model family process, formed by three main level factors: parent, dyad, and family (here family functioning is just one of its parts). This integral model incorporates processes of an adolescent, his or her parents and his or her family context, which has to a certain level an impact in the internalized problems of the adolescent. A set of family variables such as communication, social support, and parenting practices has been related to positive and negative outcomes (e.g., anxiety, depression, aggressive behavior) [73, 74].

In contrast with risk factors, family support (parental) often offered by the mother, is a source of protection for those adolescents with psychosocial risks and due to its protective character is also one of the strongest predictors of resilience [28, 73, 75]. Although a good part of the evidence that family connectedness are one of the strongest protective factors in mental health, comes from the U.K., Canada, and U.S., this phenomena is being confirmed in other cultures [24]. Our findings about family functioning perceived social support and resilience in poor Mexican youth [76] showed significant main effects of both, family functioning ($F = 18.60$; $p < 0.01$) and perceived social support ($F = 11.71$; $p < 0.05$) on resilience. In concordance with previous data [14, 28, 73, 75], mother's level of education, father's occupation, adolescent's daily spending money, conflict family, and friend perceived social support were predictors of resilience by using logistic regression analyses.

A cross-sectional study aimed to assess the influence of gender in psychopathology in adolescents attending a public mental health institution was carried [77]. Data was obtained from 67 adolescents (M_{age} 14 years, $SD = 1.49$) who answered the YSR [78] and a sociodemographic questionnaire. It was hypothesized that age and gender effects would be related to psychopathology, however, only gender main effects were found. Adolescent girls reported more anxiety/depression ($F = 6.186$, $p = 0.016$) and internalizing problems ($F = 2.740$; $p = 0.050$) at a significant level than boys. To evaluate the contribution of parent's rearing style in adolescent mental health problems, another correlational and predictive study [79] was carried in 117 low-income adolescents (12–years), attending mental health centers ($M_{age} = 14.02$; $SD = 1.70$). Participants completed a sociodemographic schedule, the YSR and the EMBU-A. Multiple regression analysis showed that the Rejection and Control of both parents were positive predictors whereas the Mother's Warmth predicted negatively: Internalizing ($R^2= 0.297$; $p = 0.035$), Externalizing ($R^2 = 0.275$; $p = 0.001$) and Mixed Syndromes ($R^2= 0.289$; $p = 0.000$). Preliminary conclusion suggests that negative parenting leads to negative outcomes as internalized problems, whereas positive parenting is a predictor of better psychological adjustment as has been reported previously [72–75].

In summary, linking family functioning, as well as parental rearing style is highly relevant in research. There is a need of cross-country studies of parenting constructs and adolescent (mental) health.

5. Conclusion

An ecological-transactional perspective encompasses a theoretical and methodological framework for a comprehensive understanding of youth outcomes. Although adolescents are regarded as healthy, the pressures of the globalized world imply multiple challenges and threats to their well- being. An increasing number of youth people suffer mental health problems and a gap between the needs and resource availability exists. Although most of the knowledge about the risk and protective factors arises from developed countries research is needed in the resilience field, particularly in developing countries where most adolescents live.

Poverty is linked to a number of adversities including stressful life events. However, the protective role of family factors and coping styles and strategies are just starting to be studied in these countries. The interplay between stressful life events, coping, and family factors should be the basis to undertake research initiative as much as preventive intervention. Developmental trajectories in high-risk settings moving to well-being and mental health or to psychopathology may be the result of this interplay.

Author details

Blanca Estela Barcelata-Eguiarte[1]* and Maria Elena Márquez-Caraveo[2]

*Address all correspondence to: bareg7@hotmail.com

1 Department of Psychology, National Autonomous of Mexico, Mexico City, Mexico

2 Child Psychiatric Hospital "Dr. Juan N. Navarro", Mexico City, Mexico

References

[1] Garmezy N. Children in poverty: Resilience despite risk. Psychiatry. 1993;56:127–136.

[2] Rutter R. Resilience as a dynamic concept. Development and Psychopathology. 2012; 24:335–344.

[3] Werner E, Smith R. Overcoming the Odds. New York: Cornell University Press; 1992.

[4] Garmezy N, Rutter M. Acute reaction to stress. In: Rutter R, Hersov, L., editors. Child and Adolescent Psychiatric. Oxford, Edimburgo: Blackwell Scientific Publication; 1985. pp. 38–56.

[5] Von Bertalanffy L. General System Theory. New York: Braziller; 1968.

[6] Bronfenbrenner U, Morris P. The bioecological model of human development. In: Cicchetti D, Cohen D, editors. Developmental Psychopathology. Vol. 3: Risk, Disorder and Adaptation. New York: John Wiley & Sons, Inc.; 2006. pp. 129–201.

[7] Luthar S. Resilience in development: A synthesis of research across five decades. In: Cicchetti D, Cohen D, editors. Developmental Psychopathology. Vol. 3: Risk, Disorder and Adaptation. New York: John Wiley & Sons, Inc.; 2006. pp. 739–795.

[8] Masten A. Global perspectives on resilience in children and youth. Child Development. 2014;85(1):6–20.

[9] Sameroff A, Rosenblum K. Psychosocial constraints on the development of resilience. Annuary of New York Academy Science. 2006;1094:116–124.

[10] Cicchetti D. Resilience under conditions of extreme stress: A multilevel perspective. World Psychiatry. 2010;9(3):145–154.

[11] Fergusson D, McLeod. F, Horwood L. Childhood sexual abuse and adult developmental outcomes: Findings from 30-years longitudinal study in New Zeland. Child Abuse and Neglect. 2013;37:664–674.

[12] Gureje O, Oladeji B, Hwang I, Chiu WT, Kessler RC, Sampson NA, et al. Parental psychopathology and the risk of suicidal behavior in their offspring: Results from the world mental health surveys. Molecular Psychiatry. 2011;16:1221–1233.

[13] Meyers SA, Millers C. Direct, mediated, moderated, and cumulative relations between neighborhood characteristic and adolescents outcomes. Adolescence. 2004;39(153):121–144.

[14] Conger R, Conger K. Resilience in midwestern families: Selected findings from the first decade of a prospective, longitudinal study. Journal of Marriage and Family. 2002;64:361–373.

[15] Hunter C. Is resilience still a useful concept when working with children and young people? Child Family Community Australia. Melbourne: Australian Institute of Family Studies; 2012.

[16] Lerner R, Schmid K. Relational developmental systems theories and the ecological validity of experimental design. Human Development. 2013;56:372–380. DOI: 10.1159/000357179

[17] Flouri E, Tzavidis N, Constantinos K. Adverse life events, socioeconomic disadvantage, and psychopathology and resilience in young children: The importance of risk factors' accumulation and protective factors' specificity. European Child and Adolescent Psychiatry. 2010;19(6):535–546.

[18] Jaffee S, Caspi A, Moffit T, Polo-Tomás M, Taylor A. Individual, family, and neighborhood factors distinguish resilient from non-resilient maltreated children: A cumulative stressors model. Child Abuse and Neglect. 2007;31:231–253.

[19] Reuchkin VV, Koposov RA, Eisemann M, Hägglöf B. Alcohol use in delinquent adolescents from Northern Russia: The role of personality, parental rearing and family history of alcohol abuse. Personality and Individual Differences. 2002;32:1139–1148.

[20] Trudeau L, Mason W, Randall G, Spoth R, Ralston E. Effects of parenting and deviant peers on early to mid-adolescent conduct problems. Journal of Abnormal and Child Psychology. 2012;40(8):1249–1264. DOI:10.1007/s10802-012-9648-1

[21] Rutter M. Annual research review: Resilience-clinical implications. Journal of Child Psychology and Psychiatry. 2013;54(4),474–487.

[22] Wadsworth M, Raviv T, Santiago C, Etter E. Testing the adaptation to poverty-related stress model: Predicting psychopathology symptoms in families facing economic hardship. Journal of Clinical Child and Adolescent Psychology. 2011;40(4),646–657.

[23] United Nations Children's Fund (UNICEF). The state of the world's children in an urban world. New York: United Nations Children's Fund; 2012.

[24] Viner RM, Ozer EM, Denny S, Marmot M, Resnick M, Fatusi A, Currie C. Adolescence and the social determinants of health. The Lancet. 2012;379(9826):1641–1652.

[25] Braveman PA, Cubbin C, Egerter S, Chideya S, Marchi KS, Metzler M, Posner S. Socioeconomic status in health research: One size does not fit all. The Journal of the American Medical Association. 2005;294(22):2879–2888.

[26] Walker S, Wachs T, Grantham-McGregor S, Black M, Nelson C, Huffman S, et al. Inequality in early childhood: Risk and protective factors for early child development. The Lancet. 2011;378(9799),1325–1338.

[27] Aguilera R, Salgado N, Romero M, Medina-Mora M. Paternal absence and international migration: Stressors and compensators associated with mental health of Mexican teenagers of rural origin. Adolescence. 2004;39(156):711–723.

[28] Gómez R, McLaren S. The association of avoidance coping style, and perceived mother and father support with anxiety/depression among late adolescents: Applicability of resiliency models. Personality and Individual Differences. 2006;30(6):1165–1176.

[29] Ager A. Annual research review: Resilience and child well-being-public policy implications. Journal of Child Psychology and Psychiatry. 2013;54(4):488–500.

[30] World Health Organization (WHO). Impact of Economic Crises on Mental Health. Copenhagen, Denmark: WHO Regional Office for Europe; 2012

[31] Hambrick EP, McCord DM. Proactive coping and its relation to the five-factor model of personality. Individual Differences Research. 2010;8(2):67–77.

[32] World Health Organization. Child and adolescent mental health policies and plans. Geneva: World Health Organization; 2005.

[33] Substance Abuse and Mental Health Services Administration – SAMHSA, Center for Mental Health Services. Promotion and Prevention in Mental Health: Strengthening Parenting and Enhancing Child Resilience. DHHS Publication No.CMHS-SVP-0175. USA: Rockville, MD. 2007.

[34] Patton GC, Coffey C, Cappa C, Currie D, Riley L, Gore F, Degenhardt L, Richardson D, Astone N, Sangowawa A, Ferguson J. Health of the world's adolescents: a synthesis of internationally comparable data. Lancet. 2012;379(9826):1665–75.

[35] Kieling Ch, Baker-Henningham H, Belfer M, Conti G, Ertem I, Omigbodun O, Rohde LA, Srinath S, Ulkuer N, Rahman A. Child and adolescent mental health worldwide: evidence for action. The Lancet. 2011;378(9801):1515–1525. DOI:10.1016/S0140-6736(11)60827-1

[36] Polanczyk G, Salum A, Sugaya LS, Caye A, Rohde LA. Annual research review: A meta-analysis of the worldwide prevalence of mental disorders in children and adolescents. Journal of Child Psychology and Psychiatry. 2015;56(3):345–365. DOI:10.1111/jcpp.12381

[37] McLauglin KA, Costello EJ, Leblanc W, Sampson NA, Kessler RC. Socioeconomic status and adolescent mental disorders. American Journal of Public Health. 2012;102(9):1742–1750.

[38] Benjet C, Borges G, Medina-Mora ME, Zambrano J, Aguilar-Gaxiola S. Youth mental health in a populous city of the developing world: Results from the Mexican Adolescent Mental Health Survey. Journal of Child Psychology and Psychiatry. 2008;2:1–10.

[39] Merikangas KR, He JP, Burstein M, Swendsen J, Avenevoli S, Case B, Olfson M. Service utilization for lifetime mental disorders in US adolescents: Results of the National Comorbidity Survey–Adolescent Supplement (NCS-A). Journal of the American Academy of Child & Adolescent Psychiatry. 2011;50(1):32–45.

[40] Costello EJ, He JP, Sampson, NA, Kessler RC, Merikangas KR. Services for adolescents with psychiatric disorders: 12-month data from the National Comorbidity Survey–Adolescent. Psychiatric Services. 2014;65(3):359–366.

[41] OECD Better Life Initiative. "Cómo va la vida en México" [Internet]. 2015. Available from: www.oecd.org/statistics/Hows-Life-2015-country-notes-data.xlsx [Accessed: 2016-07-28]

[42] Connor-Smith J, Compas B. Coping as a moderator of relation between reactivity to interpersonal stress, health status, and internalizing problems. Cognitive and Therapy Research. 2004;28(3):347–368. DOI:10.1023/B:COTR.0000031806.25021.d5

[43] Frydenberg E, Eacott Ch, Clark N. From distress to success: Developing a coping language and programs for adolescents. The Prevention Researcher. 2008;15(4):8–12.

[44] Seiffge-Krenke I, Aunola K, Nurmi JE. Changes in stress perception and coping during adolescence: The role of situational and personal factors. Child Development. 2009;80 (1):259–279. DOI:10.1111/j.1467-8624.2008.01258.x

[45] Lazarus R. From psychological stress to the emotions: A history of changing outlooks. Annual Review Psychological. 1993;44:1–21. DOI: 0066-4308/93/0201-0001 $02.00

[46] Eggum N, Sallquist J, Eisenberg N. "Then it will be good": Negative life events and resilience in Ugandan youth. Journal of Adolescent Research. 2011;26(6):766–796.

[47] Hjemdal O, Friborg O, Stiles TC, Rosenvinge JH, Martinussen M. Resilience predicting psychiatric symptoms: A prospective study of protective factors and their role in adjustment to stressful life events. Clinical Psychology and Psychotherapy. 2006;13:194–201.

[48] Patterson J. Integrating family resilience and family stress theory. Journal of Marriage and Family. 2002;64(2):349–360.

[49] Petterson S, Burke A. Effects of poverty and maternal depression on early child development. Child Development. 2001;72(6):1794–1813.

[50] Wadsworth M, Berger L. Adolescents coping with poverty-related family stress: Prospective predictors of coping and psychological symptoms. Journal of Youth and Adolescence. 2006;35(1):57–70.

[51] Benjet C, Borges G, Medina-Mora M.E, Zambrano J, Cruz C, Méndez E. Descriptive epidemiology of chronic childhood adversity in Mexican adolescents. Journal of Adolescent Health, 2009;45(5):483–489.

[52] Seiffge-Krenke I. Coping with relationship stressors: A decade review. Journal of Research Adolescence. 2011;21(1):196–210. DOI: 10.1111/j.1532-7795.2010.00723.x

[53] Hernández Q, Lucio E. Assessment of suicidal risk and associated stress in Mexican adolescent students. Mexican Journal of Psychology. 2006;23(1):55–62.

[54] Linage M, Lucio E. The relationship between youth substance abuse and coping strategies. Journal of Behavior, Health and Social Issues, 2012;4(1):55–66. DOI: 10.5460/JBHSI.V4.1.32971

[55] Barcelata B, Durán C, Lucio E. Subjective assessment of stressful life events in two adolescent's groups from marginalized areas. Mental Health. 2012;36(6):513–520.

[56] Barcelata B, Ramirez A. Perceived social support in early and late adolescence: Linking with stress and adaptation in high-risk population In: 33rd STAR International Conference. July, 2012. Palma di Mallorca, Spain.

[57] Lucio E, Durán C. Life Events Questionnaire for Adolescents. México: El Manual Moderno; 2003.

[58] Lucio E. Minnesota Multiphasic Personality Inventory for Adolescents -MMPI-A-. México: El Manual Moderno; 1998.

[59] Barcelata B, Lucio E. The impact of stressful life events and social support perceived on resilience among students on economical adversity. In: 33rd STAR International Conference. July, 2012. Palma di Mallorca, Spain.

[60] Wadsworth M, Raviv MA, Compas B, Connor-Smith J. Parent and adolescent responses to poverty related stress: Tests of mediated and moderated coping models. Journal of Child and Family Studies. 2005;14(2):283–298.

[61] Santiago C, Etter E, Wadswoth M, Raviv T. Predictors of responses to stress among families coping with poverty-related stress. Anxiety, stress, and coping development. Child Development. 2012;72(6):1794–1813.

[62] Barcelata B, Durán C, Lucio E. Coping strategies as predictors of resilience in adolescents with economic hardship. In: Moore K, Kaniasty K, Buchwald P, editors. Stress and Anxiety: Application to Economic Hardship Occupational Demands, and Developmental Challenges. Berlin: Logos Verlag; 2012. pp. 7–17.

[63] Seiffge-Krenke I, Pakalniskiene V. Who shapes whom in the family: Reciprocal links between autonomy support in the family and parents' and adolescents' coping behaviors. Youth Adolescence. 2011;40:983–995. DOI: 10.1007/s10964-010-9603-9

[64] Auerbach P, Abela J, Zhu X, Yao Sh. Understanding the role of coping in the development of depressive symptoms: Symptom specificity, gender differences, and cross-cultural applicability. British Journal of Clinical Psychology. 2010;49:547–561. DOI:10.1348/014466509X479681

[65] Barcelata B, Coppari N, Marquez-Caraveo ME. Gender and age effects in coping: A comparison between Mexican and Paraguayan adolescents. In: Kaniasty K, Moore K,

Howard S, Buchwald P, editors. Stress and Anxiety. Application to Social and Environmental Threats, Psychological Well-being, Occupational Challenges, and Developmental Psychology. Berlin: Logos Verlag; 2014. pp. 249–260.

[66] Barcelata B, Márquez-Caraveo ME, Granados A. Exploring the relationship between coping and internalizing and externalizing behaviours in adolescents at social risk. In: 9th International Conference on Child and Adolescent Psychopathology. July, 2014. Roehampton, London.

[67] Barcelata B, Rodríguez R, Marquez-Caraveo M. Coping, perceived control, positive thinking, self-control and social support as predictors of adolescent outcomes in marginalized settings. In: 37th Annual Conference Stress and Anxiety Research Society. July, 2016. Zagreb, Croacia.

[68] Pinkerton J, Dolan P. Family support, social capital, resilience, and adolescent coping. Child and Family Social Work. 2007;12:219–228.

[69] Jadue G. Family transformations in Chile: present increasing risk in the emotional, psychosocial and educational development of children. Estudios Pedagógicos. 2003;2:115–126.

[70] Razavi M, Razavi T. Family functioning components as predictors of internalizing and externalizing disorders in children. International Journal of Applied Behavioural Sciences. 2014;1(2):45–49.

[71] Repetti R, Taylor E, Seeman T. Risky families: Family social environments and the mental and physical health of offspring. Psychological Bulletin American Psychological Association. 2002;12(8):330–366.

[72] Schleider J, Weisz J. Family process and youth internalizing problems: A triadic model of etiology and intervention. Development and psychopathology. 2016;april6:1–29.

[73] Rodriguez EM, Nichols SR, Javdani S, Emerson E, Donenberg G R. Economic hardship, parent positive communication, and mental health in urban adolescents seeking outpatient psychiatric care. Journal of Child and Family Studies. 2015;24(3):617–627.

[74] Smokowski PR, Bacallao ML, Cotter KL, Evans CB. The effects of positive and negative parenting practices on adolescent mental health outcomes in a multicultural sample of rural youth. Child Psychiatry and Human Development. 2015;46(3):333–345.

[75] Bokszczanin A, Makowsky S. Family economic hardship, parental support and social anxiety in adolescents. In: Roussi P, Vassilaki E, Kaniasty K, Baker J, editors. Stress and Psychosocial Resources. Coping with life changes, occupational, demands, educational challenge, and threats to physical and emotional wellbeing. Berlin: Logos-Verlag; 2007. pp. 57–69.

[76] Barcelata B, Villaseñor M, Granados. Family functioning, perceived social support, and adolescent resilience in poverty condition. In: 20th IACAPAP World Congress Neuropsiquiatric de l'enfance et de l'adolescence. 21–25 July, 2012. IACAPAP, Paris, France.

[77] Marquez ME, Barcelata B, Barron V. Gender and age main effects on adolescent psychopathology in clinical settings. 8a. Conference of Child and Adolescent Psychopathology. July, 2013. Roehampton, London.

[78] Achenbach T, Rescorla L. Manual for the ASEBA School-age Forms and Profiles. Burlington, VT: ASEBA; 2001.

[79] Marquez ME, Barcelata B, Parental rearing style as a predictor of mental health problems in a low-income clinical sample. In: 22th International Association for Child and Adolescent Psychiatry and Allied Professions (IACAPAP) and 36th Annual Conference for the Canadian Academy of Child and Adolescent Psychiatry (CACAP). Calgary, Canada, 18-22, September, 2016.

10

Peer Bullying in Schools: A Cognitive Behavioral Intervention Program

Füsun Gökkaya

Abstract

Students face few problems in schools. Some of these conflicts may be defined with the bullying concept. The concept of bullying is defined as "to repetitively expose a student/ students to negative effects of another student or students." "Negative effects" includes students getting disturbed as well as getting hurt from the same kind of negative behavior; it also may be done by attempting to hurt someone, deliberately harming someone verbally or physically. Bullying behavior should include an "inequivalent power" between opponents and this needs to be "permanent" and "intentional." Bullying at school affects lots of students around the schools who witness bullying behavior in different dimensions; thus, it is an important problem that needs to be prevented. While some of the studies encompass interventions toward the whole school system, some studies were conducted by determining separate groups and working on those. In this paper, first, some whole school approach–based prevention programs and the effectiveness of these programs and then intervention programs for groups, which are provided to reduce and intervene bullying, will be explained. Second, cognitive behavioral therapy and its use in preventing bullying will be briefly explained. Finally, the context of a cognitive-behavioral based peer bullying intervention program.

Keywords: peer bullying, intervention program, cognitive behavioral therapy, school bullying, prevention program

1. Introduction

Students encounter various problems in the school environment and some of those are experienced among friends. Cases termed as "bullying," which is one of the problems encountered among friends, have certain characteristics that differ from cases of violence. This concept is defined as "a student/students repeatedly exposing another student/students to negative effects multiple times" [1]. This "negative effect" may range from disturbance to actual injury and can be done verbally or physically in order to attempt to do harm or deliberately harm another. In bullying behavior, certain characteristics should be present, such as an "unequal power relationship" between the sides, the situation having a "continuous" characteristic and the acts being carried out "on purpose" [1].

Research has shown that approximately 15–20% of all students are affected by peer bullying at school [2–6]. Peer bullying can be performed directly or in an indirect manner. While direct bullying is performed openly against the bullied student, indirect bullying may well range into the realm of purposeful exclusion from the social group because of discrimination [1]. Generally, peer bullying has been grouped into physical bullying, verbal bullying and social exclusion. While physical and verbal bullying are elements of direct bullying, social exclusion is in the scope of indirect bullying. Physical bullying encompasses behavior such as hitting, pushing, spitting, kicking, pulling hair and tripping, whereas verbal bullying encompasses behavior such as use of foul language, giving nicknames and insulting. Social exclusion encompasses behavior that aims to harm the social relations of the students such as gossiping, exclusion from the friend group, ignoring and not accepting the student into games. The shape of peer bullying has changes throughout the years. In recent years, the developing Internet and communication technologies have created the concept of cyber bullying [7]. Writing various things under the photographs of friends in social network sites through the Internet, spreading unfounded rumors on them, disturbing them thorough phone messages and E-mails, taking inappropriate pictures via cameras and spreading them through the Internet are all defined as cyber bullying. Additionally, although these behaviors are conducted in environments outside the school, their effects are more pronounced at school. Sexual harassment/disturbance behavior has also been discussed as a type of peer bullying with a different motivation. For this reason, sexual bullying, which encompasses sexual behavior (lifting skirts, taking pictures under skirts, pulling down pants, etc.), has been defined as a separate category.

While discussing peer bullying, students are generally grouped into bullies, victims, bully-victim and bystanders [1, 8]. Bullying at school affects bullies, victims and bystanders who witness bullying behavior in different dimensions. Victims of bullying encounter problems such as anxiety, feelings of anger and desperation, unhappiness, ostracism and loneliness [9–11]. Alongside possibilities such as disciplinary action and exclusion from academic life, children who exhibit bullying behavior during school years have high risks of having their experiences affect their adult life negatively and carry their behavior into adulthood. Longitudinal studies have shown that children and adolescents who exhibit bullying behavior at school get mixed up in acts of violence in adulthood, have impulsive behavior, lead unsuccessful lives with lower job positions and have substance abuse problems [12–15]. These findings have made interventions to prevent and reduce bullying gain importance.

In many countries (Australia, Finland, the UK, Ireland, Sweden, Italy, Norway), it can be seen that programs toward preventing peer bullying have been applied for years and country wide studies on the subject have been performed [16, 17]. Stopping bullying behavior at school can be carried out through prevention or intervention programs [16, 18, 19].

Studies researching the reasons behind bullying behavior at school have shown that the personal characteristics of the students, parental attitudes, family relationships, school atmosphere, teacher attitudes, friendship relations and cultural factors may all have effects on the subject [20–22]. For this reason, studies on reducing bullying at schools can be said to have different focal points. While some of the studies encompass interventions toward the whole school system, some studies were conducted by determining separate groups and working on those.

In this chapter first, some whole school approach-based prevention programs and the effectiveness of these programs then intervention programs for groups, which are provided to reduce and intervene bullying will be explained. Second, cognitive-behavioral therapy and its use in preventing and intervening bullying will briefly explain. Finally, the context of a cognitive-behavioral based peer bullying intervention program.

2. Whole school approach studies to prevent peer bullying at schools and their effectiveness

Whole school approach programs to prevent peer bullying at schools are applied on school, classroom and individual levels [1]. Interventions toward bullying aim at all of the students at the school developing an attitude against bullying and are applied to decrease bullying events within the school. Interventions at the school level are student and teacher questionnaires, school conference days aimed at developing a positive school environment, parent-teacher meetings, telephone interviews with parents and the regulation of school playgrounds. Classroom efforts include forming classroom rules against bullying, information being given to raise awareness, the formation of a positive environment and meetings with parents and teachers. Programs applied on an individual level include interventions such as having serious meetings with bullies and victims, having meetings with the parents of children involved in bullying, receiving help from unbiased children, providing help and support for parents, forming discussion groups with the families of bullies and victims and changes in schools and classrooms [1]. The programs summarized in this section are some of the most widely used studies.

2.1. Olweus bullying prevention program (BPP)

The first school-based program to prevent bullying, the BPP aims to change the social norms that see bullying behavior as acceptable. Within the context of this goal, it first tries to create awareness on bullying. First, the rates of bullies, bully-victims, victims, bystanders and exposure to bullying are determined through a scanning effort in the school. Then, school wide conferences, meetings with school staff, teacher trainings, family trainings, small group efforts with the families, classroom studies and individual meetings with bullies and victims are performed [1].

Alongside many studies where Olweus' program was applied and its effectiveness was researched, Olweus himself has made effectiveness evaluations regarding the application. The results of the first studies found a 50% decrease in bullying behavior [1] and later evaluations have shown the change to be between 21 and 38% [23, 24].

2.2. Creating a peaceful school learning environment (CAPSLE)

The program, developed in 1994, aims to prevent bullying and create a positive school environment through ensuring that students learn ways to solve their problems without aggression and the social skills necessary to communicate positively [14]. The program consists of four basic and two supporting elements. The first basic element is to create a positive atmosphere at school by "zero" tolerance to all bullying. The second element is the formation of a disciplinary plan to provide appropriate behavior. In the process of doing this, the importance of social skills not only among the students but also with adults in the school was stressed. The third element is a classroom management plan. For this, the aim is to raise awareness on the dynamics of bullying and develop the appropriate disciplinary measures to ensure the change of these behaviors. The fourth basic element is a unique physical training program. In this program, the focus is on self-defense sports that may help students develop self-regulation skills. Additionally, in this stage, the aim is to provide counseling in a manner that will help to prevent bullying through an appropriate counseling program for children and adults. The first supportive element of the program is changing the language used at school to increase cognitive skills and the awareness of a person of his/her role in the bullying phenomenon. The second supportive element is to focus on psychopathology instead of penalty applications in the bully-victim-bystander triangle to direct toward treatment and making the necessary referrals [9, 25]. In the program, study groups with families as well as the children are arranged to increase their awareness on the subject.

Twemlow et al. [26], who developed and applied the program, which was generally found to decrease victimization, aggressiveness and aggressive bystanders, performed a longitudinal study with a control group. The applications were performed by showing zero tolerance to bullying at the school where the program was applied. In the control group, only regular psychiatric consultation was provided. The results were evaluated by taking data on disciplinary cases and school success from those two schools. The increase in academic success and the decrease in disciplinary events in the school where the program was applied were found to be significantly different compared to the school in the control group [26].

2.3. Steps to respect

The program consists of three stages: the first stage starts with building a school bullying management team that encompasses the whole school. This team makes observations regarding bullying behavior. The antibullying strategies and procedures and the consequences that those who apply bullying behavior will face are determined and the expectations on the subject are communicated to the whole school. In the second stage, the whole school staff is trained according to the reports of the students. During school personnel training, counselors, classroom teachers and foreign personnel are all trained for awareness on the subject. Some selected school personnel are trained to work directly with children involved in bullying. The families are included in this stage. In the third stage, classroom efforts where the classroom teachers give skill trainings last 11 hours. Classroom level efforts are aimed toward increasing the socioemotional skills of the students so that they can form positive relationships. Emotion regulation, recognizing emotions, resisting certain emotions and reporting bullying behavior are all among skills taught during training. Additional aims include being able to enter a group, being able to discern bullying behavior from others and adding responsibility to bystanders [27].

The results of studies on the effectiveness of the program have shown a significant decrease in the bullying approval behavior of bystander students in the intervention group compared to the control group. Additionally, an improvement in the taking responsibility to stop bullying behavior of the bystanders in the intervention group was reported [28]. According to the results of another study, students have reported 33% less physical bullying, teachers have reported 35% decrease in fights and 20% of school staff stated that the school environment had a more positive atmosphere [29].

2.4. Bully busters

This program was prepared by Newman et al. [30]. The "Bully Busters" program is a teacher training focused psychoeducational intervention program aimed at preventing violence. The program includes both individual and environmental factors regarding a child. The aim is to ensure that especially teachers learn bullying and victimization prevention and intervention strategies, skills and techniques. The training, which starts with high priority awareness training on bullying, continues by teaching bully and victim recognition, bully and victim intervention, stress management, relaxation and coping skills. Through teacher support groups, trainings on activities to be applied in the classroom are taught to teachers. The teachers are given handbooks and CDs. The special aims of the program are increasing the coping skills of the students through strong role models, decreasing aggressive behavior and creating a more positive school atmosphere. Additionally, the program forms a discussion environment in the classroom so that students understand factors regarding being bullies and victims and aims at the provision of the necessary alternative social skills for conflict resolution.

Study results have shown that the Bully Busters program increases the knowledge of teachers on the subject and their intervention skills [31, 32], increases their personal sufficiency regarding bullying prevention [31], and decreases the bullying events among students and disciplinary problems [31, 33].

2.5. Bully prevention in positive behavioral interventions and supports: BP-PBIS

The BP-PBIS is a school-based prevention program focused on the positive behavior of students and school staff. It is a program where bullying behavior is followed for the prevention of gossiping, inappropriate behavior and cyber bullying that encompasses the whole school curriculum and aims at providing social responsibility awareness. It was prepared using a developmental approach [30].

BP-PBS teaches all of the students in a school the concept of "being respectful" and aims at adopting a three-stage response (do not talk, stop, walk) when they encounter disrespectful behavior. The program is designed to train the personnel to make the correct interventions to the problematic behavior of students by teaching the correct behavior after the three-stage response is used.

Around the school, the PBS is organized around a three-layered prevention model. In the first layer, the aim is to make the school a safe and positive environment for students around the clock. For this reason, the behavior expected from them is taught to all of the students in the form of structured rules, the appropriate behaviors are ensured to be accepted in social environments, the results of problematic behavior are made to be predictable and the punishments to be met are made clear. In the second layer, the students under risk who do not receive enough support in the first layer are provided additional support. This layer includes interventions made to the students in small groups. Bullying is tried to be eliminated using social rewards. Last, the third layer includes students who do not respond to the first and second layers and consistently act negatively to be examined and worked with separately [34].

This program is supported, in addition to subjects included in the school curriculum, activities performed by students on the Internet. The effectiveness of the program is evaluated through questionnaires and the observations of supervisors [30].

Studies evaluating the effectiveness of the program have shown that children in the schools where the program was applied encountered less peer rejection and bullying compared to schools where the program was not applied [35], and that there was a decrease in problematic behavior, especially 65% decrease in physical and verbal aggression [34].

2.6. Kiusaamista Vastaan: against bullying: KiVa

This program, which was developed in Finland, has international characteristics. In the program, it is suggested that teachers and students should form group norms in their schools through individual and group discussion. Content is presented through various materials prepared for teachers, students and parents. For example, in order to make students develop antibullying attitudes, antibullying video games are used. The whole of the program takes 20 hours and the courses are given by the teachers. In the courses, discussions, group studies, short films on bullying and role playing techniques are used to conduct the program. After each course, a classroom rule appropriate for the theme of the subject of the day is adopted. Another important factor of the program is teacher training. Teachers supervise during play time in the school playground. In the teacher training, they are taught to recognize the signals of bullying, which starts at the playground and reflects into the school and intervene appropriately. Additionally, an electronic forum environment where teachers from different schools can communicate is formed. In this electronic environment, teachers inform each other on the bullying events and interventions they encounter and make suggestions. Additionally, support groups for bullying victims are formed. Last, families are sent a handbook containing information on bullying and what they can do to prevent bullying [13].

When the effectiveness of the KiVa program was evaluated, 79.4% of the students stated that bullying stopped completely, 18.5% stated that it decreased, 0.9% stated that it stayed the same and 03% stated that it increased, while an increase in liking school and decreases in depression and anxiety were found [36]. Additionally, bullying was found to decrease in groups where bullies where characterized as having medium or little popularity [37].

3. Group studies toward intervening in peer bullying and their effectiveness

Some of the programs toward intervening in peer bullying are conducted in a classroom level while some are only toward the target student group [13]. Target-focused programs are intervention efforts made toward bullies, victims, bully-victims, or mixed groups. Since peer bullying is not a psychological disorder that is evaluated and classified according to certain diagnosis criteria, the studies performed with students with high bullying inclination were named not as therapeutic applications but as preventive group efforts in this section. In this section, although the number of the group studies made with high bullying tendencies is not much in the literature, especially the studies made with these bully students will be evaluated. For example, effort to increase the self-respect of victims, similar victim-based intervention studies and classroom-based training studies will not be discussed.

In a study performed with male adolescents displaying bullying behavior [38], the aim was to decrease bullying by using behavioral techniques. The experimental study was conducted with 54 male bullies at age 16 studying at 3 middle schools in South Africa in three groups. The results of the study were evaluated using pretest, posttest and follow-up measurements (1 month). The program was based on the social interactive model which explains the development of aggression in its theoretical basis and the behavioral approach, which is thought to be appropriate for the prevention of bullying. The program was performed by psychology students at school during school hours twice a week in nonconsecutive 10 weeks with sessions that took a total of 20 hours. In the behavioral program applied, the homework, self-monitoring, role-playing and token economy methods were used to provide positive behavior. For behavior change in rewarding nonbullying behavior, the "Wonderland Game" tokens, chocolates and movie tickets were used to utilize token economy. In each session, a topic was discussed in a manner allowing feedback on the behavior of students and role-playing, drawings and games were utilized. During role-playing, each member chose a "partner" to use the observations of the partner in "self-monitoring sessions." With the program, a small decrease in bullying behavior that was not statistically significant was achieved. The nature and shortness of the program were thought to be the reason.

In another study, the aim was to provide outpatient treatment to young people with demonstrating bullying behavior, decrease the anger of young people and to improve their interpersonal relationships and health behavior related to quality of life [39]. For this reason, 22 young people received 6 months of family therapy and 22 young people were included in the control group. Weekly sessions for 90 min were held in the first 2 months and these sessions were made once a fortnight in the following months. In the sessions, elements of systematical therapy, dynamic therapy, gestalt therapy, psychodrama therapy and behavioral therapy were used. The therapy focused on interfamilial relationships. Topics such as communication, interfamilial rules and the freedoms of family members were discussed and "family games" changing familial balance were used to raise awareness and form new family rules. Two trained therapists conducted the sessions. Once every 2 weeks, the scales used in the study were applied to the members to evaluate improvement. A year after the study, follow-up measurements were taken. The results of the study showed that the family therapy decreased the aggression and bullying behavior of young males with bullying behavior in a statistically significant manner and that the therapies increased health behavior related to quality of life.

In another study conducted with male students who engaged in bullying behavior, short-term strategic family therapy was conducted [40]. The anger and health behavior related to quality of life of male adolescents who engage in bullying were tried to be changed. Of 72 students demonstrating bullying behavior, 36 were assigned to 12-week short-term strategic family therapy and 36 were assigned to the control group. After 12 weeks of treatment, decreases in the bullying behavior of the study group, increases in anger control and increases in health behavior related to quality of life were all found to be statistically significant.

In a study where art was used to decrease bullying, the effectiveness of an opera watched by the students in decreasing bullying was evaluated using pretest and posttest measurements [41]. The opera, named Elijah's Kite, was found to be more effective compared with the results of previous studies through social-emotional learning, improving both social skills and life skills. The subject of the opera, which tried to emerge emotions through music, movement, order and dance, was the recognition of bullying, understanding the feelings of the victim and giving information on what to do in event of bullying. The study was performed with fourth and fifth graders formed from 57 males and 47 females and the opera was staged 6 weeks (3 schools) after the pretest measurements. In the results, the information of the students regarding bullying was found to be increased and reports of victimization were found to significantly decrease. Alongside these, while reports of bullying decreased with time in males, it increased in females.

In a study conducted in Turkey (Konya), the pressure exerted by high school students exerting peer pressure was tried to be decreased [42]. The study was conducted with 24 male students from among freshmen from a high school. In the study, the group psychological counseling applications developed by the researchers with an eclectic approach took 8 weeks. In the sessions, the subjects of having information on peer pressure and understanding basic concepts, sharing experiences regarding peer pressure, what the group members considered peer pressure, why they acted as such, what they feel when they exert or receive pressure, coping methods for feelings of anger, communication skills, conflict resolution training, emotion training and what the situations and automatic negative thoughts were when exerting or receiving peer pressure in daily life and how these could be changed, in respective order. As a result of the application, the program was found to be effective in decreasing peer pressure.

In another study, the elements of cognitive behavioral therapy were used in a program for bullying intervention [43]. The effects of contingency management and cognitive self-instruction on bullying behavior were examined. The sample of the study consisted of 120 randomly selected bully students from 3 schools in 3 settlements in Nigeria. The study was conducted with 2 study (self-instruction and contingency management) and one control group and each group consisted of 40 people (20 male and 20 female). The intervention groups took 1-hour trainings once a week for 6 weeks. In each session, 15 min were allocated to the discussion of the previous session, 30 min to discussion/lesson and 15 min to summarizing and assigning homework for the next session. In the intervention group that received self-instruction training, the method of using positive self-concepts instead of negative ones such as "I should overcome bullying" and "I should think twice before bullying" was used. In the contingency management group, reinforcers for positive behavior were given. In the placebo control group, trainings on subjects such as time management and the importance of keeping notes were given. Results based on pretest and posttest evaluation showed that contingency management and self-instruction had significant effects in decreasing bullying behavior. Self-instruction was found to be more effective than contingency management. The effectiveness of the treatment did not show difference according to the religion or age of the participants.

4. A general overview of cognitive behavioral therapy (CBT) and peer bullying preventions with CBT

According to cognitive model, the ways people interpret the events affect their emotions and actions. Cognitive behavioral therapy is based on two principles: one of them is our cognitions (thoughts) that determine our emotions and actions and the other one is the way we act that shows some strong effects on our thoughts and feelings. According to CBT, every single psychological disorders and problematic behaviors have an underlying mechanism as distortional and dysfunctional thoughts that affect people's psychological mental health and their actions. Evaluation and changing them cause some improvements and recruitments on emotions and actions. Briefly, fundamental assumption of CBT is changing emotions and actions by finding the negative automatic thoughts and reframing them. Cognitive and behavioral techniques are used while working on changing thoughts and emotions. These techniques are briefly emotional education, mindfulness education, cognitive restricting, role-playing and exposure techniques.

Examination of peer bullying prevention and intervention programs reveals that cognitive and behavioral techniques are frequently used although not all components of the cognitive behavioral therapy methods are employed. For instance, Olweus' [1] bullying prevention program aims to alter bullying-related cognitions at schools. Attempts at altering bullying-related cognitions involve changing these cognitions with positive thoughts, such as "children are okay with this" versus "bullying must be stopped/no child can be educated like this" or "bullying is a great opportunity" versus "I can stop bullying when I confront it."

In the Bully-Busters bullying prevention program, components of cognitive behavioral therapy are used. The program's manual teaches children to change their negative bullying-related cognitions with positive alternatives and to plan various actions against bullying. Anger management, emotion training, empathy training, cognitive training, social skills training, problem solving skills training and conflict resolution training are among other cognitive behavioral elements used in the Bully-Busters program [44].

In a bullying prevention program which used behavioral techniques involved self-monitoring, role playing and token economy [38]; while in another program which used cognitive behavioral techniques involved self-instruction and contingency management [43]. During the studies, the researchers employed the cognitive reframing technique and tried to establish positive thoughts such as "I must overcome bullying" and "I should think twice before bullying someone."

In conclusion, despite the abundance of efficacy studies on cognitive behavioral therapy programs aimed at reducing aggression among youth, studies that use cognitive behavioral interventions in youth who bully peers are limited [38, 43]. As explained above from a cognitive behavioral approach, it can be postulated that psychological disorders derive from dysfunctional thought patterns or the lack of positive-appropriate behavioral coping strategies. In this treatment approach, it is aimed to restructure effective coping strategies and problem solving skills as well as reducing cognitive bias or distortions [45].

In this context, an intervention program which included cognitive behavioral therapy elements was prepared for middle school students with high bullying tendencies. The efficacy of the program was tested in an experimental study which investigated the pretest, posttest and follow-up measures of experiment, placebo control and control (no intervention) groups. It was found that this cognitive behavioral therapy program that aimed to reduce bullying tendencies was effective in changing bullying related cognitions and in reducing bullying behavior [46].

5. Introduction of a cognitive Behavioral intervention program aimed at decreasing bullying

The cognitive behavioral intervention program was prepared according to the principles of cognitive behavioral therapy. In summary, it consists of certain techniques, namely psychoeducation, which entails understanding what bullying behaviors are, the difference between joking and conflict, how bullying harms people in the short and long terms (to encourage change and motivate the group) and feelings and thoughts that accompany bullying behavior; self-awareness training, which helps a person recognize their valuable aspects and supports positive self-perception; cognitive restructuring, which entails changing the thoughts accompanying bullying; coping techniques, which entail stopping bullying behavior and replacing them with alternative behavior; self-instruction, which entails finding slogans and internal discourses to remind of stopping bullying and repeating them to oneself; and role-playing, which is applied to use the techniques learned in hypothetical situations. Additionally, a reward system to reinforce positive behavior was used.

5.1. The process of the program, duration and content

The group application consisted of 13 120-min sessions, once a week. The first 15 min of each session is allocated to forming connections to the previous session and the discussion of homework, if present. Later, the daily subject was discussed for 20–30 min. After a 15-min break, the second half of the session was started and the subject was reinforced with an appropriate game (table game, enactment) (15–20 min). Later, free play time was given (15–20 min). At the end of the games, the reward schematics were recorded. Last, a review of the day was performed, feedback on the session was received and the session was ended.

5.1.1. Environment

The applications were made in an empty room seen appropriate by the school management (library, counselor's room, etc.). An environment where the students could comfortably sit in a circle, come to a table when needed, which was wide enough that free games and role plays could be played and which would not be used during group hours for other reasons was tried to be ensured. To use rewards, sometimes the schoolyard was also used. In each session, the pages of the program handbook were given to the students as written materials and written-table games were prepared for the subjects.

Use of rewards: in order to support members' participation, compliance with group rules, completion of assignments and positive interaction, the use of rewards is very important. In this study, a reward table was used for rewards. The reward table was recorded at the end of each session. These rewards were arranged as individual and group rewards.

5.1.2. The content of the sessions

According to the plan outlined above, the goals and general summary of each session was given below.

5.1.2.1. Sessions 1–3: psychoeducation

5.1.2.1.1. Introduction

The leader started by introducing themselves. The reason for the group gathering and the group process was explained to the students and an introduction game was played. Group rules were discussed and the contracts on compliance with group rules were given as two copies to the students to be signed. Then the aims of the study, rewards, study type and study days were explained. In order to ensure group motivation, the students were told to think of a group name until the nest session.

5.1.2.1.2. Awareness on bullying behavior

In order to make peer bullying more understandable, examples of bullying and nonbullying behavior were given in hypothetical situations and the differences between these behavior types were discussed. What peer bullying is was explained.

5.1.2.2. Sessions 4 and 5: emotional training

In order to recognize emotions, understanding someone else's emotions by bodily cues and the fact that more than one emotion can be experienced in an event were studies using emotion posters and emotion guessing games. In order to make students realize that emotions can change, different people having different emotions in various situations and the emotions that occur during bullying were studied using the experiences of the students recorded at home by homework and the prepared worksheets.

5.1.2.3. Sessions 6–10: cognitive restructuring

In these sessions, the concepts of thought, connections between thought-emotion-behavior, recognizing thoughts related to bullying, making the connections between thoughts and emotions related to bullying behavior and replacing thoughts that cause bullying with new thoughts were studied. Card games prepared beforehand were used to reinforce the subject.

In this process, awareness training was given so that group members could recognize their own positive characteristics. The needs underlying one's bullying behavior were checked, the needs for perceiving oneself as strong, valuable and leading were identified and positive personality characteristics that would make one such a person without bullying were emphasized. Additionally, what the alternatives to bullying behavior could be was discussed.

5.1.2.4. Session 11: self-instruction training

Finding slogans and internal discourses to change the thought that may cause bullying and remind of the alternative behavior and rewarding oneself when bullying behavior is stopped were studied. In order to replace bullying behavior with new behavior, behavioral experiments that would remind one of the slogans were performed. In this stage, self-instruction and role playing techniques were used.

5.1.2.5. Sessions 12 and 13: reviewing all of the techniques and conclusion

In these sessions, all of the techniques that were learned were reviewed and alternative behavior to stop bullying behavior and slogan reminding were reinforced through role playing. The efforts of the students to reward themselves when they stopped bullying behavior were supported.

6. Discussion

In the prevention of peer bullying, whole school approach programs that encompass all groups whether bully, victim, or bystander and that are applied to the school system as a whole are known to be effective [1, 13]. These programs generally contain education efforts done in large groups. However, when the risks exhibited by bullying children regarding their adult lives are considered, it was thought that these children should be the subject of separate interventions with more comprehensive techniques and thus a cognitive behavioral intervention program aimed at reducing or eliminating these behavior was prepared and its effectiveness was tested [46]. This program is not thought to be an alternative approach to prevention programs toward the school system as a whole, but as an additional application that may lead to more effective results in the reduction of bullying.

Author details

Füsun Gökkaya

Address all correspondence to: fusungokkaya@hotmail.com

Ministry of Education, İzmir, Turkey

References

[1] Olweus D. Bullying at School. 9th ed. Oxford: Blackwell; 2004.

[2] Ayas T, Piskin M. Investigation of bullying among high school students with regard to sex, grade level and school type. Elementary Education Online. 2011; 10(2): 550–568.

[3] Batsche GM, Knoff HM. Bullies and their victims: understanding a pervasive problem in the schools. School Psychology Review. 1994; 23: 165–175.

[4] Espelage D, Swearer S. Bullying in American Schools—A Social-Ecological Perspective on Prevention and Intervention. New Jersey: Lawrence Erlbaum Associates; 2004.

[5] Genç G. Bullying and management in general high school [thesis]. Malatya: Inönü University Institute of Social Sciences; 2007.

[6] Pellegrini AD. School bullies, victims and aggressive victims: factors relating to group affiliation and victimization in early adolescence. Journal of Educational Psychology. 1999; 91(2): 216–224.

[7] Wong JS. No bullies allowed understanding peer victimization, the impacts on delinquency and the effectiveness of prevention programs [thesis]. Pardee RAND Graduate School; 2009.

[8] Piskin M. Examination of peer bullying among primary and middle school children in Ankara. Ankara Education and Science. 2010; 35: 175–189.

[9] Jacops A. Components of evidence-based interventions for bullying and peer victimization. In: Steele RG, Elkin TD, Robert MC, editors. Handbook of Evidence-based Therapies for Children and Adolescents. Kansas: Springer; 2008. pp. 261–279.

[10] Gökler R. Peer bullying in schools. Journal of Human Sciences. 2009; 6(2): 511–537.

[11] Menesini E, Modena M, Tani F. Bullying and victimization in adolescence: concurrent and stable roles and psychological health symptoms. The Journal of Genetic Psychology. 2009; 170(2): 115–133.

[12] Bender D, Löseli F. Bullying at school as a predictor of delinquency, violence and other anti-social behaviour in adulthood. Criminal Behaviour and Mental Health. 2011; 21: 99–106.

[13] Farrington D P, Ttofi M M. School-based programs to reduce bullying and victimization. Campbell Systematic Reviews 2009:6 10.4073/csr.2009.6

[14] Kim MJ, Catalano RF, Haggerty KP, Abbott RD. Bullying at elementary school and problem behaviour in young adulthood: a study of bullying, violence and substance use from age 11 to age 21. Criminal Behaviour and Mental Health. 2011; 21: 136–144.

[15] Olweus D. Bullying at school and later criminality: findings from three Swedish community samples of males. Criminal Behaviour and Mental Health. 2011; 21: 151–156.

[16] Rigby K, Smith PK, Pepler PK, Smith D, Pepler K. Working to prevent school bullying: key issues. In: Rigby D, editors. Bullying in Schools: How Successful can Interventions Be? Cambridge: Cambridge University Press; 2004. pp. 1–13.

[17] Smith PK, Brain P. Bullying in schools: lessons from two decades of research. Aggressive Behavior. 2000; 26: 1–9.

[18] Mishna F, Saini M, Solomon S. Ongoing and online: Children and youth's perceptions of cyber bullying. Children and Youth Services Review. 2009; 31: 1222–1228.

[19] Rigby K. What can schools do about cases of bullying? Pastoral Care in Education. 2011; 29(4): 273–285.

[20] Doğan A. Ecological systems model as a framework for bullying. Turkish Journal of Child and Adolescent Mental Health. 2010; 17(3): 149–162.

[21] Garbarino J. An ecological perspective on the effects of violence on children. Journal of Community Psychology. 2011; 29(3): 361–378.

[22] Rodkin P, Hodges E. Bullies and victims in the peer ecology: four questions for psychologists and school professionals. School Psychology Review. 2003; 32(3): 384–400.

[23] Bauer NS, Lozano P, Rivara F. Prevention in public middle schools: a controlled trial. Journal of Adolescent Health. 2007; 40: 266–274.

[24] Black S. Evaluation of the Olweus bullying prevention program: how the program can work for inner city youth. In: Proceedings of Persistently Safe Schools, The 2007 National Conference on Safe Schools; October 29–31, 2007, Washington, DC.

[25] Twemlow SW, Sacco FC. Creating a Peaceful School Learning Environment A Training Manual for Elementary Schools. Agawam: T & S Publishing Group. [Internet]. 1999. Available from: http://www.backoffbully.com/PDF%20files/PeacefulSchools/manual.pdf [Accessed: 2016-08-15]

[26] Twemlow SW, Fonagy P, Sacco FC, Gies ML, Evans R, Ewbank R. Creating a peaceful school learning environment: a controlled study of an elementary school intervention to reduce violence. The American Journal of Psychiatry. 2001; 158: 808–810.

[27] Committee for Children. A bullying prevention program. Stop bullying: create a safe and safe respectful learning environment. [Internet]. 2014. Available from: www.writehabit.org/StR_Brochure.pdf. [Accessed: 2016-08-15]

[28] Frey KS, Hirchstein MK, Snell JL, Van Schoiack Edstrom L, MacKenzie EP, Broderick CJ. Reducing playground bullying and supporting beliefs: an experimental trial of the steps to respect program. Developmental Psychology. 2005; 41(3): 479–491.

[29] Brown EC, Low S, Smith BH, Haggerty KP. Outcomes from a school randomized controlled trial of steps to respect: a school bullying prevention program. School Psychology Review. 2011; 40(3): 423–443.

[30] Serwacki M, Nickerson AB, editors. Guide to School Wide Bullying Prevention Programs, Alberti Center for Bullying Abuse Prevention. Graduate School of Education University at Buffalo, the State University of New York. [Internet]. 2012. Available from: http://gse.buffalo.edu/gsefiles/documents/alberti/Bullying%20Prevention%20Program%20Guide%20-%20FINAL%203.16.12_0.pdf [Accessed: 2016-08-15]

[31] Bell CD, Raczynski KA, Horne AM. Bully busters abbreviated: evaluation of a group-based bully intervention program. Group Dynamics: Theory, Research and Practice. 2010; 14(3): 257–267.

[32] Newman Carlson D, Horne AM. Bully Busters: A psychoeducational intervention for reducing bullying behavior in middle school students. Journal of Counseling and Development. 2004; 82: 259–267.

[33] Carney AG. No vacation from bullying: A summer camp intervention pilot study. Education. 2008; 129(1): 163–184.

[34] Ross SW, Horner R H. Bully prevention in positive behavior support. Journal of Applied Behavior Analysis. 2009; 42(4): 747–759.

[35] Waasdorp TE, Bradshaw C P, Leaf P J. The impact of school wide positive behavioral interventions and supports on bullying and peer rejection: a randomized controlled effectiveness trial. Archives of Pediatrics and Adolescent Medicine. 2012; 166(2): 149–156.

[36] Laitinen K. Children's rights and safe learning environment. KiVa—A national anti-bullying program for Finnish schools. Finnish National Board of Education, Pestalozzi. Opetushallitus, Osaamisen Ja Sivistyksen Parhaaksi. [Internet]. 2012. Available from: http://www.oph.fi/download/143565_Kristiina_Laitinen_Pestalozzi_KiVa_04_10_2012.pdf [Accessed: 2016-08-15]

[37] Garandeau CF, Lee IA, Salmivalli C. Differential effects of the KiVa anti-bullying program on popular and unpopular bullies. Journal of Applied Developmental Psychology. 2014; 35: 44–50.

[38] Meyer N, Lesch E. An analysis of the limitations of a behavioural programme for bullying boys from a subeconomic environment. Southern African Journal of Child and Adolescent Mental Health. 2000; 12(1): 59–69.

[39] Nickel M, Krawczyk J, Nickel C, Forthuber P, Kettler C, Leiberich P, et al. Anger, interpersonal relationships and health-related quality of life in bullying boys who are treated with outpatient family therapy: a randomized, prospective, controlled trial with 1 year of follow-up. Pediatrics. 2005; 116(2): 247–253.

[40] Nickel M, Muehlbacher M, Kaplan P, Krawczyk J, Buschmann W, Kettler C, et al. Influence of family therapy on bullying behaviour, cortisol secretion, anger and quality of life in bullying male adolescents: a randomized, prospective, controlled study. The Canadian Journal of Psychiatry. 2006; 5: 355–362.

[41] Haner D, Pepler D, Cummings J, Vaughan AR. The role of arts-based curricula in bullying prevention: Elijah's kite—a children's opera. Canadian Journal of School Psychology. 2010; 25(1): 55–69.

[42] Sargın N, Çetinkaya B. The effectiveness of group counseling in reducing peer pressure. Journal of Social Sciences Institute of Selcuk University. 2010; 23: 185–192.

[43] Eweniyi G, Adeoye A, Ayodele K. O, Raheem A. The effectiveness of two psycho-social behavioural interventions on adolescents' bullying behaviour among Nigerian adolescents. Journal of Studies in Social Sciences. 2013; 4(2): 246–261.

[44] Doll B, Swearer SS. Cognitive behavioral interventions for participants in bullying and coercion. In: Mennuti R, Freeman A, Christner R, editors. Cognitive-Behavioral Interventions in Educational Settings. New York: Routledge; 2006.

[45] O'Connor T, Creswell C. Cognitive-behavioural therapy for children and adolescents. Psychiatry. 2005; 4(9): 123–125.

[46] Gökkaya F. Developing a cognitive behavioral intervention program to reduce bully tendencies in primary school children and the program effectiveness. [Unpublished doctoral dissertation]. Izmir: Ege University Social Science Institute; 2015.

11

Integrative Approach to Child and Adolescent Mental Health

Seungpil Jung

Abstract

The prevalence of mental disorders between children and adolescents is 10–20% worldwide. Research has shown that most mental disorders begin at childhood and adolescence. Neurodevelopmental disorders are classified by which the development of the central nervous system is disturbed and are associated with varying degrees of consequences in one's mental, emotional, physical, and economic states. Recently, research in mental health, neurobiology, and early childhood development supported the case for early intervention and prevention. The causes of mental disorders in children and adolescents are not currently known, but research suggests that a combination of factors that include heredity, biology, psychological trauma, spiritual well-being, and environmental stress might be involved. There are many factors that play into child and adolescent mental health and disorders; therefore, individualized, personalized, and integrative approaches are necessary in therapeutic interventions and prevention. Thus, by ensuring that the needed mental health care competencies are made available in each primary health care team and by assuring fully integrated mental health and other types of health care, primary health care teams would best provide early, efficient, effective, and optimal recovery-based care.

Keywords: child and adolescent mental health, neurodevelopmental disorder, integrative mental health

1. Introduction: growth and development of the brain

The nervous system is derived from the ectoderm—the outermost tissue layer—of the embryo. The neuroectoderm appears in the third week of fetal development and forms the neural plate that is the source of the majority of neurons and glial cells in the mature human [1]. This is called the neural tube which later gives rise to the brain, the spinal cord, and the telencephalon, which eventually encompasses the two lateral ventricles, which in turn develops into the areas of the brain known as the basal ganglia and the limbic system [2]. Over time, cells cease division and begin to differentiate into neurons and glial cells, creating the main cellular components of the brain. The newly created neurons migrate to various parts of the brain to differentiate into the different brain structures. The fetal brain develops from neurons moving outward from early precursor cells [3]. After the neurons migrate, they grow extensive dendrites (a neuron's input) and axons (a neuron's output), components that allow communication with other neurons via synapses. Synaptic "discussions" lead to the establishment of functional neural circuits that mediate sensory and motor processing, as well as underlying behavior. This establishment is crucial, as the human brain develops the most in the first 20 years of one's life, and development is driven mostly by genetics and environmental factors (GxE hypothesis). At birth, the infant has many more neurons and synapses than it will use as an adult [4]. The strong bond and attachment of infants to their parents are crucial at a young age since their physical and social environments aid to strengthen the neurons that are used repeatedly. As the infant continues to develop, those neurons that keep up active "discussions" develop to perform better and efficiently. Several clinical and animal studies have shown that providing a child in developmental stages an enriched physical or social environment can significantly improve learning and memory, encourage exploration, and decrease fearful responses to new and unfamiliar experiences [5–10]. It can also reduce the impact of genetic or environmental risk matters. Despite these experimental and clinical researches, it is hard to know the relationship between the particular mechanisms of brain development and mental activities. Psyche is a function of the brain, and psychic phenomena and disorders may have neurobiological correlation. According to a longitudinal study, children as young as 18 months may suffer from mental illness as older children do. Risk factors and predictors of mental illness could be identified in the first 10 months of life, and the association of risks found in studies of older children seems to operate already from birth [11]. Even though there is plenty of research, it would be necessary to have further evidence between mental illness and risk factors of children at a young age.

2. Causes of neurodevelopmental disorders

Ten to twenty percent of children and adolescents experience mental disorders worldwide [12]. Research has shown that most mental disorders begin at childhood and adolescence [13, 14]. Neurodevelopmental disorders are classified by which the development of the central nervous system is disturbed and are associated with varying degrees of consequences in one's mental, emotional, physical, and economic states. Developmental brain dysfunction, which can manifest as neuropsychiatric problems or impaired motor function, learning, language, or non-verbal communication are also characterized by abnormal behavioral or cognitive phenotypes originating either *in utero* or during early postnatal life. The causes of mental disorders in children and adolescents are not currently known, but research suggests that a combination of factors that include heredity, biology, psychological trauma, and environmental stress might be involved [15].

A large cohort study of neurodevelopmental disorders showed a direct association of the severity of the physical condition with most classes of mental disorders. It also showed a strong overlap between physical and mental conditions and their impact on the severity of functional impairment in youth [16]. Specific patterns of comorbidity have important implications for the etiology. Prospective tracking of cross-disorder morbidity will be important to establishing more effective mechanisms for the prevention and intervention of mental disorders [16]. Genomic technology has shown great advances in gathering evidence that the current paradigm of psychiatric research needs to be updated. These studies provided converging evidence across a number of different levels, supporting the hypothesis that genetic risk factors are shared between disorders and challenging the validity of the classification systems currently used in research and clinical practice [17]. Through genomic technology, the growing list of genes that contribute to early onset developmental disorders is in its hundreds. That increasing number is further complicated by the observation that each patient can carry a unique combination of alleles of varying degree of effect that occurs *de novo* or inherited [18]. In the last 10 years, tremendous progress has been made in our comprehension of early onset developmental disorders [19–26]. To date, five main pathways have been identified as candidates for early onset neurodevelopmental disorders: chromatin remodeling, cytoskeleton dynamics, mRNA translation, metabolism, and synapse formation and function [17]. Understanding the symptoms and course of action for each individual, as well as the biology ranging from genetic and environmental risk factors to the neural circuits involved, remains a substantial challenge for geneticists and neurobiologists [27–29]. Many mechanisms of human brain development remain hidden, but neuroscientists are beginning to uncover some of these complex steps through extensive studies [30–32]. Research finds that neurons migrate from their birthplace near the ventricular walls to their final destination in the brain. As they collect together, they form each of the various brain structures and acquire specific ways of transmitting nerve messages. The result is the creation of a precise and elaborate adult network of 100 billion neurons capable of directing a movement in the body, a perception, an emotion, or other brain functions. Both genetic factors and activity-dependent factors play a role in developing the brain's architecture and circuitry.

3. Shifting paradigm in child and adolescent health

In 2000, scientific and clinical research groups were formed to create an agenda for the fifth major revision of the *Diagnostic and Statistical Manual of Mental Disorders* (*DSM-5*) [33]. These groups generated hundreds of white papers, monographs, and journal articles that provided the psychiatric field with a summary of the state of the science relevant to psychiatric diagnosis and faults within the current research in order to fortify knowledge in those fields. In 2005, the *DSM-5* Task Force was commissioned by the American Psychiatric Association (APA) to start revisions from the 1994 published *DSM-4*. The Task Force was also aided by 13 different work groups tasked with focusing on various disorder areas. Despite the great advances in neuroscience and genetic research during the last 20 years, there are still too few reliable genetic or other biomarkers that can reliably guide the diagnosis of psychiatric disorders. The diagnostic criteria in the *DSM-5* is a concept of neurodevelopmental disorders, such as intellectual disability, communication disorders, autism spectrum disorders, attention-deficit/hyperactivity disorder, specific learning disorders, and motor disorders. As a diagnostic tool, the *DSM* considers different disorders as distinct entities. However, from the diagnostic perspective, such disorders do not classify neatly within their boundaries as the DSM would want it. As an alternative tool for diagnosis and research into psychiatric disorders, the U.S. National Institute of Mental Health (NIMH) introduced the Research Domain Criteria (RDoC) project. This new project strives to create an experimental classification system that can provide a first step toward precision medicine for mental disorders [34]. The RDoC stems from the Research Diagnostic Criteria (RDC), created in the 1970s in response to the problems in diagnosis that the field of psychiatry experienced as it emerged from the shadow psychological domination [35]. In the RDoC, five main "domains"—Negative Valence Systems, Positive Valence Systems, Cognitive Systems, Systems for Social Processes, Arousal/Regulatory Systems—reflect a brain system in which functioning is impaired, to different degrees, in difference psychiatric conditions [36, 37].

The RDoC framework strives to free researchers and investigators from the rigid classification system of the DSM and pursue research questions in psychopathology that take advantage of burgeoning knowledge of complex behaviors and how these relate to specific aspects of brain activity [38]. It provides a set of guidelines for evaluating the strength of hypotheses relating clinical symptoms or impairments to dimensions of behavioral functioning and neural systems. The future of the RDoC is undetermined but will depend on how well the diagnostic system can direct clinicians to concise and effective treatment or prevention strategies for each individual patient [38]. The RDoC approach to clinical research of child and adolescent psychopathology contributes to the understanding of development as an aspect of the heterogeneity within DSM disorders and commonalities across seemingly disparate disorders. Incorporating the RDoC as a diagnostic tool in this area of clinical research promises to be fruitful avenue of research into the root causes and manifestations of mental illness, eventually leading to more precise and patient-specific treatments [39].

4. Early life programming as target for prevention of child and adolescent

Behavioral and emotional mental disorders with a high prevalence frequently commence in childhood or adolescence. With some respect, the fetal origins of adult disease models explain the associations between undernutrition of the fetus and an increased risk of cardiovascular disease, diabetes, and metabolic syndrome in later life [40]. This model has been expanded to include events beginning prior to conception as well as early postnatal life [41]. Three main classes of prenatal exposure were investigated in the late 1990s for a range of general health outcomes: lifestyle factors, maternal mental health, which covers antenatal stress, anxiety, and depression, and teratogenic and neurotoxic exposures to specific toxins found in substance abuse, environmental toxins, and prescription medication [42]. Recent human epidemiological and animal studies indicate that stressful experiences *in utero* or during early life may increase the risk of neurological and psychiatric disorders, arguably via altered epigenetic regulation. Altered epigenetic regulation may potentially influence fetal endocrine programming and brain development across several generations, resulting in the added attention paid to possible transgenerational effects of stress. Based on existing evidence, it would be possible that prenatal stress, as an epigenetic factor, may become one of the most powerful influences on mental health in later life [43]. Epidemiological studies suggested that gestational exposures to environmental factors such as stress are strongly associated with an increased incidence of neurodevelopmental disorders, including attention-deficit hyperactivity disorder (ADHD), schizophrenia, autism spectrum disorders (ASD), and depression [44–47]. There is growing evidence from human studies showing that early exposures to lifestyle factors and maternal mental health are predictive of child behavioral, emotional, and learning outcomes. Already a number of successful programs have been developed, such as nurse visitation in the perinatal period [48]. Recent emerging evidence shows that current interventions aiming to prevent postnatal depression in women are beneficial and effective not only for women with depression but also for those suffering from anxiety and high stress disorders [49–51].

Fetal programming refers to the way in which environmental events alter the course of fetal development, resulting in lasting modifications in the structure and function of biological systems. Programming refers to the influence of a specific environmental factor at a specific point in development. There are exposures during pregnancy such as maternal mental health, lifestyle factors, and potential teratogenic and neurotoxic exposures on child outcomes. Outcomes of interest are common child and adolescent mental disorders such as hyperactive, behavioral, and emotional disorders. The preconception and perinatal periods offer opportunities for the prevention of harmful fetal exposures. Therefore, it is imperative that during the perinatal period maternal mental health prevention efforts should be most strongly advocated and developed. Interventions developed with evidence-based advisement for the perinatal period could later be instituted into the public health system and grow toward universal and targeted interventions. In the course of time, such interventions are likely to have lifelong effects on mental and physical health [52].

5. The role of inflammation in child and adolescent mental health

Data from human and laboratory animals provide compelling evidence that stress-relevant neurocircuitry and immunity form an integrated system that evolved to protect organisms from a wide range of environmental threats [53]. In particular, the fetal inflammatory response to intrauterine infection seems to contribute to neonatal brain injury and subsequent neurological disability [54]. The preconception and perinatal periods are important because deleterious fetal exposures can be prevented during those periods. Therefore, future mental health prevention efforts must be focused on the critical period as well as prevention models should be developed focusing on the perinatal period. Interventions based on evidence-based recommendations for the perinatal period may occur as the form of public health, interventions that are universal and more targeted. If successful, such interventions can have enduring, lifelong effects on (mental) health. Extensive experimental studies are being conducted on the precise mechanisms of how latent or persistent inflammation negatively affects neurochemical and neurobiological abnormalities related to schizophrenia and/or autism. By further clarifying such mechanisms, novel immunomodulatory interventions that help prevent abnormal brain development and long-term mental illness suffered by people with prenatal infectious/inflammatory histories can be established [44].

The quality of the fetal environment can be compromised in several ways. Indirect stresses such as endocrine, metabolic, or immune responses of toxins like nicotine or alcohol produces vascular restrictions, thereby impeding oxygen and nutritional supply to the fetus. Direct transfer of maternal glucocorticoids or other agents across the placenta are the other stresses. These stresses include neuro-immune factors that are now being recognized as playing important roles in the etiology of neurological and neuropsychiatric disorders, including immunological processes that target the developing brain and prenatal mental infection. Recent data have elucidated the mechanisms by which the innate and adaptive immune systems interact with neurotransmitters and neuronal circuits to influence the risk for depression. Responses of stress mediated via activation of the inflammasome to secrete inflammatory cytokines, heightened serotonin metabolism, and reduced neurotransmitter availability together with hypothalamic-pituitary-adrenal axis hyperactivity. If this intricate neuro-immune communication network is dysregulated during pregnancy, the maternal milieu can be modified, which enhances the emergence of depressive symptoms, as well as negative obstetric and neuropsychiatric outcomes [55].

There are multiple pathways through which inflammatory cytokines can lead to reduced synaptic availability of the monoamines, which can be believed to be a fundamental mechanism in the pathophysiology of depression. Brain regions that regulate motor and motivation activity (promoting social avoidance and energy conservation) in addition to arousal, alarm, and anxiety (promoting hypervigilance and protection against attack) are involved in the primary cytokine targets in the CNS. Dopamine is fundamental to motivation and motor activity, and cytokines have been found to decrease the dopamine release in the basal ganglia together with decreased effort-based motivation and reduced activation of reward circuitry in the basal ganglia, specifically the ventral striatum [56–59]. Pathogen infection and food antigen penetration across gastro-intestinal barriers are means by which environmental factors might affect immune-related neurodevelopment [60]. The proteins gluten and casein are hydrolyzed in the GI tract into peptides, some of which have been shown to have opioid-like properties and are referred to as exorphins [61, 62]. The immunomodulatory potential of these exorphins is not well-understood, with observations that among the repertoire of digested peptides, some have pro-inflammatory and others have anti-inflammatory effects [63]. A study suggested that a strictly supervised and restricted elimination diet can improve the symptom scores of children with ADHD [64], but up to now, there is neither evidence for food-associated mental diseases nor recommendation for dietary therapies besides the experimental stage. A longitudinal study proposed an association between allergic disorder in early childhood and the development of ADHD in later life [65]. Polymorphisms in the C-reactive protein (CRP) gene were associate both with increased peripheral blood concentrations of CRP and symptoms of post-traumatic stress disorder, especially increased arousal for individuals exposed to civilian trauma [66].

Currently, it is discussed whether this association is an epiphenomenon or a consequela of the inner-psychic events. The role of hormonal signals operating in pregnancy or early postnatal interactions that is able to alter the sensitivity of certain target tissues, often via altered expression of hormone receptors, to these same hormones in later development [67]. There is also an increasing recognition of mechanisms of resilience that, ranging from effector T cells producing IL-4 to $T\text{-}_{Reg}$ cells with anti-inflammatory properties, there is a variety of T cell responses and their neuroprotective effects. For the development of new anti-depressant therapies, a better understanding of such neuroprotective pathways and of the inflammatory mechanisms, ranging from inflammasome activation to cell trafficking to the brain, would be important [68].

6. Integrative approaches to improve child and adolescent mental health

Human beings, in health and disease, are complex systems of dynamically interacting biological, psychological, social, energetic, intellectual, and spiritual processes. There are many factors that play into child and adolescent mental health and disorders; therefore, individualized, personalized, and integrative approaches are necessary in therapeutic interventions and prevention. Complex, interrelated causes, and consequences are understood to be parts of adolescent mortality, sexually transmitted disease, pregnancy, substance abuse, and depression. Therefore, categorical programs targeting only single type of problem behavior and seeking simple solutions are not adequate [69]. Prospective follow-up studies on youth have shown that child and adolescent mental disorders are related to a wide array of adverse outcomes [70]. Recent epidemiological studies have shown that about one fourth of youth experience a mental disorder in the previous year, and approximately one third across their lifetimes. For children, anxiety disorders were most frequent, followed by behavior disorders, mood disorders, and substance use disorders in that order. The difference in rates across the world can be explained by both methodologic factors and true cultural differences in childhood disorders and their magnitude [71]. Recently, research in mental health, neurobiology, and early childhood development supported the case for early intervention and prevention. For instance, according to epidemiologic surveys, some mental health disorders had an early age of onset while an association between increased risk of mental health disorders as an adult and early symptoms was found in other studies [72]. Another research emphasized recognizing the importance of early developmental screening and interventions, in addition to issuing related anticipatory guidance for pediatricians [73]. The other research also increased the understanding of how cognitive and emotional developments in older children and adolescents were related. Newly found evidence on age of onset, risk factors, and effective prevention strongly suggest that early identification and intervention in the primary care environment is important. The range of primary care practice includes a wide variety of activities, such as promoting well-being, preventing illness, and diagnosing and treating illness. A practice to meet children's mental health needs must have a similarly wide scope of activities. This comprehensive approach should consider the full scope and intensity of social, emotional, and behavioral problems influencing children and adolescent. Such an approach needs strategies targeted to different levels of need and coordinated between the systems serving children. Three levels of intervention exist in mental health—namely, prevention and health promotion, early intervention, and treatment, and using validated and standardized tools for screening and assessment used to identify and treat emotional and behavioral problems earlier.

The way people receive health care is being transformed by the technology in new and exciting ways. Electronic and mobile devices for mental health are available for various conditions, but implementation into clinical practice is low [74]. Also, there is no evidence that using novel media is promoting mental health, but new diagnostic entities have been introduced in the DSM-5, such as Internet addiction. Also, service providers can deliver cost-effective and innovative care to geographically distant areas. Still issues have to be solved with regard to data integrity and security [75].

E-mental health care is defined as mental health services through the Internet and related technologies [76]. E-health is a broader concept which has an information and communication technology (ICT) to connect patients and physicians in real time [77]. According to systematic reviews of the computerized treatments of common mental health problems (therapist-assisted and self-directed), E-mental health treatments were shown to be more effective than zero treatment and equally effective as face-to-face treatment [78]. A clinical study has shown that the effect of computerized interventions for children and adolescents with depression and anxiety [79].

E-therapy is an emerging and fast developing field of research and practice that involves the application of digital technologies to assist or deliver psychotherapy. Currently, a vast majority of E-therapy programs have been developed for adults. It is imperative to find a more suitable and user-friendly method to treat children and adolescents. E-therapy programs for children and adolescents need to take in to account developmental considerations. Also, evidence-based research and further discussion would be needed to determine the optimal forms of delivery and efficiency of E-therapies in clinical environment.

Virtual reality (VR) involves a computer-generated simulation of a three-dimensional image or environment. The use of a VR platform offers an effective treatment option for improving social impairments commonly found in autism spectrum disorder [80]. VR appears to be a promising and motivating platform to safely practice and rehearse social skills for children with ASD. New virtual reality games dealing with motor coordination were tested with children having developmental coordination disorder [81]. The findings will offer essential information on whether such electronic games would have a positive impact on the children's physical and mental health [81]. Mental disorders and substantive mental health problems in children and adolescents are complex phenomena with regard to the pathoetiology, social, and clinical expressions and in the interventions that can ameliorate, modify, or prevent onset, effects, or negative outcomes [82]. On the other hand, it needs to be investigated which interventions are effective, separating these from the ones without effect or adverse effects. To meet the mental health care needs of young people and their families, convergence, not isolation, of professional identities is required. This change is affected by advances in scientific knowledge and clinical therapeutics, as well as changes in social forces and importance of convergence. Thus, by ensuring that the needed mental health care competencies are made available in each primary health care team and by assuring fully integrated mental health and other types of health care, primary health care teams would best provide early, efficient, effective, and optimal recovery-based care [83].

Author details

Seungpil Jung

Address all correspondence to: spjung@yu.ac.kr

Department of Family Medicine, Yeungnam University, College of Medicine, South Korea

References

[1] Saladin KS. *Anatomy & physiology: the unity of form and function*. 6th ed. New York: McGraw-Hill; 2011. p. 514.

[2] Carlson NR. *Physiology of behavior*. 11th ed. Boston: Pearson; 2013. p. 76.

[3] Walsh CA, Morrow EM, Rubenstein JL. Autism and brain development. *Cell*. 2008;135:396-400. doi: 10.1016/j.cell.2008.10.015.

[4] Kalia M. Brain development: anatomy, connectivity, adaptive plasticity, and toxicity. *Metabolism*. 2008;57(Suppl 2):S2-S5. doi: 10.1016/j.metabol.2008.07.009.

[5] Blair C, Razza RP. Relating effortful control, executive function, and false belief understanding to emerging math and literacy ability in kindergarten. *Child Dev*. 2007;78:647-663. DOI: 10.1111/j.1467-8624.2007.01019.x.

[6] Fox SE, Levitt P, Nelson CA 3rd. How the timing and quality of early experiences influence the development of brain architecture. *Child Dev*. 2010;81:28-40. doi: 10.1111/j.1467-8624.2009.01380.

[7] Eisenberg N, Vidmar M, Spinrad TL, Eggum ND, Edwards A, Gaertner B, et al. Mothers' teaching strategies and children's effortful control: a longitudinal study. *Dev Psychol*. 2010;46:1294-1308. doi: 10.1037/a0020236.

[8] Paus T. How environment and genes shape the adolescent brain. *Horm Behav*. 2013;64:195-202. doi: 10.1016/j.yhbeh.2013.04.004.

[9] Postma IR, Groen H, Easterling TR, Tsigas EZ, Wilson ML, Porcel J, et al. The brain study: cognition, quality of life and social functioning following preeclampsia; an observational study. *Pregnancy Hypertens*. 2013;3:227-234. doi: 10.1016/j.preghy.2013.06.003.

[10] Schlotz W, Godfrey KM, Phillips DI. Prenatal origins of temperament: fetal growth, brain structure, and inhibitory control in adolescence. *PLoS One*. 2014;9(5):e96715. doi: 10.1371/journal.pone.0096715.

[11] Skovgaard AM. Mental health problems and psychopathology in infancy and early childhood. An epidemiological study. *Dan Med Bull*. 2010;57(10):B4193.

[12] Kieling C, Baker-Henningham H, Belfer M, Conti G, Ertem I, Omigbodun O, et al. Child and adolescent mental health worldwide: evidence for action. *Lancet*. 2011;378(9801):1515-1525. doi: 10.1016/S0140-6736(11)60827-1.

[13] National Institute of Mental Health. *Any disorder* [Internet]. Bethesda: NIMH; [2010] [cited 2016 Aug 15]. Available from: https://www.nimh.nih.gov/health/statistics/prevalence/file_148474.pdf.

[14] Kessler RC, Amminger GP, Aguilar-Gaxiola S, Alonso J, Lee S, Ustün TB. Age of onset of mental disorders: a review of recent literature. *Curr Opin Psychiatry*. 2007;20:359-364. doi:10.1097/YCO.0b013e32816ebc8c.

[15] Norman RE, Byambaa M, De R, Butchart A, Scott J, Vos T. The long-term health consequences of child physical abuse, emotional abuse, and neglect: a systematic review and meta-analysis. *PLoS Med*. 2012;9(11):e1001349.

[16] Merikangas KR, Calkins ME, Burstein M, He JP, Chiavacci R, Lateef T, et al. Comorbidity of physical and mental disorders in the neurodevelopmental genomics cohort study. *Pediatrics*. 2015;135:e927-e938. doi: 10.1542/peds.2014-1444.

[17] Doherty JL, Owen MJ. Genomic insights into the overlap between psychiatric disorders: implications for research and clinical practice. *Genome Med*. 2014;6:29. doi: 10.1186/gm546.

[18] Bourgeron T. The genetics and neurobiology of ESSENCE: the third Birgit Olsson lecture. *Nord J Psychiatry*. 2016;70:1-9. doi: 10.3109/08039488.2015.1042519.

[19] Peça J, Feliciano C, Ting JT, Wang W, Wells MF, Venkatraman TN, et al. Shank3 mutant mice display autistic-like behaviours and striatal dysfunction. *Nature*. 2011;472(7344):437-442. doi: 10.1038/nature09965.

[20] Won H, Lee HR, Gee HY, Mah W, Kim JI, Lee J, et al. Autistic-like social behaviour in Shank2-mutant mice improved by restoring NMDA receptor function. *Nature*. 2012;486(7402):261-265. doi: 10.1038/nature11208.

[21] Schmeisser MJ, Ey E, Wegener S, Bockmann J, Stempel AV, Kuebler A, et al. Autistic-like behaviours and hyperactivity in mice lacking ProSAP1/Shank2. *Nature*. 2012;486(7402):256-260. doi: 10.1038/nature11015.

[22] Tabuchi K, Blundell J, Etherton MR, Hammer RE, Liu X, Powell CM, et al. A neuroligin-3 mutation implicated in autism increases inhibitory synaptic transmission in mice. *Science*. 2007;318(5847):71-76. doi:10.1126/science.1146221.

[23] Jamain S, Radyushkin K, Hammerschmidt K, Granon S, Boretius S, Varoqueaux F, et al. Reduced social interaction and ultrasonic communication in a mouse model of monogenic heritable autism. *Proc Natl Acad Sci U S A*. 2008;105:1710-1715. doi: 10.1073/pnas.0711555105.

[24] Varoqueaux F, Aramuni G, Rawson RL, Mohrmann R, Missler M, Gottmann K, et al. Neuroligins determine synapse maturation and function. *Neuron*. 2006;51:741-754. doi:10.1016/j.neuron.2006.09.003.

[25] Baudouin SJ, Gaudias J, Gerharz S, Hatstatt L, Zhou K, Punnakkal P, et al. Shared synapticpathophysiology in syndromic and nonsyndromic rodent models of autism. *Science* 2012;338(6103):128-132. doi: 10.1126/science.1224159.

[26] Boissart C, Poulet A, Georges P, Darville H, Julita E, Delorme R, et al. Differentiation from human pluripotent stem cells of cortical neurons of the superficial layers amenable to psychiatric disease modeling and high-throughput drug screening. *Transl Psychiatry*. 2013;3:e294. doi: 10.1038/tp.2013.71.

[27] Willsey AJ, Sanders SJ, Li M, Dong S, Tebbenkamp AT, Muhle RA, et al. Coexpression networks implicate human midfetal deep cortical projection neurons in the pathogenesis of autism. *Cell*. 2013;155:997-1007. doi: 10.1016/j.cell.2013.10.020.

[28] Parikshak NN, Luo R, Zhang A, Won H, Lowe JK, Chandran V, et al. Integrative functional genomic analyses implicate specific molecular pathways and circuits in autism. *Cell*. 2013;155:1008-1021. doi: 10.1016/j.cell.2013.10.031.

[29] Gokhale A, Larimore J, Werner E, So L, Moreno-De-Luca A, Lese-Martin C, et al. Quantitative proteomic and genetic analyses of the schizophrenia susceptibility factor dysbindin identify novel roles of the biogenesis of lysosome-related organelles complex 1. *J Neurosci*. 2012;32(11):3697-3711. 10.1523/JNEUROSCI.5640-11.2012.

[30] Isshiki M, Tanaka S, Kuriu T, Tabuchi K, Takumi T, Okabe S. Enhanced synapse remodelling as a common phenotype in mouse models of autism. *Nat Commun*. 2014;5:4742. doi: 10.1038/ncomms5742.

[31] Hou ST, Jiang SX, Smith RA. Permissive and repulsive cues and signaling pathways of axonal outgrowth and regeneration. *Int Rev Cell Mol Biol*. 2008;267:125-181. doi: 10.1016/S1937-6448(08)00603-5.

[32] Swayne LA, Bennett SA. Connexins and pannexins in neuronal development and adult neurogenesis. *BMC Cell Biol*. 2016;17(Suppl 1):10. doi: 10.1186/s12860-016-0089-5.

[33] American Psychiatric Association. *Diagnostic and statistical manual of mental disorders: DSM-5*. 5th ed. Washington, DC: American Psychiatric Association; 2013.

[34] Bruce NC. Research domain criteria: toward future psychiatric nosologies. *Dialogues Clin Neurosci*. 2015;17(1):89-97.

[35] Spitzer RL, Endicott J, Robins E. Research diagnostic criteria: rationale and reliability. *Arch Gen Psychiatry*. 1978;35:773-782. doi:10.1001/archpsyc.1978.01770300115013.

[36] Casey BJ, Craddock N, Cuthbert BN, Hyman SE, Lee FS, Ressler KJ. DSM-5 and RDoC: progress in psychiatry research?. *Nat Rev Neurosci*. 2013;14:810-814. doi: 10.1038/nrn3621.

[37] National Institute of Mental Health. *Development and definitions of the RDoC domains and constructs* [Internet]. Bethesda: NIMH; [2016] [cited 2016 Aug 15]. Available from: https://www.nimh.nih.gov/research-priorities/rdoc/development-and-definitions-of-the-rdoc-domains-and-constructs.shtml.

[38] Cuthbert BN. Research domain criteria: toward future psychiatric nosologies. *Dialogues Clin Neurosci*. 2015;17:89-97.

[39] Garvey M, Avenevoli S, Anderson K. The national institute of mental health research domain criteria and clinical research in child and adolescent psychiatry. *J Am Acad Child Adolesc Psychiatry*. 2016;55:93-98. doi: 10.1016/j.jaac.2015.11.002.

[40] Barker DJ. The wellcome foundation lecture, 1994. The fetal origins of adult disease. *Proc Biol Sci.* 1995;262(1363):37-43. doi:10.1098/rspb.1995.0173.

[41] Gluckman PD, Hanson MA. The developmental origins of health and disease: the breadth and importance of the concept. In: Marelyn Wintour E, Owens JA, editors. *Early life origins of health and disease.* New York: Springer Science+Business Media; 2006. pp. 1-7.

[42] Nathanielsz PW. *Life in the womb: the origin of health and disease.* Ithaca, N.Y.: Promethean Press; 1999.

[43] Babenko O, Kovalchuk I, Metz GA. Stress-induced perinatal and transgenerational epigenetic programming of brain development and mental health. *Neurosci Biobehav Rev.* 2015;48:70-91. doi: 10.1016/j.neubiorev.2014.11.013.

[44] Meyer U, Feldon J, Dammann O. Schizophrenia and autism: both shared and disorder-specific pathogenesis via perinatal inflammation?. *Pediatr Res.* 2011;69(5 Pt 2):26R-33R. doi: 10.1203/PDR.0b013e318212c196.

[45] Howerton CL, Bale TL. Prenatal programing: at the intersection of maternal stress and immune activation. *Horm Behav.* 2012;62:237-242. doi: 10.1016/j.yhbeh.2012.03.007.

[46] Bale TL, Baram TZ, Brown AS, Goldstein JM, Insel TR, McCarthy MM, et al. Early life programming and neurodevelopmental disorders. *Biol Psychiatry.* 2010;68:314-319. doi:10.1016/j.biopsych.2010.05.028.

[47] Brown AS. Epidemiologic studies of exposure to prenatal infection and risk of schizophrenia and autism. *Dev Neurobiol.* 2012;72:1272-1276. doi: 10.1002/dneu.22024.

[48] Olds DL, Sadler L, Kitzman H. Programs for parents of infants and toddlers: recent evidence from randomized trials. *J Child Psychol Psychiatry.* 2007;48:355-391. DOI: 10.1111/j.1469-7610.2006.01702.x

[49] Dennis CL. Psychosocial and psychological interventions for prevention of postnatal depression: systematic review. *BMJ.* 2005;331(7507):15. doi:10.1136/bmj.331.7507.15.

[50] Fisher JR, Wynter KH, Rowe HJ. Innovative psycho-educational program to prevent common postpartum mental disorders in primiparous women: a before and after controlled study. *BMC Public Health.* 2010;10:432. doi: 10.1186/1471-2458-10-432.

[51] Lumley J, Austin MP, Mitchell C. Intervening to reduce depression after birth: a systematic review of the randomized trials. *Int J Technol Assess Health Care.* 2004;20:128-144.

[52] Lewis AJ, Galbally M, Gannon T, Symeonides C. Early life programming as a target for prevention of child and adolescent mental disorders. *BMC Med.* 2014;12:33. doi: 10.1186/1741-7015-12-33.

[53] Pace TW, Mletzko TC, Alagbe O, Musselman DL, Nemeroff CB, Miller AH, et al. Increased stress-induced inflammatory responses in male patients with major depression and increased early life stress. *Am J Psychiatry.* 2006;163:1630-1633. DOI:10.1176/ajp.2006.163.9.1630.

[54] Leviton A, Allred EN, Kuban KC, Hecht JL, Onderdonk AB, O'shea TM, et al. Microbiologic and histologic characteristics of the extremely preterm infant's placenta predict white matter damage and later cerebral palsy. The ELGAN study. *Pediatr Res.* 2010;67:95-101. doi: 10.1203/PDR.0b013e3181bf5fab.

[55] Leff-Gelman P, Mancilla-Herrera I, Flores-Ramos M, Cruz-Fuentes C, Reyes-Grajeda JP, García-Cuétara Mdel P, et al. The immune system and the role of inflammation in perinatal depression. *Neurosci Bull.* 2016;32:398-420. doi: 10.1007/s12264-016-0048-3.

[56] Schatzberg AF, Nemeroff CB. The American Psychiatric Publishing textbook of psychopharmacology. 4th ed. Washington, DC: American Psychiatric Publishing; 2009. pp. 903-944.

[57] Capuron L, Pagnoni G, Drake DF, Woolwine BJ, Spivey JR, Crowe RJ, et al. Dopaminergic mechanisms of reduced basal ganglia responses to hedonic reward during interferon alfa administration. *Arch Gen Psychiatry.* 2012;69:1044-1053. doi: 10.1001/archgenpsychiatry.2011.2094.

[58] Eisenberger NI, Berkman ET, Inagaki TK, Rameson LT, Mashal NM, Irwin MR. Inflammation-induced anhedonia: endotoxin reduces ventral striatum responses to reward. *Biol Psychiatry.* 2010;68:748-754. doi: 10.1016/j.biopsych.2010.06.010.

[59] Felger JC, Mun J, Kimmel HL, Nye JA, Drake DF, Hernandez CR, et al. Chronic interferon-α decreases dopamine 2 receptor binding and striatal dopamine release in association with anhedonia-like behavior in nonhuman primates. *Neuropsychopharmacology.* 2013;38(11):2179-2187. doi: 10.1038/npp.2013.115.

[60] Severance EG, Alaedini A, Yang S, Halling M, Gressitt KL, Stallings CR, et al. Gastrointestinal inflammation and associated immune activation in schizophrenia. *Schizophr Res.* 2012;138:48-53. doi: 10.1016/j.schres.2012.02.025.

[61] Lachance LR, McKenzie K. Biomarkers of gluten sensitivity in patients with non-affective psychosis: a meta-analysis. *Schizophr Res.* 2014;152:521-527. doi: 10.1016/j.schres.2013.12.001.

[62] Reichelt KL, Hole K, Hamberger A, Saelid G, Edminson PD, Braestrup CB, et al. Biologically active peptide-containing fractions in schizophrenia and childhood autism. *Adv Biochem Psychopharmacol.* 1981;28:627-643.

[63] Kamiński S, Cieslińska A, Kostyra E. Polymorphism of bovine beta-casein and its potential effect on human health. *J Appl Genet.* 2007;48:189-198. doi:10.1007/BF03195213.

[64] Pelsser LM, Frankena K, Toorman J, Savelkoul HF, Dubois AE, Pereira RR, et al. Effects of a restricted elimination diet on the behaviour of children with attention-deficit hyperactivity disorder (INCA study): a randomised controlled trial. *Lancet.* 2011;377(9764):494-503. doi:10.1016/S0140-6736(10)62227-1.

[65] Chen MH, Su TP, Chen YS, Hsu JW, Huang KL, Chang WH, et al. Is atopy in early childhood a risk factor for ADHD and ASD? a longitudinal study. *J Psychosom Res.* 2014;77:316-321. doi: 10.1016/j.jpsychores.2014.06.006.

[66] Michopoulos V, Rothbaum AO, Jovanovic T, Almli LM, Bradley B, Rothbaum BO, et al. Association of CRP genetic variation and CRP level with elevated PTSD symptoms and physiological responses in a civilian population with high levels of trauma. *Am J Psychiatry*. 2015;172:353-362. doi: 10.1176/appi.ajp.2014.14020263.

[67] Meaney MJ, Szyf M, Seckl JR. Epigenetic mechanisms of perinatal programming of hypothalamic-pituitary-adrenal function and health. *Trends Mol Med*. 2007;13:269-277. doi: 10.1016/j.molmed.2007.05.003.

[68] Miller AH, Raison CL. The role of inflammation in depression: from evolutionary imperative to modern treatment target. *Nat Rev Immunol*. 2016;16:22-34. doi: 10.1038/nri.2015.5.

[69] Ooms T, Herendeen L. Integrated approaches to youths' health problems: federal, state and community roles. Wisconsin Family Impact Seminars. Madison: Policy Institute for Family Impact Seminars; 1989.

[70] Buka SL, Monuteaux M, Earls F. The epidemiology of child and adolescent mental disorders. In: Tsuang MT, Tohen M, editors. Textbook in psychiatric epidemiology. 2nd ed. New York, NY: John Wiley and Sons Inc; 2002. pp. 629-655.

[71] Merikangas KR, Nakamura EF, Kessler RC. Epidemiology of mental disorders in children and adolescents. *Dialogues Clin Neurosci*. 2009;11:7-20.

[72] O'Connell ME, Boat TF, Warner KE. *Preventing mental, emotional, and behavioral disorders among young people: progress and possibilities*. Washington, DC: National Academies Press; 2009.

[73] Shonkoff JP, Phillips DA. *From neurons to neighborhoods: the science of early childhood development*. Washington, DC: National Academy Press; 2000.

[74] Whitfield G, Williams C. If the evidence is so good–why doesn't anyone use them? A national survey of the use of computerized cognitive behaviour therapy. *Behav Cogn Psychother*. 2004;32(1):57-65. doi: 10.1017/S1352465804001031.

[75] Kylie B, Anthony JB, Kathleen MG. Security considerations for E-mental health interventions. *J Med Internet Res*. 2010;12(5):e61. doi: 10.2196/jmir.1468.

[76] Lal S, Adair CE. E-mental health: a rapid review of the literature. *Psychiatr Serv*. 2014;65:24-32. doi: 10.1176/appi.ps.201300009.

[77] Sood S, Mbarika V, Jugoo S, Dookhy R, Doarn CR, Prakash N, et al. What is telemedicine? A collection of 104 peer-reviewed perspectives and theoretical underpinnings. *Telemed J E Health*. 2007;13:573-590.

[78] Ginsburg S, Foster S. *Strategies to support the integration of mental health into pediatric primary care* [Internet]. 2009 [cited 2016 Aug 15]:1-36. Available from: http://www.nihcm.org/pdf/PediatricMH-FINAL.pdf.

[79] Stasiak K, Fleming T, Lucassen MF, Shepherd MJ, Whittaker R, Merry SN. Computer-based and online therapy for depression and anxiety in children and adolescents. *J Child Adolesc Psychopharmacol*. 2016;26:235-245. doi: 10.1089/cap.2015.0029.

[80] Didehbani N, Allen T, Kandalaft M, Krawczyka D, Chapmana S. Virtual reality social cognition training for children with high functioning autism. *Comput Human Behav.* 2016;62:703-711. doi: http://dx.doi.org/10.1016/j.chb.2016.04.033.

[81] Straker LM, Campbell AC, Jensen LM, Metcalf DR, Smith AJ, Abbott RA, et al. Rationale, design and methods for a randomised and controlled trial of the impact of virtual reality games on motor competence, physical activity, and mental health in children with developmental coordination disorder. *BMC Public Health.* 2011;11:654. doi: 10.1186/1471-2458-11-654.

[82] Rutter M, Stevenson J. Developments in child and adolescent psychiatry over the last 50 years. In: Rutter M, Bishop D, Pine D, editors. *Rutter's child and adolescent psychiatry.* 5th ed. Malden, MA: Blackwell Publishing; 2008. pp. 3-17.

[83] Kutcher S, Davidson S, Manion I. Child and youth mental health: integrated health care using contemporary competency-based teams. *Paediatr Child Health.* 2009;14:315-318.

12

Internet Addiction Disorder

Pabasari Ginige

Abstract

Internet addiction (IA) was introduced as a new disorder in mid-1990s. Since then, there is growing concern about the addictive nature of the Internet. This chapter is a comprehensive review of published seminal, research and review papers, meta-analyses and book chapters/books on IA in adolescents. The conceptualization of IA, epidemiology, phenomenology, screening, diagnoses, treatment and prevention are discussed with relevant references. The concept of IA is at fetal level with no consensus on definition, norms or clinical criteria. Asian countries such as China and South Korea are affected most. A multination meta-analysis estimated an overall prevalence of 6% for IA. Most of the research identifies IA in gaming, gambling, social networking and cybersex. A few assessment tools have been used with no comparability or cultural sensitivity. Diagnostic criteria are proposed based on those used for substance abuse and pathological gambling. The treatments are mainly psychological with a lot of emphasis on cognitive behavior therapy. The Internet is a very versatile and useful tool for children and adolescents, and it is not advisable to ban it totally. The review highlights education of them on sensible Internet use and supports inclusion of IA in international disease classifications.

Keywords: Internet addiction, children and adolescents, epidemiology, management

1. Introduction

The Internet evolved from early 1980s to the modern day revolutionizing the broadcasting, information sharing and connecting individuals worldwide. Today, it has become an in-built part of daily lives of people including children and adolescents. The Internet can be used for many purposes: educational such as teaching, learning and research; business, such as monetary/document exchanges and conference meetings; recreational such as games, online gambling and watching sexually explicit material, and as a mode of connecting people via texting, calling, social websites, chat applications and e-mails. Research has found increasing number of students are using the Internet for their academic activities, for example, one US study showed an increase in the Internet use among students from 24.5% in 1996 to 79.5% in 2001 [1]. However, together with the many benefits come the risks that are inevitably intertwined due to the innate qualities of the Internet.

There is growing concern about the addictive quality of the Internet, and pioneering researchers have introduced the concept of addiction (IA) in mid-1990s [2, 3]. IA has attracted the attention of media and general public increasingly, with the speedy growth in computer use and the Internet access [4]. The Internet today has reached not only the computer, but also the mobile phone and even the wristwatch with many more sophisticated high-tech apparatus with the Internet facility being introduced to the world, incessantly. It is common to find children and adolescents coming from a reasonable socioeconomical background, around the globe, using a personal digital devise like a smart phone, tablet or a laptop with the Internet. It is important to look into how it is like to grow up with such a vast degree of stimulating and inviting attractions from the cyber world on the developing brain.

This chapter explores the conceptualization of IA as an evolving novel theme [3, 5], describes the types of Internet addiction disorders (IAD) and looks into available epidemiology and etiology. Then, a proposal of a neurobiological basis for IA in the developing brain is introduced based on the current knowledge on more established dependences of substances/behaviors such as gambling of the maturing brain. Identification of high-risk children and adolescents and association of IA with other psychiatric disorders such as depression are discussed next followed by an account of the symptoms and signs of varying clinical presentations of IA and diagnosis. Then a review of treatment modalities, proposed so far, and prognosis of and finally prevention strategies for this, most probably, a fastest growing addiction disorder of the world is discussed.

2. The concept of Internet addiction and its controversies

IA was introduced as a disorder by Young in her seminal paper "Internet Addiction: The emergence of a new clinical disorder" in 1996 [2]. She proposed diagnostic criteria for IA based on the existing Diagnostic and Statistical Manual of Mental Disorders 4th edition (DSM-4) criteria for substance dependence [6]. In 1999, David Greenfield too proposed IA to be a form of addictive disorder [7]. These researchers highlighted that the tolerance and withdrawal symptoms of Internet use and those of substance use have similar features. There are others who suggest that IA is an impulse control disorder or even an obsessive-compulsive disorder. But the symptom overlap with substance and known behavioral addictions supports the notion that IA is an addiction—a behavioral one—for that matter.

An increasing incidence of IA together with its high cooccurrence with other established psychiatric disorders was pointed out later [8]. The proposal to include "Internet addiction disorder" in the 5th edition of Diagnostic and Statistical Manual of Mental Disorders (DSM-5) was brought forward. DSM-5 acknowledged the growing concern about the Internet use and related problems, but they claimed there is "insufficient peer-reviewed evidence to establish the diagnostic criteria and course descriptions" to identify the behavior as a mental disorder.

However, DSM-5 has introduced the condition Internet gaming disorder with some proposed criteria under "Emerging Measures and Models" heading for future study. The DSM-5 work group has reviewed many articles about online gaming, and they found some behavioral similarities of Internet gaming to other addiction behaviors which are established as disorders, namely gambling disorder and substance use disorders. The proposed criteria for Internet gaming disorder focus on preoccupation and behaviors, which mainly consume most aspects of life, withdrawal, tolerance, lack of control of use and marked deterioration of the function. The criteria are mostly as proposed by early researches on Internet addiction disorder [2].

Lack of consensus on a definition for IA, which is even blurred subcategory of Internet use (i.e., gaming, social media, cybersex, etc.), makes it difficult to derive prevalence data. Also, there is little or no knowledge of natural histories of cases. Thus, limited scientific research from around the globe has hindered IA earning a place as a disorder in DSM-5 [6].

However, in parts of the world where Internet gaming has an apparent high prevalence, relevant governments such as Chinese have accepted Internet gaming as an established "addiction" and South Korea have identified IA as a problem at governmental level and declared it a serious public health hazard [8]. Such highly affected Asian countries have developed separate treatment units for Internet gaming addiction, in hospitals (e.g., China, Korea). There are an increasing number of researchers looking into the diagnosis of IA, and many researchers agree that the criteria to identify Internet addiction are like in any addiction with craving and compulsion to use despite the knowledge of the harm, loss of control in terms of initiation, continuation and conclusion of the use and withdrawal features such as mood symptoms and distress. In the case of children, however, the knowledge of harm may not be relevant due to the level of cognitive development. For example, a Taiwanese study has proposed diagnosis criteria for Internet addiction and when tested on a group of adolescents found them to be of high specificity and sensitivity [9]. The criteria of Ko et al. are more organized than what is introduced by Young in 1998 [10] with the former following the pattern of International Classification of Diseases 10th version (ICD 10) by World Health Organization (WHO) [11]. However, we need larger multicenter international collaborative studies to understand the prevalence, etiology and the course of IA before we adopt criteria proposed based on local studies as the validity and reliability of the diagnostic criteria have to be ensured. Mental healthcare professionals in many countries particularly in Asia and Europe are increasingly urging the authorities such as World Health Organization to identify IA as an independent disorder [12].

3. Controversies

The Internet is undoubtedly a very useful commodity. Can we consider liberal use of the Internet as an illness at all? Is it unwanted pathologization of changing times? A disadvantage of such a labeling could be the stigmatization of the Internet, which has many important and versatile uses. One may wonder whether there is any underlying pharmaceutical company agenda in pushing this as a diagnosis!

One controversial view is based on the argument that there is no "chemical substance" as such, to get addicted to. However, American Society of Addiction Medicine (ASAM) has defined addiction as a chronic brain disorder, which is not limited to substance use [13].

A strong argument against an independent disorder of IA is brought up by some researchers who believe existing and well-established disorders such as depression or social anxiety are the root causes of driving people to misuse the Internet [14, 15]. They argue that IA therefore is not a new disorder but a consequence of a more primary problem in mental health. Others (e.g., Some Forensic Psychiatrists) suggest that we should consider problematic Internet use, and the same way we consider the online gamblers as gamblers but not as Internet addicts [16].

More and more younger age groups are using the Internet with wider prevalence of the availability of the Internet. It is wondered how young is too young for children to go online. Some question the demarcation between passionate high involvement and problematic use or addiction [17]. Some experts in the field bring the argument whether we are pathologizing a common behavior [18, 19]. It is also relevant to keep in mind the discrepancies in cultural beliefs and attitudes toward the Internet use in different parts of the world. In southeast Asia, for example, parents appear to believe any behavior that takes time away from family or educational pursuits as abnormal [20]. This may partly explain the highly inflated prevalence rates of IA in countries such as Taiwan and South Korea [21].

4. Terminology in Internet addiction

Currently, some have settled into a less controversial term for the problem of IA, the "problematic Internet use" (PIU) [22, 23]. A large European Union-funded multicountry study used the terms Internet addictive behavior (IAB) for IA and dysfunctional Internet behavior (DIB) for problematic use of the Internet [24]. Compulsive Internet use (CIU) is another term used [25]. A more recent European study involving 11 countries has adopted the terms pathological Internet use (PtIU) and maladaptive Internet use (MIU) [26]. The salient features of addiction and problem use are more or less the same though the terminology used by different researchers is different. Addiction to the Internet basically implied a craving for the Internet use for uncontrollably long periods with impairment of functionality in the absence of any other disorders accounting for the condition and problem use was when one not meeting addictive features but nevertheless there are problems in bio psychosocial aspects in life. This chapter uses the terms IA and problem use for simplicity and clarity.

5. Types of Internet addiction disorders

One very common online activity among adolescents is recognized as online gaming. Many attractive single- and multiplayer games are being marketed among the youth worldwide. (e.g., World of Warcraft Clash of Clans, Slither.io, Clash Royale, Pokemon). Virtual communities created by some of the games could be more appealing for an adolescent than the real communities; the gamer can become an avatar of anybody he or she wishes; some games are designed in such a way gamers can buy cars and mansions and have a virtual second life. People spend/invest a whole lot in the second life at the cost of a deteriorating real life. Author, going by her clinical experience, wonders whether the adolescents with low self-esteem who are not recognized in real life might gain a lot of recognition from other fellow gamers in the online community as great warriors. However, this hypothesis needs to be explored through proper research. A US study has found Internet gaming to be associated with alcohol and recreational drug abuse and poor interpersonal relationships with no gender differences [27]. Research has found online gaming addiction to be associated with aggression, low sociability and self-efficacy, and a lower satisfaction with life [24]. The gamers with these risk factors engage in intense use and are of all age groups. It should be interesting to see the nature of these associations, whether these negative characteristics in the adolescents lead to IA or IA results in these traits. Such knowledge can provide us with interventions in terms of prevention of IA. No clear answer is evident from available data at present.

Another type of internet use, which is popular among adolescents, is social networking using applications such as viber, whatsapp, instagram, facebook, twitter, my space etc. and chat rooms/e-mail. A child or an adolescent will be very much overwhelmed by the amount of online connections he or she can have through these connecting apps. Notifications popping up will invariably distract the youth from homework or any other academic activity. Being connected with around the world friends 24 × 7 could be an around the clock distraction and disturbance. Author recalls one of her patients, a 16-year-old schoolgirl who receives 14,000+ text messages via Viber per day. Her life revolved around receiving and sending texts to her boyfriend and friends and would become aggressive toward family and property when the parents attempted to limit the Internet time. Another grave risk involved in social media sites is children and adolescents getting exposed to unknown adults who may abuse the "online friendship" and bring harm on the young.

Cybersex is also an attractive type of Internet activity among adolescents. Premature exposure to various aspects of sexuality and exposure to adverse sexual activity may hinder the healthy psychosexual development in children and adolescents. Problem use of Internet pornography by adolescents has been associated with alcohol, illicit drugs, greater number of sexual partners, poor interpersonal real-life relationships with partners and poor self-worth [27].

Online gambling is the most studied type of IA. It is found to be highly addictive among adults, yet there are not enough studies to know the situation among adolescents. However, it is reasonable to state that going by available data and author' s clinical experience, social networking and gaming are strongly associated with problem use of the Internet.

Watching videos/movies was not related to problem use of the Internet according to one study [24]. Yet the evidence is not conclusive to derive a definite idea about this type of Internet activity.

Males are found to have been engaging in gaming significantly more compared to females, whereas more females tend to spend time in social media at a significantly higher rate than males. Children and adolescents tend to indulge in these online attractions at the expense of their school work and real-life relationships with friends/family and sports. Researchers have found that IA or problem use can arise from involvement in a range of online activities [2, 23, 28–30].

6. Epidemiology of Internet addiction

Researchers have looked into the prevalence of IA. As discussed above, being an evolving concept there are very few empirical studies and even fewer meta-analyses on IA. Further, it is difficult to compare and contrast available studies due to the vast differences in the methodology as a result of the ill-defined and poor consensual concept of IA. The considerable lack of unanimity in terminology is apparent in studies, and prevalence rates mentioned here are from studies that use many different terms for IA.

IA is reported more commonly in Asian countries and in males aged 12–20. The available research on game addiction centers mostly on young males worldwide. There is some evidence to believe that the onset of IA is probably in late childhood/early adolescence [31]. There are many reports in countries such as China and South Korea. A few European and American studies are also available. The researchers who make an effort to educate the authorities and public in USA claim that IA is a silent epidemic in United States, at present. There are a fewer African studies mainly from South Africa that indicate a lower prevalence estimate compared to other countries of the world. One study reported the figure as 1.67–5.29% [32]. A meta-analysis from 31 nations from seven world regions (North America, Oceania, North & West Europe, South & East Europe, Middle East, Asia and South America) revealed an overall prevalence estimate of 6% in IA. The results showed that the adverse real-life living conditions such as poor satisfaction with life, greater overall pollution, lower national income and greater time spent in traffic were directly proportional to the IA. Middle East had the highest individual world region prevalence estimate of IA, the figure being 10.9% [33].

The far eastern countries such as China report 10.2% of moderate users and 0.6% of severely addicted [34]: South Korea have found 1.6% [35], 3.5% [36], 4.3% [37], 10.7% [38] and 20.3% [39] of adolescents with IA. In Taiwan, 17.9% of students were found to be addicted to the Internet [40].

A European Union-funded research project was carried on among adolescents in Greece, Germany, the Netherlands, Iceland, Poland, Romania and Spain [24]. The Internet addiction was detected in 1.2% of the total sample, and 13.9% have been found to have problematic Internet use. Less affluent countries of the sample, Spain, Romania and Poland, have showed a higher prevalence of problem use, while Germany and Iceland have shown the lowest. The problem use was associated more commonly with boys, older adolescents and those who had parents with low level of education. The problem users have shown lower psychosocial well-being.

A more recent research on the prevalence of Internet addiction on a large number of adolescents from 11 European countries has showed that the overall prevalence of problematic Internet use was 4.4%, and rates were higher in males than in females (5.2% versus 3.8%) and differed between countries ($\chi(2) = 309.98$; d.f. = 20; $P < 0.001$). A significant correlation between problem use and mean hours online and male gender were found [26].

The Indian subcontinent is seemingly overtaking other nations with 53% of Indians connected to the Internet every waking hour according to a recent study conducted in 10 countries by a global management consulting firm AT Kearney Global Research based in London. India has made several attempts to contribute to available knowledge base on IA and related problems in adolescents. One 2013 cross-sectional study conducted among 987 adolescents in Mumbai has revealed 74.5% as moderate users, 24.8% as possible addicts and 0.7% as addicts. Males in comparison with females were significantly more addicted [41]. Many such local researches are available online, yet a national figure on prevalence of IA or problem use is not yet available in India where one of the leading and fastest growing information technology industries prevails.

A preliminary survey was conducted on the Internet use in a convenient sample of 179 adolescents from schools in central Sri Lanka by author and her team to derive a general idea about the Internet use among adolescents and the views of their significant adults on the Internet [42]. Sri Lanka is a middle-income developing country in South Asia where the Internet is promoted at large scale by multinational companies for competitive prices. No published studies are available on the Internet use among children and adolescents in Sri Lanka. The survey found that 91.06% of the sample was using the Internet with no sex difference; 2.79% of parents and 3.3% of teachers liked students using the Internet; and 45% of each adult group had a neutral view (**Table 1**). This is interesting as for some parents and teachers in Sri Lanka believe the Internet is a bad influence on the young that entices them into pornography and risky relationships. The Internet is not affordable to many young Sri Lankans yet, but mobile phone packages with Internet facility are coming up increasingly enabling the children and adolescents to use the Internet unsupervised by adults. Out of the sample, 68.7% used the Internet for social media and 55.6% was watching films and videos (**Table 2**).

Responses	Parents (%)	Teachers (%)
Like	2.79	3.35
Neutral	45.81	44.69
Somewhat against	43.02	44.13
Totally against	7.26	5.70
Not responded	1.12	1.12

Table 1. View of the parents and teachers about Internet usage of students [42].

Components	Number of users	Percentage (%)
Social media	112	68.7
Gossip sites	13	8
Films and videos	90	55.6
Online games	49	30.1
Educational purposes	119	73
Blogs	2	1.2
Other	11	6.7

Table 2. Purpose of Internet usage (out of 163 Internet users) [42].

7. Etiology

Many children and adolescents are engaging in the Internet use for academic pursuits as well as recreation. But not all will end up being addicted to or problem users of the Internet. The pertinent question what makes a particular adolescent becomes a victim of IA is the question we should try and find an answer. However, like the etiology of any other mental and psychosomatic disorder in psychiatry, the answer is not that simple. After reviewing the attempts made by researchers to come up with a model to understand IA and its management, the author believes that the well-known biopsychosocial model of disease is a feasible and logical explanation for IA, too.

The genetic factors play a part in addictions, and therefore, biological vulnerability is considered to contribute for IA too. The psychological component with cognitive errors, negative effects and personality traits also accounts for the condition. Here, it is noteworthy that personality is again determined by the genetic composition of the individual. Finally, the social factors such as affordability and availability of the devices and networks, the attitudes of the parents and schools about the Internet and the nature of the education system (i.e., whether students are requested to use a lot of online activities for school work as in most high schools in North America) and the inert qualities of the Internet itself that attract youngsters are also contributing for IA.

Researchers have wondered whether different types of Internet addictions (i.e., cybersex, social networking, gaming, etc.) have same underlying mechanisms or not. Apparently, all the types have common features of the well-established signs and symptoms of addiction, pleasure generating quality and the ability to go anonymous if necessary. Yet it is only speculation until scientific evidence is available on underlying pathophysiology.

8. The neurobiological basis of the Internet addiction

It is known that the developing brains of children and adolescents are more vulnerable to get addicted to rewarding activities. Adolescent period is a period of heightened neuroplasticity that makes this age more susceptible to the effects of addictive drugs [43]. Internet addiction and other similar addictive behaviors too can reasonably be considered to have the same effect as drugs on these vulnerable brains. Based on the available knowledge of neurobiology of addiction, scientists have proposed a neurobiological theory for Internet addiction. The "reward center" or "pleasure pathway" of the brain is responsible for the pleasure experienced by an individual. Neurochemicals associated with pleasure such as dopamine, morphine, like endorphins, and others are released when the brain areas such as nucleus accumbens of the pleasure pathway are activated [44, 45]. Substances of addiction or similar behaviors of addictions are found to activate the pleasure pathway. The receptors involved gets affected when exposed to the chemicals over time, and tolerance and withdrawal develop like in any addiction, needing more and more online input to achieve the same stimulation or "kick" together with continuous engagement in the behavior to avoid withdrawal features

[46]. Some activists working on education of public against hazards of the Internet argue, in the genetically vulnerable adolescent or child, lack of love care and affection by the significant adults in his or her life leads to no or minimal activation of pleasure pathways. The children are left alone to fill the emptiness from outside pleasures such as the Internet. That is a theory worth more research as it can be utilized to prevent Internet addiction.

The Internet offers a strong reinforcement for addiction like any other addiction as depicted in Dr. Kimberly Young's Hand Book on Internet Addiction [47]. In gambling, as psychologists found through their extensive research, a variable ratio reinforcement schedule (VRRS) operates giving the gambler the suspension of unpredictability and varying rewards. It is proposed what happens in Internet addiction is also the same. The computer applications are increasingly developed to engage the user fully and incessantly. The coupling of the online activity with pleasure generating themes (sex, sense of connection through social networks, etc.) will heighten the reinforcement leading to more severe addictions [48].

9. High-risk groups for Internet addiction

Qualitative research has reported how the adolescence itself is a risk factor [49].

The developing brain of adolescents has an innate quality of curiosity and a drive for adventures with risk taking. The Internet also gives answers to almost any query they have, keeps them connected and can be a load of never-ending fun at mere finger tips.

However, certain adolescents are more vulnerable to the addictive quality of the Internet than others. One with deficient real-life social skills may find it easy to have online relationships as there is no pressure of real-life eye-to-eye contacts, gestures and human touch. They may find it boosting to be liked and praised online. They may tend to overuse virtual realities offered by attractions in the Internet to fill the voids of boredom and loneliness of real life. At the press of a key, an "emoticon" expressing the due feeling could be far less distressing and comforting than all the "hard work" of trying to express emotions in real-life relationships for the shy adolescent.

Adolescents who are lacking emotional and psychological support are found to be at highest risk and so are the adolescents with identified emotional and behavioral disorders [31].

It is worth exploring the fact whether the adolescents who face tremendous academic pressure in real life tend to find temporary solace in stress-free virtual reality of being online. This may explain the high prevalence of gaming reported in Asian cultures those give priority to the education of the children even at the expense of the psychological well-being of the children. However, this theory needs empirical support.

It is found that living in metropolitan areas was associated with problem use of the Internet. It is not clear whether it is due to wider availability of the Internet by way of free WiFi in cafes, shops and malls in metropolitan area. Poor adult supervision seems a key element in high-risk adolescents. Students not living with a biological parent, low parental involvement and parental unemployment have shown the highest relative risks of both problem use and addiction of Internet.

Availability of one or several devices to log into the Internet such as smart phones, tablets and even wrist watches at present with wide spread availability of the Internet paves way for increase in the risk of IA.

The Internet-based treatment programs are trialed and used in the management of individuals with autism spectrum disorders. However, there is some concern that, despite its benefits, the Internet has the risk of addictive use in this special group of people [50].

It has been found that doing homework/research was negatively associated with problematic Internet use [24]. A positive correlation was found between Internet use for academic purposes and greater self-esteem, better relationship with parents and less use of substances of abuse [27]. Maybe the studious adolescent does not possess some of the risk factors leading to problem use of Internet to begin with, and it could be the reason for positive findings. This needs more exploration as it may lead us to understand preventive measures.

10. The association of Internet addiction with psychiatric conditions

Several authors have reported a significant comorbidity of IA and mental health disorders. Particularly, depression and anxiety disorders among adolescents may increase the vulnerability of an IA. The affected adolescents may find online activities distracting them from real life low or anxious mood and distressing cognitions [51]. Attention deficit hyperactivity disorder (ADHD) is another behavioral disorder IA is associated with making the affected children and adolescents more vulnerable to IA [52].

But some work brings about the notion whether the depressive and anxiety symptoms experienced by problem or addicted Internet users are more a consequence rather than a cause or co-occurrence [53].

A cross-sectional survey among a sample of 175 university undergraduates in Peradeniya, Sri Lanka, reported IA was positively correlated with depression, loneliness and time spent on the Internet, while it negatively correlated with healthy lifestyle [54].

11. Clinical features and diagnosis

A good detailed history from is paramount for the diagnosis of IA. The adults bring the affected child or adolescent, usually. Mostly, it is the parents who notice the changes in behavior. The clinical picture may be subtle or marked. In subtle cases, the parents or teachers may complain of a drop in school work, disinterest in extracurricular activities previously interested in and lying about the Internet usage—both about the time spent and the particular online activity (e.g., "No.... I did not spend one hour it was just a half an hour!!!!" or "No.... I was not playing Clash of Clans but just checking up something for my home work!!!!"). Denial and concealment of the extent of the Internet use are quite often seen in the clinical practice, and they complicate matters as help is then sought very late into the problem. Problem use leads to irritabilities, arguments with parents and sleepiness in daytime. However, if the condition is not intervened early, there may be a risk of the adolescent engaging in the behavior openly and resisting adult interventions more aggressively.

Dramatic or marked presentations around the Internet use may also occur. The adolescent may be caught engaging in cybersex during school hours or at home, and the school or devastated parents will bring him or her to a psychiatrist.

In some other cases, a teenager may be engaging in online gaming for excessive hours. Going by the DSM-5 proposed criteria, clinicians can have some directives in order to diagnose Internet gaming disorder. An adolescent who is sitting at a device with the Internet and spends 8–10 h or more per day and at least 30 h per week, in gaming neglecting not only academic activities but also food or sleep, may be diagnosed as a victim of Internet gaming disorder [6]. They typically get angry and agitated if parents try to prevent the addicted behavior.

Clinicians should keep in mind the close association the IA or problem use has with the mental health of the adolescent. It should be the rule to look for features of comorbid, consequent or causative psychiatric disorders such as depression or anxiety. A thorough history and a mental state examination are warranted.

Extreme cases were reported in mostly Asian countries. The world was shocked to hear the news of the young adult couple from Seoul, South Korea, neglecting their infant daughter to death in order to raise a virtual baby called Animus in a gaming community. There are many news items of individuals including teenagers dying after excessive game playing from China, Taiwan, Hong Kong and South Korea. In these extreme cases, the online game is usually a highly addictive role-playing fantasy game.

Young states not only psychological but also physical problems such as back pain, eye strain and carpal tunnel syndrome can be caused by long hours (more than 18 h a day) online [10]. It is reported that cardiopulmonary-related deaths have also occurred in addicts in Internet cafes [55]. Therefore, it is important to look for any associated physical problems.

In the absence of any DSM or ICD 10 criteria for diagnosis of IA, reader is directed to two criteria commonly used to arrive at a diagnosis of IA: Young's diagnostic questionnaire for Internet addiction [10] and Ko et al. 's proposed diagnostic criteria for Internet addiction [9].

12. Assessment tools for Internet addiction

Despite the lack of consensus in diagnostic criteria, many tools of screening and assessing the degree of the Internet-related problems have been developed and used in research around the globe. Internet addiction disorder diagnostic criteria (IAD–DC) by Goldberg in 1995 [56] is the first scale on IA, found in literature. Later a widely used 20-item, quantitative, assessment scale Internet addiction test (IAT) was developed: Young's Internet addiction test [57]. Many researchers are using IAT up-to-date due to its high reliability. Internet addiction disorder scale by Goldberg in 2000 is a qualitative 11-item scale. Readers are directed to the critical review of existing scales and their psychometric properties by Laconi et al. published in 2014, which is freely available online in the journal, Computers in Human Behaviour, for a more comprehensive in-depth review of the subject [58]. (One of the many advantages of the Internet!)

However, the assessment tools will only substantiate the clinical assessment through history and mental state in diagnosing IA.

13. Management of Internet addiction

It is understandable that there are no definitive treatments laid down for IA in light of the knowledge it is not an accepted disorder at present. However, while world health authorities are being cautious about the fundamental existence of a disorder of IA, children, adolescents and adults are increasingly reported to be facing adversities related to the Internet. Some states (e.g., China, South Korea) have gone ahead and started their own diagnoses and management systems, as they cannot afford to wait till the disease classification systems give them a label to start. Internet addiction can be detrimental to the affected individual adolescent and his or her family, and if one such adolescent walks into the clinical practice of a mental health professional, he or she should be armed with best available options of treatment.

It is important to keep in mind that it is very easy to place restrictions on a child not to use the Internet by adults, parents, teachers and therapists themselves, who grew up in a pen and paper era! The new technology evolves and societies have to keep abreast with the development for successful survival. Therefore, total banning of an adolescent from using the Internet is not the answer. In other words, total abstinence should not be the goal [59]. Instead, controlled/safe/balanced or more preferably **sensible Internet usage** should be the goal. Both the treating clinician and the affected individual should come to a consensus about the details of sensible use depending on the age, educational demands, cultural value system, etc.

14. Assessment of Internet addiction

The first step has to be a detailed history and mental state examination as in the case of any other mental health disorder.

A suitably validated assessment scale such as Young's Internet addiction test (IAT) [10] can be utilized to substantiate clinical diagnosis but not to replace it, as the gold standard in diagnosing any mental and behavioral disorder, including behavioral addictions such as IA, is the clinical diagnosis. However, the cultural differences should be considered when using a tool developed in another sociocultural background.

Comorbidities should be considered, actively looked for and intervened. For example, a social phobic or a depressed adolescent may be masking his affective status by engaging in the Internet activities that make him happy and gives the feeling of being in control. In such cases, where the IA is only secondary, treating the underlying mental health disorder should be the priority. In mild cases of secondary IA, treating the root condition itself may help the individual to refrain from misusing the Internet.

15. Treatment of Internet addiction

According to a 2011 systematic review and consort evaluation on clinical trials of Internet addiction treatment by King and his team, we are unable to come up with definitive treatment modules for Internet addiction. The evidence base available for treatment is defective with conclusions coming from anecdotal reports, small-uncontrolled studies with no randomization [60].

15.1. Psychological treatments

The clinicians and therapists have attempted to have some direction from existing treatment types mainly extrapolating methods used for more known addictions such as substance addictions. Many methods such as boot camp-style treatments, cognitive behavior therapy (CBT), family therapy, group therapy, behavior therapies such as social skills training and counseling have being used worldwide [60].

Most of the psychological treatments employed had sprung from CBT [61]. This is probably due to the fact that CBT has proven to be efficacious in many other behavioral addictions such as gambling disorder and impulse control disorder.

Dr. Young the pioneering researcher on IA in her book "Internet Addiction: Symptoms, Evaluation, and Treatment" [62] and in her study [63] offers some practical treatment strategies based on CBT. Though the clinical evidence for the efficacy of the methods is not stated, they offer some important directions in managing the individual patient until more evidence to establish them or replace them arrives. The suggestions are mainly based on practical behavioral techniques that are agreed upon by the user. The reader is referred to Dr. Young's book for a detailed account on those treatment strategies. The user's consent, willingness and high motivation are important in order to practice the suggested treatment strategies. In the case of children and adolescents, they may not be very agreeable to the suggestions as their cognitive development is not complete to understand the adverse aspect of the Internet.

A randomized controlled study used eight sessions of multimodal school-based group CBT or no treatment on 56 adolescents aged 12–17 years randomly allocated into treatment and no treatment [64]. The Internet use has decreased in both groups, while actively treated group has additionally improved in some other general constructs.

Many other investigators have found CBT-based treatment approaches being effective on the sample of adolescents they studied [65–67].

Cash and his colleagues in their summary on Internet addiction mention the importance of utilizing motivational interviewing (MI) a client-centered technique used to change adverse behaviors, as a component in treatment plans for IA (19). MI has not been used so far in the treatment of Internet addiction according to available information.

Since any problem in children and adolescence is closely associated with the family, it is warranted to consider family-based therapies for IA. Though there is not enough evidence to support for efficacy of such interventions, overall improvement in communication in the family and better monitoring of the Internet use are some of the benefits noticed [68, 69].

Many enthusiastic and innovative therapies based on behavior therapy have been put to practice to bring about a positive change in Internet addictive behaviors, such as Reality therapy (RT) [70] and Acceptance & Commitment Therapy (ACT) [71] with varying results.

Simple educational programs for children in real life or ironically online are considered to combat problem use of the Internet. One such online program follows the 12 steps self-help treatment approach used for alcoholic anonymous [60].

Some suggests that there is an important place for physical exercise in helping adolescents to reduce the use of the Internet. Sports believed to be compensating for the reduced dopamine levels in brain resulted in the decreased online use. Further, sports can be a part of CBT programs [72].

15.2. Pharmacological treatments

A few types of medications have been used, and there are some studies looking into the effectiveness of them. However, there are no adequate randomized controlled trials to derive definitive guidance to treatments.

There are several reports on the use of selective serotonin-reuptake inhibitors (SSRIs) particularly when Internet addiction is comorbid with depression and anxiety for which SSRIs have an established place as an effective treatment [73, 74]. The SSRI, escitalopram [75], non-tricyclic antidepressants, bupropion [76], psycho-stimulant, methylphenidate [77], mood stabilizers [22], antipsychotic, quetiapine [78] and opioid receptor antagonist and naltrexone [79] have been trialed as treatments. However, most of these studies were quite short term and some are case reports. Hence, no pharmacological medication can be recommended for IA per se in children and adolescents at present.

15.3. Multimodal treatments

IA being a complicated phenomenon involving many aspects of life as biological, psychological and sociocultural, a combined or a multimodal treatment approach is increasingly considered by the concerned scientific community. There are reports on group CBT, parental training, teacher education, family therapy, medication, case management and brief intervention therapies, which are combined according to the necessity [80–85]. A widely inclusive IA recovery program with mindfulness-based relapse prevention, digital detoxification and animal-assisted therapy among many other different multidisciplinary approaches is proposed in 2012 [86].

16. Tips on sensible Internet use

Author suggests, after reviewing available solutions on the Internet (You tube, Ted Talks, etc.) by activists as well as scientific reports, some simple techniques based on behavior therapy with or without cognitive component that can be utilized to use the Internet sensibly (Box 1).

- Having a prior discussion and an agreement on Internet use before a family purchase Internet facility. (healthy digital diet and digital nutrition)
- All in the household following through the plan. (Modeling by the adults)
- Setting aside devices at family/friends gatherings and meal times. (Disconnect to reconnect)
- Having a family Internet-free day probably on a Sunday so that education or work/business is not affected. (Digital Detox)
- When at studies or assignments switching of the notifications of chat sites or social networks just the way people place mobile phones on silent mode or switch them off.
- Have an assigned time for socializing on the net (by using an alarm) and setting limits on checking on social media responses, for example, only three times per day or once a week. (Checking on checking)
- Internet times to be replaced by more attractive offline activities (not offline studies!) such as getting together with friends in real life, competitive or recreational sports, aerobics, etc. (Doing it in real)
- Reward for being off Internet as planned, for example, by having a vacation every 3 months or weekend movie/dinner out. (Celebrate)

Box 1. Tips on sensible Internet use.

17. Clinical course and prognosis

Not much is known about the natural history of the condition as the concept of IA itself is at a very preliminary level. We need follow-up studies.

The experience from highly affected countries suggests that the problem of IA is quite a complex one. With the ubiquity of the Internet and its innate qualities of urging individuals to misuse despite harm, the course of IA is seemingly long term and resistant to treatment.

Prognosis of the highly addicted adolescent seems poor in general given the available information. However, clinicians should not be pessimistic in attempting to treat IA of an affected individual patient as multimodal treatment approached though not tested adequately offers some hope.

18. Prevention

IA is considered at different intensity by different countries depending on how affected their population by it. Asian countries are undoubtedly most affected and hence have come up with most solutions too.

Most of the Internet-based activities are promoted among children and adolescents. Case is particularly so in online gaming which seemingly is the most prevalent type of Internet addiction disorder that could even reach DSM-5 at least at a warning stage.

A mass awareness program on the concept of IA is important. It has to be carefully planned and implemented as a total aversion from the Internet even before it reaches most of the children and adolescents in some parts of the world would be a shame given the unbeatable wonderful positive aspects of the Internet on education, business and recreation. The reader is also reminded at this point, of the accusation by some, that a normal phenomenon is being pathologized by introducing the concept of Internet addiction.

Primary prevention is encouraged by developing a sensible Internet culture starting from the individual household. Adults should set living examples and have controlled access to the Internet following a discussion and agreement in the family upon the way of the Internet use (Box 1).

Secondary and tertiary prevention may call for drastic methods if a nation is seriously affected. For example, total ban of the Internet in certain time of the day for under 18-year-olds, developing a system to slow down the Internet if played more than a certain number of hours (South Korea) [8], restricting Internet gaming among youth by demanding a "game fatigue system" from the game operators (China) [8].

19. Summary

The Internet use is increasingly becoming an integral part of day-to-day life of all age groups around the world. The concept of "Internet addiction" remains controversial and at a fetal stage waiting to be evolved into maturity with better quality research. While IA has not reached DSM-5 or probably the future ICD 11, we cannot ignore the numbers or the seriousness of cases reported in Asian countries, neither can we ignore the individual families seeking help for problematic Internet users, children and adolescents. An internationally consensual multicenter attempt to define the concept, look into etiology, develop valid and reliable diagnostic criteria and come up with effective management strategies that involve prevention is warranted. We are gifted with the technology of Internet, and it has come to stay and will expand in new horizons we may only see in science fictions today. The children should be taught to use it with respect in a moderated and controlled but positive way. Such an approach only will win the cooperation of today's children and adolescents who are growing up with the Internet as a daily commodity.

Acknowledgments

1. Dr. Sampath Tennakoon, Senior Lecturer, Department of Community Medicine, Faculty of Medicine, University of Peradeniya, Sri Lanka.

2. Dr. Helani Alahakoon, Temporary Lecturer, Department of Psychiatry, Faculty of Medicine, University of Peradeniya, Sri Lanka.

3. Dr. Rangana Kuruwita, Temporary Lecturer, Department of Psychiatry, Faculty of Medicine, University of Peradeniya, Sri Lanka.

4. Miss. H.G Devika Malkanthi, Temporary Lecturer, Department of Psychiatry, Faculty of Medicine, University of Peradeniya, Sri Lanka.

Author details

Pabasari Ginige

*Address all correspondence to: dsen@abo.fi

Department of Psychiatry, Faculty of Medicine, University of Peradeniya, Peradeniya, Sri Lanka.

References

[1] Odell PM, Korgen KO, Schumacher P, Delucchi M. Internet use among female and male college students. Cyber Psychology & Behavior. 2000; 3(5): 855–862.

[2] Young KS. Psychology of computer use: XL. Addictive use of the Internet: a case that breaks the stereotype. Psychological Reports. 1996; 79: 899–902.

[3] Griffiths M. Behavioural addictions: an issue for everybody?. Journal of Workplace Learning. 1996; 8(3): 19–25.

[4] Shaw M, Black DW. Internet addiction: definition, assessment, epidemiology, and clinical management. CNS Drugs. 2008; 22: 353–365.

[5] Young KS. Internet addiction: the emergence of a new clinical disorder. Cyber Psychology & Behavior. 2009: 1(3), January: 237–244.

[6] American Psychiatric Association. Diagnostic and Statistical Manual of Mental Disorders (5th ed.). Arlington, VA: American Psychiatric Publishing. 2013.

[7] Greenfield D. Virtual Addiction: Help for Netheads, Cyberfreaks, and Those Who Love Them. CA: New Harbinger Publications; 1999.

[8] Block JJ. Issues for DSM-5: internet addiction. American Journal of Psychiatry. 2008; 165: 306–307.

[9] Ko CH, Yen JY, Chen CC, Chen SH, Yen CF. Proposed diagnostic criteria of Internet addiction for adolescents. Journal of Nervous and Mental Disease. 2005b; 193(11): 728–733.

[10] Young KS. Internet addiction: the emergence of a new clinical disorder. Cyber Psychology & Behavior. 1998; 1(3): 237–44.

[11] World Health Organization. (1992). The International Classification of Diseases, Tenth Revision, Classification of Mental and Behavioural Disorders: Clinical Descriptions and Diagnostic Guidelines. Geneva: World Health Organization.

[12] Flisher C. Getting plugged in: an overview of internet addiction. Journal of Paediatric Child Health. 2010; 46: 557–559.

[13] American Society of Addiction Medicine. Public Policy Statement: Definition of Addiction. 2011; http://www.asam.org/1DEFINITION_OF_ ADDICTION_LONG_4-11.pdf.

[14] Bell V. Taking an internet history. British Journal of Psychiatry. 2009; 194: 561–562.

[15] Shaffer HJ, Hall MN, Vander BJ. "Computer addiction": a critical consideration. American Journal of Orthopsychiatry. 2000; 70: 162–168.

[16] Lenihan F. Computer addiction—a skeptical view. Advances in Psychiatric Treatment. 2007; 13: 31–33.

[17] Charlton JP, Danforth IDW. Distinguishing addiction and high engagement in the context of online game playing. Computers in Human Behaviour. 2007: 23: 1531–1548.

[18] Griffiths MD, Parke J. Adolescent gambling on the Internet: a review. International Journal of Adolescent Medicine and Health. 2010; 22: 59–75.

[19] Billieux J, Schimmenti A, Khazaal Y, Maurage P, Heeren A. Are we overpathologizing everyday life? A tenable blueprint for behavioral addiction research. Journal of Behavioural Addictions. 2015; 4(3): 119–23.

[20] Griffiths, M.D. Social gambling via Facebook: further observations and concerns. Gaming Law Review and Economics. 2013; 17: 104–106.

[21] Kuss DJ, Griffiths MD, Karila L, Billieux J. Internet addiction: a systematic review of epidemiological research for the last decade. Current Pharmaceutical Design. 2014: 20: 4026–4052.

[22] Shapira NA, Goldsmith TD, Keck PE Jr, Khosla UM, McElroy SL. Psychiatric features of individuals with problematic internet use. Journal of Affective Disorders. 2000; 57(1–3): 267–272.

[23] Davis RA. A cognitive-behavioral model of pathological Internet use. Computers in Human Behavior. 2001: 17: 187–195.

[24] Tsitsika A, Tzavela E, Mavromati F, & the EU NET ADB Consortium. (Ed.). Research on Internet Addictive Behaviours among European Adolescents (EU NET ADB Project). Athens: National and Kapodestrian University of Athens; 2012.

[25] Meerkerk GJ. Owned by the internet, Explorative research into the causes and consequences of compulsive internet use. [Thesis]. Erasmus University Rotterdam, Rotterdam; 2007.

[26] Durkee T, Kaess M, Carli V, Parzer P, Wasserman C, Floderus B. et al. Prevalence of pathological internet use among adolescents in Europe: demographic and social factors. Addiction. 2012; 107: 2210–22.

[27] Padilla-Walker LM, Nelson LJ, Carroll JS et al. More than a just a game: video game and internet use during emerging adulthood. Journal of Youth and Adolescence. 2010; 39: 103–113.

[28] Beard KW. Internet addiction: a review of current assessment techniques and potential assessment questions. Cyber Psychology & Behavior. 2005; 8(1), Feb: 7–14.

[29] Griffiths M, Wood RT. Risk factors in adolescence: the case of gambling, videogame playing, and the internet. Journal of Gambling Studies. 2000; 16: 199–225.

[30] King VL, Stoller KB, Kidorf M et al. Assessing the effectiveness of an Internet-based videoconferencing platform for delivering intensified substance abuse counseling. Journal of Substance Abuse Treatment. 2009; 36: 331–338.

[31] Pridgen B. Navigating the internet safely: recommendations for residential programs targeting at-risk adolescents. Harvard Review of Psychiatry. 2010; 18: 131–138.

[32] Thatcher A, Goolam S. Development and psychometric properties of the problematic Internet use Questionnaire. South African Journal of Psychology. 2005; 35: 793–809.

[33] Cheng C, Li AY. Internet addiction prevalence and quality of (real) life: a meta-analysis of 31 nations across seven world regions. Cyberpsychology, Behavior, and Social Networking. 2014; 17(12): 755–60.

[34] Lam LT, Peng Z, Mai J, Jing J. The association between internet addiction and self-injurious behaviour among adolescents. Injury Prevention. 2009;15(6): 403–8.

[35] Kim K, Ryu E, Chon MY, Yeun EJ, Choi SY, Seo JS et al. Internet addiction in Korean adolescents and its relation to depression and suicidal ideation: a questionnaire survey. International Journal of Nursing Studies. 2006; 43(2): 185–92.

[36] Whang LS, Lee S, Chang G. Internet over-users' psychological profiles: a behavior sampling analysis on internet addiction. Cyber Psychology & Behavior. 2003; 6: 143–50.

[37] Jang KS, Hwang SY, Choi JY. Internet addiction and psychiatric symptoms among Korean adolescents. Journal of School Health. 2008; 78(3): 165–71.

[38] Park SK, Kim JY, Cho CB. Prevalence of Internet addiction and correlations with family factors among South Korean adolescents. Adolescence. 2008; 43(172): 895–909.

[39] Ha JH, Kim SY, Bae SC, Bae S, Kim H, Sim M, et al. Depression and Internet addiction in adolescents. Psychopathology. 2007; 40(6): 424–30.

[40] Tsai HF, Cheng SH, Yeh TL, Shih CC, Chen KC, Yang YC. The risk factors of Internet addiction—a survey of university freshmen. Psychiatry Research. 2009; 167(3): 294–29.

[41] Goel D, Subramanyam A, Kamath R. A study on the prevalence of internet addiction and its association with psychopathology in Indian adolescents. Indian Journal of Psychiatry. 2013; 55(2): 140–143.

[42] Ginige P, Kuruwita KAPR, Alahakoon SH, Malkanthi HGD. A survey on internet use of adolescence in a selected sample of central province in Sri Lanka. Unpublished dataset, cited with permission; 2016.

[43] Hyland EC & Chandler LJ. Adaptive plasticity of NMDA receptors and dendritic spines: implications for enhanced vulnerability of the adolescent brain to alcohol addiction. Pharmacology Biochemistry and Behavior. 2007; 86(2): 200–8.

[44] Gabor Maté. In the Realm of Hungry Ghosts: Close Encounters with Addiction: North Atlantic Books; Berkeley, CA. 2010.

[45] Bai Y-M, Lin C-C, Chen J-Y. Internet addiction disorder among clients of a virtual clinic. Psychiatric Services. [Letter]. 2001; 52(10): 1397.

[46] Ko C-H, Liu G-C, Hsiao S, Yen J-Y, Yang M-J, Lin W-C, et al. Brain activities associated with gaming urge of online gaming addiction. Journal of Psychiatric Research. 2009; 43(7): 739–47.

[47] Cooper A, Putnam DE, Planchon LA, Boies SC. Online sexual compulsivity: getting tangled in the net. Sexual Addiction & Compulsivity. 1999; 6(2): 79–104.

[48] Grohol JM. Internet addiction guide. Internet addiction guide. 1999 [updated 2005, April 16]; Available at: http: //psychcentral.com/ netaddiction/

[49] Dreier M. et al. Qualitative component of research on internet addictive behaviours among European adolescents, in Tsitsika, A. et al. (eds), Research on Internet addictive Behaviours among European Adolescents; 2012. National and Kapodistrian University of Athens, Athens: EU NET ADB. Available at www.eunetadb.eu.

[50] Finkenauer C, Pollmann MMH. Begeer, S. et al. Brief report: examining the link between autistic traits and compulsive internet use in a non-clinical sample. Journal of Autism and Developmental Disorders. 2012; 42: 2252.

[51] Lin SSJ, Tsai CC. Sensation seeking and Internet dependence of Taiwanese high school adolescents. Computers in Human Behavior. 2002; 18: 411–426.

[52] Yoo HJ, Cho SC, Ha J, Yune SK, Kim SJ, Hwang J et al. Attention deficit hyperactivity symptoms and internet addiction. Psychiatry and Clinical Neurosciences. 2004; 58(5): 487–94.

[53] Dong G, Lu Q, Zhou H, Zhao X. Precursor or sequela: pathological disorders in people with Internet addiction disorder. Public Library of Science One [serial on the Internet] 2011; 6(2) Available from:http://www.plosone.org/article/info%3Adoi%2F10.1371%2Fjournale.pone.0014703.

[54] Chamika RMA, Dias S. Relationship of internet addiction with depression, loneliness and health related lifestyle among university students. IPURSE; 2016.

[55] Choi YH. Advancement of IT and seriousness of youth internet addiction. In 2007 International Symposium on the Counseling and Treatment of Youth Internet Addiction. Seoul, South Korea: National Youth Commission; 2007: 20.

[56] Goldberg, I. (1995). Internet addictive disorder (IAD) diagnostic criteria. Retrieved July 27, 2007, from www.psycom.net/iadcriteria.html.

[57] Young KS. Caught in the Net: How to Recognize the Signs of Internet Addiction—and A Winning Strategy for Recovery. New York: Wiley; 1998.

[58] Laconi S, Rodgers RF, Chabrol H. The measurement of Internet addiction: a critical review of existing scales and their psychometric properties. Computers in Human Behavior. 2014; 41: 190–202.

[59] Grant JE, Potenza MN, Weinstein A, Gorelick DA. Introduction to behavioral addictions. The American Journal of Drug and Alcohol Abuse. 2010; 36(5): 233–41.

[60] King DL, Delfabbro PH, Griffiths MD, Gradisar M. Assessing clinical trials of Internet addiction treatment: a systematic review and CONSORT evaluation. Clinical Psychology Review. 2011; 31(7): 1110–6.

[61] Widyanto L, Griffiths MD. 'Internet addiction': a critical review. International Journal of Mental Health and Addiction. 2006; 4(1): 31–51.

[62] Young KS. Internet Addiction: Symptoms, Evaluation, and Treatment. Innovations in Clinical Practice [serial on the Internet]. 1999; 17: Available from: http://treatmentcenters.com/downloads/internet-addiction.pdf.

[63] Young KS. Cognitive behavior therapy with Internet addicts: treatment outcomes and implications. Cyber Psychology & Behavior. 2007; 10(5): 671–9.

[64] Du Y, Jiang W, Vance A. Longer term effect of randomized, controlled group cognitive behavioral therapy for Internet addiction in adolescent students in Shanghai. Australian and New and Journal of Psychiatry. 2010; 44: 129–134.

[65] Cao L, Su L-Y, Gao XP. Control study of group psychotherapy on middle school students with Internet overuse. Chinese Mental Health Journal. 2007; 21(5): 346–9.

[66] Li G, Dai XY. Control study of cognitive-behavior therapy in adolescents with Internet addiction disorder. Chinese Mental Health Journal. 2009; 23(7): 457–70.

[67] Zhu T-m, Jin R-j, Zhong X-m. Clinical effect of electro acupuncture combined with psychological interference on patient with Internet addiction disorder. Chinese Journal of Integrated Traditional & Western Medicine. 2009; 29(3): 212–4.

[68] Yen JY, Ko CH, Yen CF, Wu HY, Yang MJ. The comorbid psychiatric symptoms of Internet addiction: attention deficit and hyperactivity disorder (ADHD), depression, social phobia, and hostility. Journal of Adolescent Health. 2007; 41(1): 93–8.

[69] Peukert P, Sieslack S, Barth G, Batra A. Internet- and computer game addiction: Phenomenology, comorbidity, etiology, diagnostics and therapeutic implications for the additives and their relatives. Psychiatrische Praxis. 2010; 37(5): 219–24.

[70] Kim J-U. A reality therapy group-counseling program as an Internet addiction recovery method for college students in Korea. International Journal of Reality Therapy. 2007; 26(2): 3–9.

[71] Twohig MP, Crosby JM. Acceptance and Commitment Therapy as a treatment for problematic Internet pornography viewing. Behavior Therapy. 2010; 41(3): 285–95.

[72] Lanjun Z. The applications of group mental therapy and sports exercise prescriptions in the intervention of Internet addiction disorder. Psychological Science (China). 2009; 32(3): 738–41.

[73] Arisoy O. Internet addiction and its treatment. Psikiyatride Guncel Yaklasimlar. 2009; 1(1): 55–67.

[74] Huang X-Q, Li M-C, Tao R. Treatment of Internet addiction. Current Psychiatry Reports. 2010; 12(5): 462–70.

[75] Dell'Osso B, Hadley S, Allen A, Baker B, Chaplin WF, Hollander E. Escitalopram in the treatment of impulsive-compulsive Internet usage disorder: an open-label trial followed by a double-blind discontinuation phase. Journal of Clinical Psychiatry. 2008; 69(3): 452–6.

[76] Han DH, Hwang JW, Renshaw PF. Bupropion sustained release treatment decreases craving for video games and cue-induced brain activity in patients with Internet video game addiction. Experimental and Clinical Psychopharmacology. 2010; 18(4): 297–304.

[77] Han DH, Lee YS, Na C, Ahn JY, Chung US, Daniels MA, et al. The effect of methylphenidate on internet video game play in children with attention-deficit/hyperactivity disorder. Comprehensive Psychiatry. 2009; 50(3): 251–6.

[78] Atmaca M. A case of problematic Internet use successfully treated with an SSRI-antipsychotic combination. Progress in Neuro Psychopharmacology & Biological Psychiatry. [Letter]. 2007; 31(4): 961–2.

[79] Bostwick JM, Bucci JA. Internet sex addiction treated with naltrexone. Mayo Clinic Proceedings. 2008; 83(2): 226–30.

[80] Orzack MH, Voluse AC, Wolf D, Hennen J. An ongoing study of group treatment for men involved in problematic Internet-enabled sexual behavior. Cyber Psychology & Behavior. 2006; 9(3): 348–60.

[81] Du Y-s, Jiang W, Vance A. Longer term effect of randomized, controlled group cognitive behavioural therapy for Internet addiction in adolescent students in Shanghai. Australian and New Zealand Journal of Psychiatry. 2010; 44(2): 129–34.

[82] Fang-ru Y, Wei H. The effect of integrated psychosocial intervention on 52 adolescents with Internet addiction disorder. Chinese Journal of Clinical Psychology. 2005; 13(3): 343–5.

[83] Rong Y, Zhi S, Yong Z. Comprehensive intervention on Internet addiction of middle school students. Chinese Mental Health Journal. 2005; 19(7): 457–9.

[84] Shek DTL, Tang VMY, Lo CY. Evaluation of an Internet addiction treatment program for Chinese adolescents in Hong Kong. Adolescence. 2009; 44(174): 359–73.

[85] Bai Y, Fan FM. The effects of group counseling on Internet dependent college students. Chinese Mental Health Journal. 2007; 21(4): 247–50.

[86] reSTART: Internet Addiction Recovery Program. First detox center for Internet addicts opens its doors: Creates solutions for computer related addictive behaviors. 2009. [cited 2011 August 21]; Available from: http://www.netaddictionrecovery.com.

Permissions

All chapters in this book were first published in HAA, by InTech Open; hereby published with permission under the Creative Commons Attribution License or equivalent. Every chapter published in this book has been scrutinized by our experts. Their significance has been extensively debated. The topics covered herein carry significant findings which will fuel the growth of the discipline. They may even be implemented as practical applications or may be referred to as a beginning point for another development.

The contributors of this book come from diverse backgrounds, making this book a truly international effort. This book will bring forth new frontiers with its revolutionizing research information and detailed analysis of the nascent developments around the world.

We would like to thank all the contributing authors for lending their expertise to make the book truly unique. They have played a crucial role in the development of this book. Without their invaluable contributions this book wouldn't have been possible. They have made vital efforts to compile up to date information on the varied aspects of this subject to make this book a valuable addition to the collection of many professionals and students.

This book was conceptualized with the vision of imparting up-to-date information and advanced data in this field. To ensure the same, a matchless editorial board was set up. Every individual on the board went through rigorous rounds of assessment to prove their worth. After which they invested a large part of their time researching and compiling the most relevant data for our readers.

The editorial board has been involved in producing this book since its inception. They have spent rigorous hours researching and exploring the diverse topics which have resulted in the successful publishing of this book. They have passed on their knowledge of decades through this book. To expedite this challenging task, the publisher supported the team at every step. A small team of assistant editors was also appointed to further simplify the editing procedure and attain best results for the readers.

Apart from the editorial board, the designing team has also invested a significant amount of their time in understanding the subject and creating the most relevant covers. They scrutinized every image to scout for the most suitable representation of the subject and create an appropriate cover for the book.

The publishing team has been an ardent support to the editorial, designing and production team. Their endless efforts to recruit the best for this project, has resulted in the accomplishment of this book. They are a veteran in the field of academics and their pool of knowledge is as vast as their experience in printing. Their expertise and guidance has proved useful at every step. Their uncompromising quality standards have made this book an exceptional effort. Their encouragement from time to time has been an inspiration for everyone.

The publisher and the editorial board hope that this book will prove to be a valuable piece of knowledge for researchers, students, practitioners and scholars across the globe.

List of Contributors

Anneliese Dörr, Sandra Viani and María Elena Gorostegui
Psychiatry and Mental Health Department, University of Chile, Santiago, Chile

Miranda Novak and Josipa Mihić
Department of Behavioral Disorders, Prevention Research Laboratory, Faculty of Education and Rehabilitation Sciences, University of Zagreb, Croatia

Francesca Giordano
Department of Psychology, Resilience Research Unit, Università Cattolica del Sacro Cuore, Milan, Italy

Isabel Hernández-Otero
Department of Child and Adolescent Psychiatry, University Hospital Virgen de la Victoria, Málaga, Spain

Carlos Gómez Sánchez-Lafuente and Cecilia Hernández González
University Hospital Virgen de la Victoria, Málaga, Spain

Martin H. Maurer
University of Heidelberg, Heidelberg, Germany

Roshni Sondhi
Department of Mental Health and Behavioral Sciences, Fortis Healthcare, New Delhi, India

Claudia Juárez-Portilla and Rossana Citlali Zepeda
Biomedical Research Centre, University of Veracruz, Xalapa, Veracruz, Mexico

Tania Molina-Jiménez
Faculty of Chemical Pharmaceutical Biologist, and Faculty of Biology, University of Veracruz, Xalapa, Veracruz, Mexico

Jean-Pascal Morin and Gabriel Roldán-Roldán
Department of Physiology, Faculty of Medicine, National Autonomous University of Mexico, Mexico City, Mexico

Nat Kendall-Taylor and Allison Stevens
Frame Works Institute, Washington, D.C., USA

Blanca Estela Barcelata-Eguiarte
Department of Psychology, National Autonomous of Mexico, Mexico City, Mexico

Maria Elena Márquez-Caraveo
Child Psychiatric Hospital "Dr. Juan N. Navarro", Mexico City, Mexico

Füsun Gökkaya
Ministry of Education, İzmir, Turkey

Seungpil Jung
Department of Family Medicine, Yeungnam University, College of Medicine, South Korea

Pabasari Ginige
Department of Psychiatry, Faculty of Medicine, University of Peradeniya, Peradeniya, Sri Lanka.

Index

www.ingramcontent.com/pod-product-compliance
Lightning Source LLC
LaVergne TN
LVHW081024210926
848485LV00004B/945

* 9 7 8 1 6 3 9 8 7 1 0 4 9 *